IDKD Springer Series

Series Editors

Juerg Hodler, Former Chairman of Radiology
University Hospital of Zürich
Zürich, Switzerland

Rahel A. Kubik-Huch, Department of Radiology
Cantonal Hospital of Baden
Baden, Switzerland

Justus E. Roos, Department of Radiology and Nuclear Medicine
University Teaching and Research Hospital, Hospital of Lucerne
Lucerne, Switzerland

The world-renowned International Diagnostic Course in Davos (IDKD) represents a unique learning experience for imaging specialists in training as well as for experienced radiologists and clinicians. IDKD reinforces his role of educator offering to the scientific community tools of both basic knowledge and clinical practice. Aim of this Series, based on the faculty of the Davos Course and now launched as open access publication, is to provide a periodically renewed update on the current state of the art and the latest developments in the field of organ-based imaging (chest, neuro, MSK, and abdominal).

Juerg Hodler • Rahel A. Kubik-Huch
Justus E. Roos
Editors

Musculoskeletal Diseases 2026–2029

Diagnostic Imaging

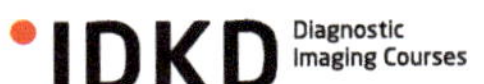

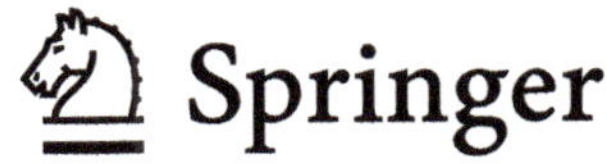

Editors
Juerg Hodler
Former Chairman of Radiology
University Hospital of Zurich
Hedingen, Switzerland

Rahel A. Kubik-Huch
Department of Radiology
Cantonal Hospital of Baden
Baden, Switzerland

Justus E. Roos
Radiology and Nuclear Medicine
University Teaching and Research Hospital
Lucerne, Lucerne, Switzerland

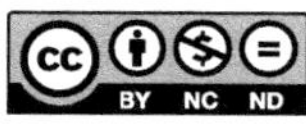

ISSN 2523-7829 ISSN 2523-7837 (electronic)
IDKD Springer Series
ISBN 978-3-032-17039-2 ISBN 978-3-032-17040-8 (eBook)
https://doi.org/10.1007/978-3-032-17040-8

Foundation for the Advancement of Education in Medical Radiology. This work was supported by Foundation for the Advancement of Education in Medical Radiology.

This Springer imprint is published by the registered company Springer Nature Switzerland AG
The registered company address is: Gewerbestrasse 11, 6330 Cham, Switzerland

Preface

The International Diagnostic Course in Davos (IDKD) is a unique learning experience based on interactive workshops. They are of interest to radiologists, nuclear physicians, and clinicians interested in imaging. The course is useful for various levels of experience, from residents preparing for their board's examination to experienced imaging experts. Clinicians wishing to update their knowledge to the current state of the art in imaging appreciate the course as well.

The IDKD workshop teachers are internationally renowned experts. They are all contributing to this issue of the IDKD book series with the current topic of musculoskeletal imaging. It includes relevant pediatric/adolescent aspects. All relevant imaging modalities are covered, including MRI, CT, ultrasound, PET, and standard radiographs.

The IDKD books were originally started as a syllabus for the IDKD courses. They have developed into outstanding publications over the years. We reach large number of readers from all over the world with impressive download numbers of the online version. IDKD books are featured in the PubMed database.

Great emphasis has been put on the design of this book in order to improve readability and for quick orientation. Important aspects are highlighted in the form of learning objectives, key points, tables, take-home messages, and summaries.

Additional information on IDKD courses can be found on the IDKD website: www.idkd.org.

Hedingen, Switzerland — Juerg Hodler
Baden, Switzerland — Rahel A. Kubik-Huch
Lucerne, Switzerland — Justus E. Roos

Contents

1 Shoulder: Instability

Christian W. A. Pfirrmann and Klaus Woertler

Learning Objectives

- To identify the various forms of glenohumeral instability and recognize the anatomical contributors
- To know the principles behind the glenoid track concept and the mechanics of an engaging Hill-Sachs lesion
- To interpret the MR imaging features of SLAP lesions and anatomic variants that may mimic pathology
- To know the concepts of microinstability and anterosuperior and posterosuperior glenoid impingement (ASI & PSI)

1.1 Glenohumeral Instability

Glenohumeral instability is defined as the inability of the humeral head to remain centered within the glenoid cavity. This condition can be categorized based on etiology and direction of instability. There are three forms of dislocation: static, dynamic, and voluntary [6].

Static instability arises from structural abnormalities of the shoulder, such as glenoid dysplasia or massive rotator cuff tears. These abnormalities result in persistent decentering of the humeral head.

In contrast, dynamic instability is the more common presentation. It is often triggered by trauma and is often accompanied by labrum injuries, glenohumeral ligament injuries, or glenoid rim fractures. Generalized ligamentous laxity may also contribute to dynamic instability.

From an imaging standpoint, it is essential to distinguish between traumatic and atraumatic instabilities. Both forms may present with recurrent dislocations. However, traumatic instability is frequently associated with identifiable structural damage, such as labral tears, ligamentous disruption, and osseous defects. Atraumatic instability, on the other hand, may occur without any discernible injury [14].

Key Point

In cases of atraumatic instability, imaging studies may reveal a structurally intact glenohumeral joint without evident abnormalities.

Instability can manifest in one direction—either anterior or posterior—or in multiple planes, as in multidirectional instability, which affects a smaller group of patients.

Joint stability is maintained by a combination of soft tissue and bone elements, including the glenoid labrum, glenohumeral ligaments, and bone architecture. Although the labrum is often the focus of imaging studies, it contributes only about 10% to joint stability. Therefore, a complete diagnostic evaluation must also include the ligamentous structures and bone anatomy.

1.2 Anterior Instability

1.2.1 Anterior Labral Injuries Associated with Glenohumeral Instability

Bankart Lesion First introduced by A. S. Blundell Bankart in the *British Medical Journal* in 1923 [1], the Bankart lesion involves a complete detachment of the anteroinferior labrum along with the adjacent periosteum. On axial MR images, the

C. W. A. Pfirrmann (✉)
MRI – Medical Radiological Institute, Zurich, Zurich, Switzerland
e-mail: christian.pfirrmann@pfirrmann.ch

K. Woertler
Institute for Diagnostic and Interventional Radiology, Musculoskeletal Radiology Section, TUM University Hospital Rechts der Isar, Munich, Germany
e-mail: klaus.woertler@tum.de

J. Hodler et al. (eds.), *Musculoskeletal Diseases 2026-2029*, IDKD Springer Series,
https://doi.org/10.1007/978-3-032-17040-8_1

labrum appears displaced and floats away from the glenoid margin, reflecting its loss of anchorage (Fig. 1.1).

Perthes Lesion Described earlier in 1906 [5], the Perthes lesion features a separation of the anteroinferior labrum from the glenoid rim, while the periosteal layer remains intact. Despite the labrum often appearing near-normal on imaging, its functional contribution to joint stability is compromised (Fig. 1.2).

ALPSA Lesion In 1993, Neviaser [16] characterized the anterior labroligamentous periosteal sleeve avulsion (ALPSA) lesion as a distinct entity in shoulder instability. Here, the labrum is avulsed but the periosteum connecting it to the glenoid remains intact. The labral tissue migrates medially and inferiorly, eventually healing along the scapular neck, altering its biomechanical role (Fig. 1.3).

GLAD Lesion Also described by Neviaser in 1993 [17], the GLAD lesion—short for glenolabral articular disruption—combines a superficial tear of the anteroinferior labrum with damage to the adjacent glenoid articular cartilage. Unlike other lesions, the labrum remains attached and in correct position. Patients typically present with anterior shoulder pain but retain overall joint stability (Fig. 1.4).

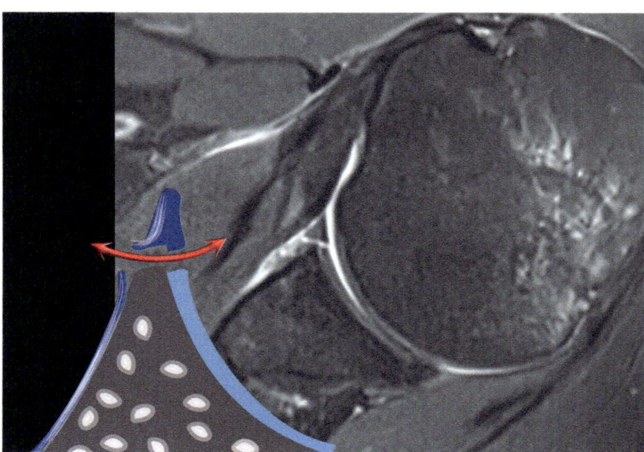

Fig. 1.1 Bankart lesion. Axial MR arthrography using fluid-sensitive, fat-saturated sequences demonstrates a Bankart lesion (red arrow), characterized by a tear of the anteroinferior labrum. Both the labrum and the adjacent periosteum are fully detached, resulting in a labrum that appears displaced and floating away from the glenoid rim

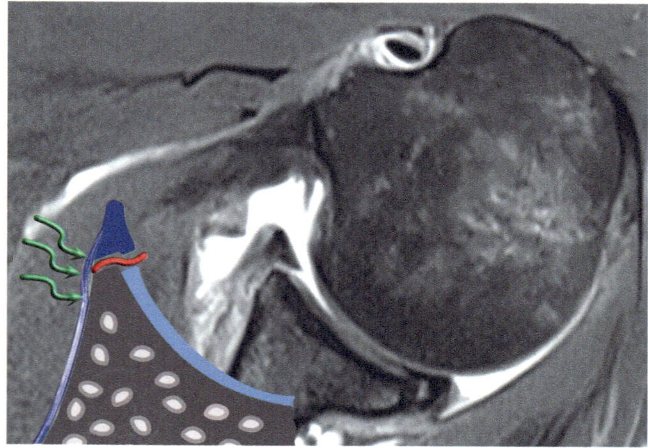

Fig. 1.2 Perthes lesion. On axial fluid-sensitive fat-saturated MR arthrography, the anteroinferior labrum (red arrow) is seen separated from the glenoid margin, yet it remains adherent to an intact periosteal layer

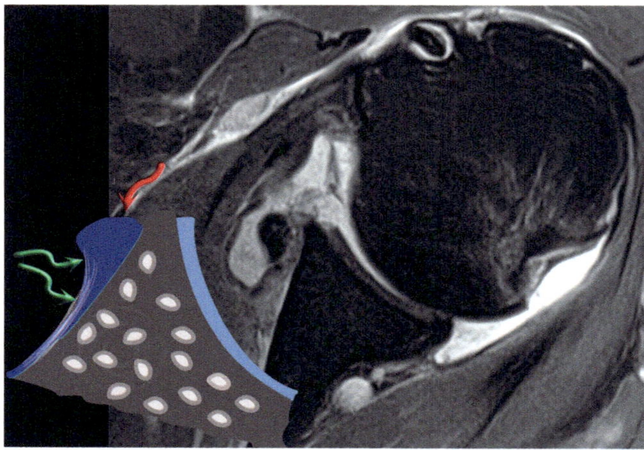

Fig. 1.3 ALPSA lesion. This axial MR arthrography image reveals an ALPSA lesion (red arrow), where the labrum is avulsed and displaced medially

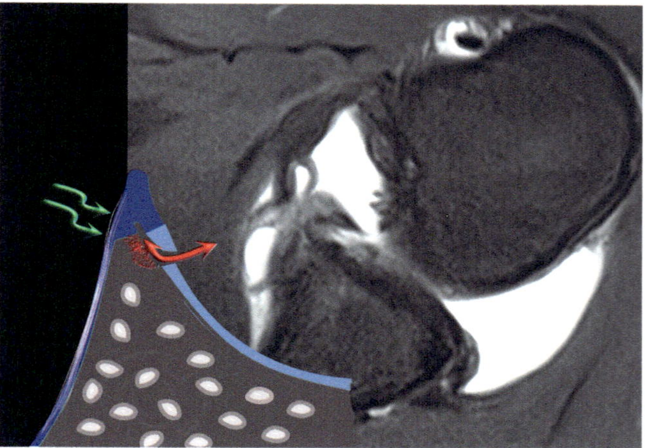

Fig. 1.4 GLAD lesion. Axial fluid-sensitive fat-saturated MR arthrography illustrates a GLAD lesion. There is an avulsion of the anterior-inferior glenoid articular cartilage accompanied by a partial tear of the labrum. Notably, the labrum remains in place and is neither detached nor dislocated

1.2.2 Ligamentous Injuries in Anterior Glenohumeral Instability

Among the key stabilizing structures of the shoulder, the inferior glenohumeral ligament (IGHL) plays a central role. Spanning from the glenoid to the humerus, the IGHL resembles a hammock, comprising robust anterior and posterior bands that support joint integrity.

Two anatomical variants of IGHL attachment to the glenoid have been described [4]. In the majority of cases (approximately 80%), the ligament anchors directly to the labrum, with some fibers extending onto the glenoid neck. In the remaining 20%, the IGHL inserts solely onto the glenoid neck without labral involvement. Consequently, detachment of the labrum typically implies disruption of the IGHL in most cases as well.

IGHG failure most commonly occurs at its glenoid insertion. When the ligament avulses from the humeral side, the injury is referred to as a **humeral avulsion of the glenohumeral ligament (HAGL)** lesion. These lesions can be challenging to detect arthroscopically. On MR arthrography, suggestive findings include the **J sign**, where the normally U-shaped axillary recess adopts a J-shaped configuration, and the presence of axillary fluid extravasation.

However, caution is warranted: false-positive interpretations of HAGL lesions on MRI are not uncommon [15]. Extravasation of contrast may also be seen in cases with an intact IGHL or in midsubstance tears, underscoring the importance of correlating imaging findings with clinical and surgical assessment.

Key Point

In the majority of shoulders, the inferior glenohumeral ligament (IGHL) inserts directly into the labrum. As a result, labral avulsion typically implies concurrent disruption of the IGHL at its glenoid attachment.

1.2.3 Bony Lesions in Anterior Instability

1.2.3.1 Glenoid

Osseous deficiency of the anterior glenoid rim is widely recognized as a critical contributor to glenohumeral joint instability. When the osseous defect exceeds 50% of the glenoid's maximal anteroposterior diameter, the shoulder loses substantial resistance to dislocation. In such cases, soft tissue repair—such as Bankart repair or labral reconstruction—may be insufficient to restore stability. Surgical augmentation of the glenoid, typically via a Latarjet procedure or bone grafting, is often required to reestablish joint congruency.

Glenoid bone loss may arise from various causes: it can be congenital, result from an acute rim fracture, or develop progressively due to chronic instability. Recurrent anterior subluxations of the humeral head can erode the glenoid margin over time, which is termed "glenoid bone loss," even in the absence of a discrete bony fragment.

1.2.3.2 Humerus

The characteristic groove-like defect of the humeral head, now known as the Hill-Sachs lesion, was first documented by Harold A. Hill and Maurice D. Sachs in *Radiology* in 1940. Its presence is considered a hallmark of anterior glenohumeral instability. Although Hill-Sachs lesions are frequently encountered, only approximately 7% require specific treatment [13]. For clinical decision-making, it is essential to evaluate the lesion's size, position, and its relationship to the glenoid.

Certain morphological features increase the likelihood of a Hill-Sachs lesion becoming "engaging," thereby contributing to recurrent instability. These include lesions that are large and broad, those located more medially on the humeral head, and those oriented obliquely when the humerus is in a neutral position. When an engaging Hill-Sachs lesion coexists with a substantial glenoid defect, the condition is referred to as a **bipolar lesion** and often necessitates surgical intervention to restore joint stability.

1.2.3.3 Glenoid Track Concept

When the shoulder is placed in abduction and external rotation (ABER), individuals with anterior glenohumeral instability often experience subluxation accompanied by a distinct sense of apprehension. Apprehension is defined as the fear of the patient of imminent dislocation in this vulnerable position.

The **glenoid track** refers to the zone of contact between the glenoid surface and the posterosuperior aspect of the humeral head during ABER (Fig. 1.5). This contact region spans approximately 84% of the glenoid's transverse diameter, while the remaining 16% interfaces with the medial edge of the rotator cuff footprint [9].

This biomechanical framework allows classification of Hill-Sachs lesions based on their relationship to the glenoid track:

- **On-track**: The Hill-Sachs defect remains confined within the glenoid track and does not pose a risk for engagement.
- **Off-track**: The Hill-Sachs defect extends medially beyond the glenoid track, increasing the likelihood of engagement and recurrent instability.

Understanding this relationship is critical for surgical planning, particularly in cases where a Hill-Sachs defect and glenoid bone loss coexist.

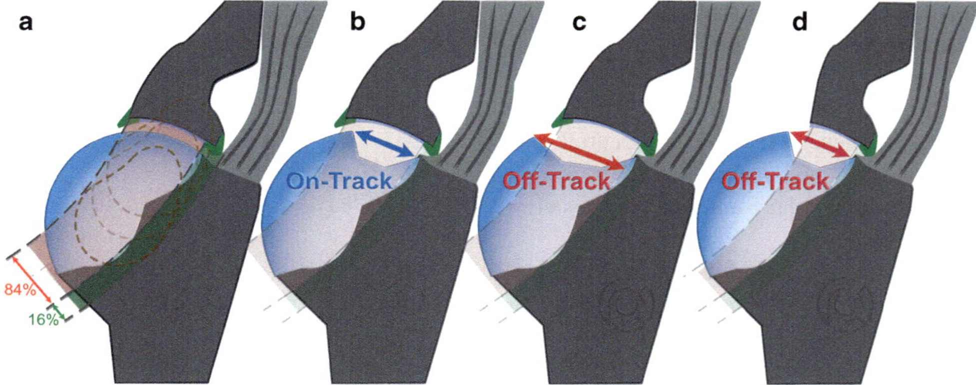

Fig. 1.5 Glenoid track theory, on-track situation and off-track situation. (**a**) The glenoid track represents the area of contact between the glenoid surface and the posterosuperior humeral head in the ABER position. (**b**) In an on-track configuration, the Hill-Sachs lesion remains confined within the glenoid track and does not engage. (**c**) In an off-track scenario, the Hill-Sachs defect extends medially beyond the glenoid track, increasing the risk of engagement. (**d**) When a glenoid rim defect is present, the glenoid track is narrowed. If the Hill-Sachs lesion extends beyond this reduced track medially, it becomes engaging

> **Key Point**
> Factors that contribute to an "off-track" lesion include an extensive Hill-Sachs defect that extends far medially on the humeral head and/or is accompanied by anterior glenoid bone loss.

1.3 Posterior Glenohumeral Instability

1.3.1 Labral Lesions in Posterior Instability

Posterior instability of the shoulder is frequently encountered in physically active individuals, particularly among young men, such as those in military service. This form of instability is commonly attributed to repetitive microtrauma affecting the posterior capsule and labral structures.

Activities that involve repeated loading of the shoulder—such as pushups, pullups, and heavy bench pressing—can predispose to posterior instability. Similar stress patterns are observed in sports like swimming and golf, where repetitive motion places strain on the posterior stabilizers of the glenohumeral joint.

Anatomical predispositions contributing to posterior glenohumeral instability include increased retroversion of the glenoid, augmented retroversion of the humeral head, and structural abnormalities such as posterior glenoid dysplasia, which may be associated with conditions like brachial plexus birth palsy [19].

> **Key Point**
> The following anatomical factors contribute to structural predispositions that lead to posterior glenohumeral instability:
>
> - Increased glenoid retroversion
> - Increased humeral head retroversion
> - Posterior glenoid dysplasia (brachial plexus birth palsy)

The Kim lesion refers to an avulsion of the posteroinferior portion of the glenoid labrum [12]. This type of labral injury is frequently subtle and may be difficult to detect on imaging. Adjacent to the tear, a marginal lesion at the chondrolabral junction is often present, typically resulting from repetitive posterior subluxations of the humeral head (Fig. 1.6).

This constellation of findings—known as Kim's triad—comprises a concealed posteroinferior labral tear, a marginal chondral defect, and increased glenoid retroversion, all of which contribute to posterior shoulder instability.

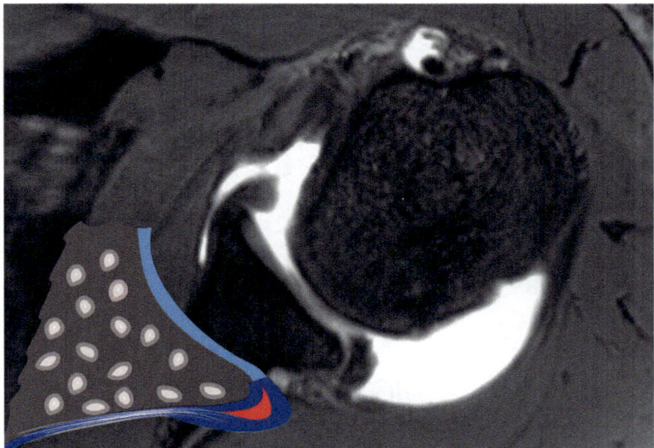

Fig. 1.6 Kim's lesion. Axial fluid sensitive fat-saturated MR arthrography image shows a posteroinferior labrum avulsion lesion (red arrow)

1.4 Superior Labral Anterior-to-Posterior (SLAP) Lesions

SLAP lesions of the shoulder are injuries of the superior glenoid labrum and biceps anchor that extend in an anterior to posterior direction. In arthroscopic series, these tears show a variable prevalence of up to 38%, largely depending on the patient population. The inter- and intraobserver variability with regard to the arthroscopic diagnosis of SLAP lesions is however substantial, even among experienced shoulder surgeons [8, 21].

Typical mechanisms of injury include a fall on an outstretched arm or a flexed elbow, chronic overuse due to repetitive torsion of the biceps anchor in overhead sports ("peelback mechanism"), and anterior dislocation of the shoulder. Following anterior shoulder dislocation, a SLAP lesion ultimately represents a superior extension of an anteroinferior labral tear [26].

The original classification by Snyder [21] describes four types of SLAP lesions:

Type 1—degenerative fraying of the superior labrum
Type 2—avulsion of the superior labrum and biceps anchor from the glenoid
Type 3—bucket-handle tear of the superior labrum with preserved biceps anchor
Type 4—bucket-handle tear of the superior labrum involving the long head of biceps tendon

Whereas type 1 lesions are of little clinical relevance, type 2 and 4 lesions impair the stabilizing function of the biceps insertion and therefore can provoke glenohumeral instability. In type 3 lesions, the biceps anchor is stable. The concept of surgical treatment of patients with SLAP lesions has recently changed. Anatomical repair is no more recommended in persons older than 25 years, and therefore, most patients are nowadays treated by biceps tenodesis.

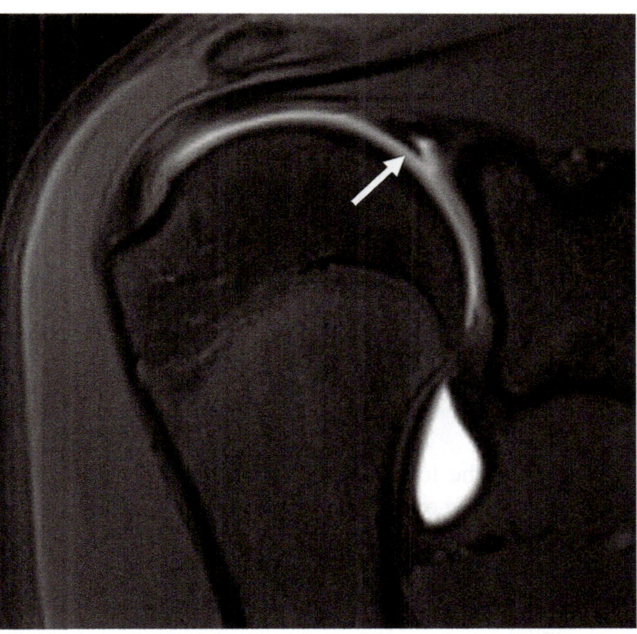

Fig. 1.7 SLAP type 2 lesion. Coronal oblique T1-weighted MR arthrogram with fat suppression shows laterally oriented linear extension of contrast media into the biceps anchor (arrow)

Conventional MR imaging shows limited sensitivity in detection of SLAP lesions. With high sensitivity, specificity, and inter- and intraobserver agreement, MR arthrography represents the diagnostic modality of choice [10, 23]. Most SLAP lesions are best depicted on MR images oriented in the coronal oblique plane. SLAP type 1 lesions may cause increased signal intensity and irregular contours of the superior labrum but can only be diagnosed infrequently on MR imaging. SLAP type 2 lesions (most common type) exhibit linear extension of fluid or contrast media into the superior labrum and biceps anchor (Fig. 1.7). If the cleft is oriented vertically or curves laterally, the diagnosis of a tear is obvious. If the cleft extends medially, a type 2 lesion must be distinguished from sublabral recess, which represents a common anatomic variant. In this regard, criteria for a SLAP type 2 lesion are irregular margins, a wide separation between the superior labrum and the glenoid, and extension of the cleft over the supraglenoid tubercle. SLAP type 3 and 4 lesions are bucket-handle tears with variable degrees of caudad fragment displacement. In a type 3 lesion, the labral fragment typically appears triangular and separated from the intact biceps tendon on coronal oblique MR images. In type 4 lesions, the bucket-handle fragment is composed of the superior glenoid labrum as well as portions of the biceps tendon, and thus the horizontal portion of the tear extends into the biceps tendon [10, 23, 26].

Key Point
Criteria for differentiation of a SLAP type 2 tear from a sublabral recess are the following:

- Superior or lateral extension
- Irregular margins, broad cleft, and/or extension over supraglenoid tubercle in case of medial extension

1.5 Biceps Tendon Instability

Instability of the long head of biceps tendon (LHBT) can cause subluxation or dislocation of the tendon in a medial or, rarely, in a lateral direction. Whereas subluxation means partial or transient loss of contact, dislocation is defined as complete and permanent loss of contact between the tendon and the bicipital groove of the humeral head. Abnormal mobility usually leads to biceps tendinopathy, which is characterized on MR imaging by thickening and irregularity of the LHBT as well as increased signal intensity on images obtained with short echo times [22, 25].

1.5.1 Medial Instability of the Long Head of Biceps Tendon

Medial instability of the LHBT can be observed as an isolated finding or in association with other shoulder pathologies. The underlying cause is a lesion of the stabilizing biceps pulley system, formed by the superior glenohumeral ligament (SGHL), the coracohumeral ligament (CHL), the subscapularis (SSC) tendon, and the supraspinatus (SSP) tendon [7, 8]. If the LHBT dislocates medially, it can slip into an intratendinous, intraarticular, or extraarticular position [22].

Intratendinous dislocation can occur in presence of a combined defect of the SGHL and the superior portion of the SSC tendon. The LHBT then cuts into the SSC tendon defect and may promote progression to complete tendon detachment (Fig. 1.8). If the entire SSC tendon is detached from the lesser tuberosity, the LHBT is allowed to dislocate into the glenohumeral joint. Extraarticular dislocation of the LHBT is less common. It describes medial displacement of the LHBT superficial to the SSC tendon as a sequel of a combined tear of the CHL and the anterior portion of the SSP tendon. Intrasheath subluxation of the LHBT may be observed with isolated SGHL or isolated SSC tendon lesions. It is important to understand that medial dislocation of the LHBT seen on axial MR images is not a sign for an isolated lesion of the pulley sling. The most reliable sign for an isolated SGHL lesion is the "displacement sign" on sagittal MR images, which describes caudad displacement of the LHBT onto the SSC tendon in the mid third of the rotator interval [2, 20, 22, 25].

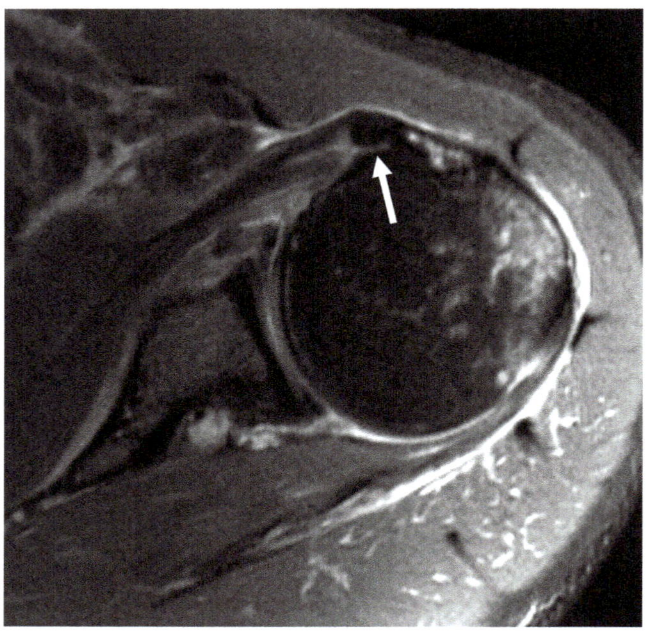

Fig. 1.8 Medial LHBT instability with intratendinous dislocation. Axial intermediate-weighted MR image with fat suppression demonstrates medial dislocation of the LHBT into an articular-sided partial tear of the SSC tendon (arrow)

1.5.2 Lateral Instability of the Long Head of Biceps Tendon

Lateral instability of the biceps tendon is very rare but may be evident following fractures of the greater tuberosity. Posttraumatic deformity with a shallow bicipital sulcus or a flattened greater tuberosity may allow the LHBT to sublux or dislocate laterally [25].

Key Point
- Medial instability of the LHBT can be a sequel of different lesions of the pulley system. The tendon can dislocate intratendinously, intraarticularly, or, rarely, extraarticularly.

1.6 Microinstability

Microinstability (functional instability, microtraumatic glenohumeral instability) is an acquired form of shoulder instability, which has been attributed to repetitive capsular microtrauma in chronic overuse without frank dislocation. It most commonly affects the dominant shoulder of athletes performing excessive abduction and external rotation movements in overhead sports, such as throwing, racket sports, handball, or swimming. Clinically, the condition manifest with pain and reduced strength and coordination. Microinstability can lead to intrinsic impingement and indirect structural damage, including capsular laxity and tears, anterior and posterior labral injuries, ganglia, SLAP lesions, and partial rotator cuff tears. Since MR arthrography has been shown to be more accurate than conventional MR imaging in the detection of these lesions, it remains the method of choice in the diagnostic workup of the athlete's shoulder [26].

1.6.1 Posterosuperior Glenoid Impingement (PSI)

The term PSI describes a mechanism of repetitive forceful contact between the undersurface of the rotator cuff and the posterosuperior glenoid in abduction and external rotation that leads to a characteristic pattern of injuries ("kissing lesions") (Fig. 1.9). It represents the classic form of intrinsic impingement in overhead athletes, who complain of posterior shoulder pain and loss of strength. The two main theories on the essential lesions in the development of PSI are chronic traumatization of the anterior joint capsule due to microinstability on the one hand and contracture of the posteroinferior capsule with a glenohumeral internal rotational deficit (GIRD) on the other hand [3, 11]. Both conditions are thought to be responsible for abnormal anterior translation of the humeral head during the cocking phase, which leads to impingement of the rotator cuff between the greater tuberosity and the glenoid.

MR imaging can show corresponding partial tears at the articular surface of the posterior portion of the SSP and/or the ISP tendon and lesions of the posterosuperior glenoid labrum (degenerative fraying, tears) that might be associated with osseous abnormalities (BME, large cysts, bone remodeling) of the greater tuberosity and the superior glenoid at the sites of excessive contact. Lesions of the anterior joint capsule are frequent findings, best demonstrated on MR arthrograms obtained in the ABER position. An association of these features with a (posterior) SLAP lesion is common [7, 26].

1.6.2 Anterosuperior Glenoid Impingement (ASI)

ASI is by far less common than PSI. It refers to squeezing of the fibers of the subscapularis tendon and the pulley sling between the anterior margin of the glenoid and the humeral head in forceful adduction and internal rotation, as it occurs during the follow-through phase of throwing or racket sports. The main symptom is anterior shoulder pain.

MR imaging can demonstrate a pulley lesion as well as sequels of LHBT instability. Lesions of the SSC tendon initially develop on the articular side of the superior portion of the tendon.

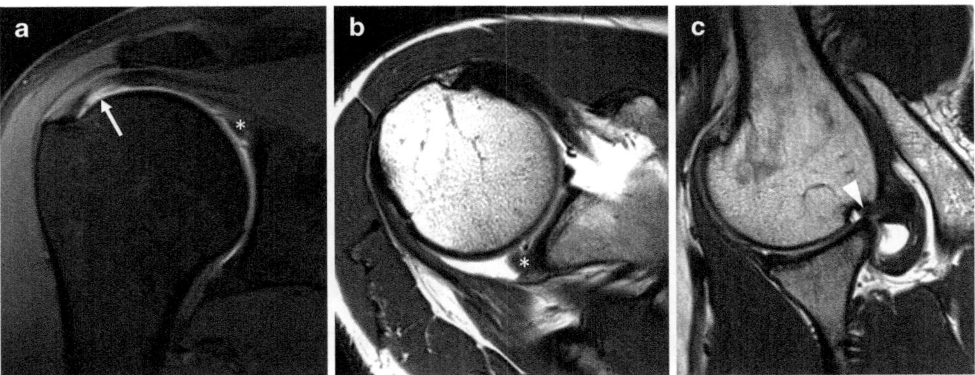

Fig. 1.9 PSI in an overhead athlete. (**a**) Coronal T1-weighted MR arthrogram with fat suppression shows an articular-sided partial tear of the posterior portion of the SSP tendon (arrow) and degenerative changes of the posterosuperior labrum (asterisk). (**b**) Corresponding axial T1-weighted MR arthrogram confirms increased signal intensity and fraying of the posterosuperior glenoid labrum (asterisk). (**c**) T1-weighted MR arthrogram obtained in the ABER position demonstrates contact (arrowhead) between the two lesions in abduction and external rotation ("kissing lesions")

Key Points
- Microinstability of the shoulder is typically seen in overhead athletes and may provoke a variety of structural lesions.
- PSI can be recognized by a typical pattern of injuries ("kissing lesions").

1.7 Normal Variants of the Glenoid Labrum

The glenoid labrum is a fibrocartilaginous rim around the entire margin of the glenoid. It is approximately 4 mm in thickness and most often appears triangular on cross section. The shape of the glenoid labrum is, however, quiet variable. Superiorly, the labrum is continuous with the biceps anchor (labral-bicipital complex), anteroinferiorly, with the inferior glenohumeral ligament (labro-ligamentous complex). There are several anatomic variants that can be confused with labral injuries and thus should be recognized on cross-sectional imaging. The most important variants include the sublabral recess, the sublabral hole, and the Buford complex [18].

1.7.1 Sublabral Recess

The sublabral recess represents a common variant of the superior labrum observed in more than 70% of individuals. It represents a synovialized cleft with a depth of up to 10 mm located under the superior labrum and biceps anchor. Unlike described in early radiological studies, a sublabral recess may well extend posterior to the biceps insertion. Anteriorly, it can be continuous with a sublabral hole. On coronal oblique MR images or arthrograms, a typical recess appears as a smooth, medially curved line of fluid or contrast media with a maximum width of 2 mm pointing at the supraglenoid tubercle. In the presence of a deep recess, the superior labrum may be meniscoid and appear hypermobile on arthroscopic examination [10, 18, 26].

1.7.2 Sublabral Hole

A sublabral hole (foramen) is the most common variant of the anterosuperior glenoid labrum with a prevalence of 7–12%. The term refers to lack of attachment of the intact labrum to the glenoid between the 1 and 3 o'clock position. The foramen usually does not extend anteroinferiorly. Therefore, location is the most important feature to distinguish a sublabral hole from a labral tear, which typically involves the anteroinferior segment of the labrum [18].

1.7.3 Buford Complex

The Buford complex is an anatomic variant characterized by complete absence of the anterosuperior labrum between the 1 and 3 o'clock position and a thickened, cord-like middle glenohumeral ligament, which may have an atypical labral insertion together with the base of the LHBT (Fig. 1.10). With a prevalence of around 2%, this anomaly is believed to be less common than the sublabral hole. On MR imaging, the Buford complex can be mistaken for a labral avulsion from the glenoid. The key to a correct diagnosis is to recognize that the assumed labral fragment is continuous with the anterior joint capsule and not with the anteroinferior labrum [18, 24].

Key Point
- Sublabral recess, sublabral hole, and Buford complex are variants of labral anatomy that may be confused with SLAP lesions or labral tears. Typical morphology and location are key features for their distinction.

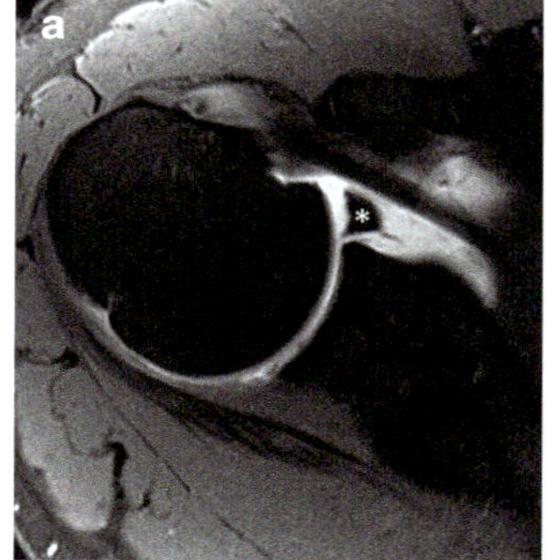

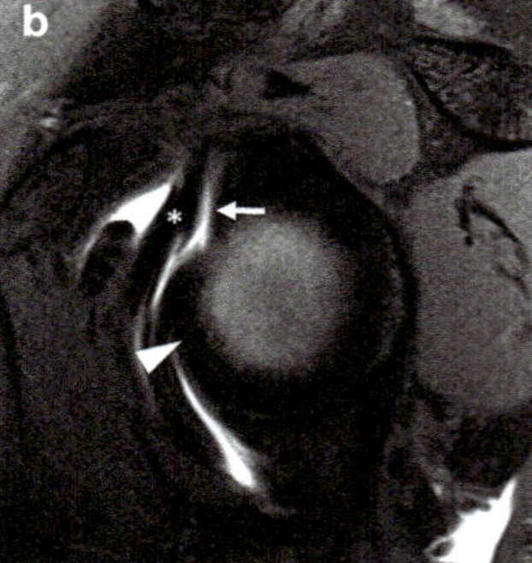

Fig. 1.10 Buford complex (**a**) Axial T1-weighted MR arthrogram with fat suppression shows thick structure of low signal intensity (asterisk) unattached to the anterior glenoid, simulating a labral tear. (**b**) Corresponding sagittal oblique image reveals continuity of this structure with the anterior capsule and thus represents a cord-like MGHL. Note absence of the anterosuperior labrum (arrow) and an intact anteroinferior labrum (arrowhead)

Take-Home Messages

- The classification in traumatic instability and atraumatic instability is very important because the examination in a patient with an atraumatic instability of the glenohumeral joint may be normal.
- All structures (labrum, ligament, bone) contributing glenohumeral instability must be addressed.
- Medial instability of the long head of the biceps tendon may result from various injuries to the pulley system.
- Sublabral recesses, sublabral holes, and the Buford complex represent normal anatomical variants of the glenoid labrum that can mimic SLAP tears or other labral injuries. Accurate differentiation relies on recognizing their characteristic shape and typical anatomical location.

Conflict of Interest Statement I/We declare no competing interests as defined by Springer Nature or other interests that might be perceived to influence results and/or discussion reported in this manuscript.

References

1. Bankart AS. Recurrent or habitual dislocation of the shoulder-joint. Br Med J. 1923;2(3285):1132–3. https://doi.org/10.1136/bmj.2.3285.1132.
2. Bennett WF. Subscapularis, medial, and lateral head coracohumeral ligament insertion anatomy. Arthroscopic appearance and incidence of "hidden" rotator interval lesions. Arthroscopy. 2001;17(2):173–80. https://doi.org/10.1053/jars.2001.21239.
3. Burkhart SS, Morgan CD, Kibler WB. The disabled throwing shoulder: spectrum of pathology part I: pathoanatomy and biomechanics. Arthroscopy. 2003;19(4):404–20. https://doi.org/10.1053/jars.2003.50128.
4. Eberly VC, McMahon PJ, Lee TQ. Variation in the glenoid origin of the anteroinferior glenohumeral capsulolabrum. Clin Orthop Relat Res. 2002;400:26–31. https://doi.org/10.1097/00003086-200207000-00004.
5. G P. Über Operationen bei habitueller Schulterluxationen. Dtsch Z Chir. 1906;85:199–227.
6. Gerber C, Nyffeler RW. Classification of glenohumeral joint instability. Clin Orthop Relat Res. 2002;400:65–76. https://doi.org/10.1097/00003086-200207000-00009.
7. Giaroli EL, Major NM, Higgins LD. MRI of internal impingement of the shoulder. AJR Am J Roentgenol. 2005;185(4):925–9. https://doi.org/10.2214/AJR.04.0971.
8. Gobezie R, Zurakowski D, Lavery K, Millett PJ, Cole BJ, Warner JJ. Analysis of interobserver and intraobserver variability in the diagnosis and treatment of SLAP tears using the Snyder classification. Am J Sports Med. 2008;36(7):1373–9. https://doi.org/10.1177/0363546508314795.
9. Gyftopoulos S, Yemin A, Beltran L, Babb J, Bencardino J. Engaging Hill-Sachs lesion: is there an association between this lesion and findings on MRI? AJR Am J Roentgenol. 2013;201(4):W633–8. https://doi.org/10.2214/AJR.12.10206.
10. Holzapfel K, Waldt S, Bruegel M, Paul J, Heinrich P, Imhoff AB, Rummeny EJ, Woertler K. Inter- and intraobserver variability of MR arthrography in the detection and classification of superior labral anterior posterior (SLAP) lesions: evaluation in 78 cases with arthroscopic correlation. Eur Radiol. 2010;20(3):666–73. https://doi.org/10.1007/s00330-009-1593-1.
11. Jobe CM. Superior glenoid impingement. Curr Concept Clin Orthop Relat Res. 1996;330:98–107.
12. Kim SH, Ha KI, Yoo JC, Noh KC. Kim's lesion: an incomplete and concealed avulsion of the posteroinferior labrum in posterior or multidirectional posteroinferior instability of the shoulder. Arthroscopy. 2004;20(7):712–20. https://doi.org/10.1016/j.arthro.2004.06.012.
13. Kurokawa D, Yamamoto N, Nagamoto H, Omori Y, Tanaka M, Sano H, Itoi E. The prevalence of a large Hill-Sachs lesion that needs to be treated. J Shoulder Elb Surg. 2013;22(9):1285–9. https://doi.org/10.1016/j.jse.2012.12.033.
14. Matsen FA 3rd, Harryman DT 2nd, Sidles JA. Mechanics of glenohumeral instability. Clin Sports Med. 1991;10(4):783–8.
15. Melvin JS, Mackenzie JD, Nacke E, Sennett BJ, Wells L. MRI of HAGL lesions: four arthroscopically confirmed cases of false-positive diagnosis. AJR Am J Roentgenol. 2008;191(3):730–4. https://doi.org/10.2214/AJR.07.3631.
16. Neviaser TJ. The anterior labroligamentous periosteal sleeve avulsion lesion: a cause of anterior instability of the shoulder. Arthroscopy. 1993a;9(1):17–21. https://doi.org/10.1016/s0749-8063(05)80338-x.
17. Neviaser TJ. The GLAD lesion: another cause of anterior shoulder pain. Arthroscopy. 1993b;9(1):22–3. https://doi.org/10.1016/s0749-8063(05)80339-1.
18. Park YH, Lee JY, Moon SH, Mo JH, Yang BK, Hahn SH, Resnick D. MR arthrography of the labral capsular ligamentous complex in the shoulder: imaging variations and pitfalls. AJR Am J Roentgenol. 2000;175(3):667–72. https://doi.org/10.2214/ajr.175.3.1750667.
19. Pfirrmann CW, Zanetti M, Hodler J. Joint magnetic resonance imaging: normal variants and pitfalls related to sports injury. Radiol Clin North Am. 2002;40(2):167–80. https://doi.org/10.1016/s0033-8389(02)00003-9.
20. Schaeffeler C, Waldt S, Holzapfel K, Kirchhoff C, Jungmann PM, Wolf P, Stat D, Schroder M, Rummeny EJ, Imhoff AB, Woertler K. Lesions of the biceps pulley: diagnostic accuracy of MR arthrography of the shoulder and evaluation of previously described and new diagnostic signs. Radiology. 2012;264(2):504–13. https://doi.org/10.1148/radiol.12112007.
21. Snyder SJ, Karzel RP, Del Pizzo W, Ferkel RD, Friedman MJ. SLAP lesions of the shoulder. Arthroscopy. 1990;6(4):274–9. https://doi.org/10.1016/0749-8063(90)90056-j.
22. Walch G, Nove-Josserand L, Boileau P, Levigne C. Subluxations and dislocations of the tendon of the long head of the biceps. J Shoulder Elb Surg. 1998;7(2):100–8. https://doi.org/10.1016/s1058-2746(98)90218-x.
23. Waldt S, Burkart A, Lange P, Imhoff AB, Rummeny EJ, Woertler K. Diagnostic performance of MR arthrography in the assessment of superior labral anteroposterior lesions of the shoulder. AJR Am J Roentgenol. 2004;182(5):1271–8. https://doi.org/10.2214/ajr.182.5.1821271.
24. Williams MM, Snyder SJ, Buford D Jr. The Buford complex--the "cord-like" middle glenohumeral ligament and absent anterosuperior labrum complex: a normal anatomic capsulolabral variant. Arthroscopy. 1994;10(3):241–7. https://doi.org/10.1016/s0749-8063(05)80105-7.
25. Woertler K. Rotator interval. Semin Musculoskelet Radiol. 2015;19(3):243–53. https://doi.org/10.1055/s-0035-1549318.
26. Woertler K, Waldt S. MR imaging in sports-related glenohumeral instability. Eur Radiol. 2006;16(12):2622–36. https://doi.org/10.1007/s00330-006-0258-6.

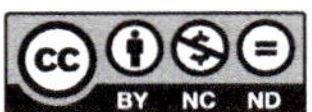
BY NC ND

Rotator Cuff

2

Tetyana Gorbachova and Eva Llopis

Learning Objectives

- Review anatomy of the rotator cuff and new anatomic concepts that improve understanding of the tear patterns.
- Describe current classifications of the rotator cuff tears.
- Emphasize imaging findings pertinent to accurate description of rotator cuff pathology on MRI that affect clinical decision-making.
- Recognize common pitfalls and mimickers in imaging evaluation of the rotator cuff.

2.1 Anatomy of the Rotator Cuff

The rotator cuff is composed of four muscles and tendons: supraspinatus, infraspinatus, teres minor, and subscapularis. In addition to their main function of enabling the movements of shoulder, rotator cuff muscles serve as dynamic stabilizers of the humeral head in the glenoid cavity. Histologically, the fibers of the rotator cuff are arranged in five layers in various fascicular orientations according to depth [1]. The rotator cable is a linear condensation of fibers located in layer 4 representing deep extension of coracohumeral ligament. The cable courses transversely from the rotator interval across the supraspinatus and infraspinatus tendons perpendicular to layers 2 and 3, acting like suspension bridge distributing the forces and limiting retraction. Region between rotator cable and tendinous insertion to the greater tuberosity is known as the rotator crescent [2].

Supraspinatus muscle originates from the supraspinatus fossa and the superior surface of the scapular spine and consists of two muscle bellies, anterior and posterior. Larger anterior belly of the supraspinatus muscle has a bipennate configuration, occupies three quarters of the supraspinatus fossa, and has a cordlike tendon with a long intramuscular course. Posterior belly of the supraspinatus is a smaller unipennate muscle with a flat and wide quadrangular-shaped tendon [3]. Infraspinatus muscle also consists of two distinct portions, a larger oblique portion that originates from the infraspinatus fossa and the smaller transverse portion arising from the inferior surface of the scapular spine. The tendon of the transverse portion is described as a thin membrane-like tissue that has a more superficial course and inserts to the deeper tendon of the oblique portion of the infraspinatus but does not reach the greater tuberosity footprint [4]. Mochizuki et al. redefined classic concept of the anatomy of the humeral insertions of the supraspinatus and infraspinatus tendons. The insertion area of the supraspinatus tendon occupies triangular area of the anteromedial half of the horizontal facet of the greater tuberosity and sometimes extends to the superior most area of the lesser tuberosity, while insertional area of the infraspinatus tendon has a wide, trapezoid shape and occupies posterior lateral half of the horizontal facet and the entire oblique facet [5]. Moser et al. described an "aponeurotic expansion" of the anterior superior supraspinatus tendon identified in approximately half of their cadaveric and clinical cases, often depicted as a tendon-like structure coursing from the anterior aspect to the supraspinatus tendon lateral to the long head of the biceps outside its synovial sheath inserting distally on the pectoralis major tendon [6].

The teres minor muscle arises from the middle portion of the lateral border of the scapula and fascia of the infraspinatus muscle. The upper ovoid portion of the teres minor tendon attaches to the vertical facet of the greater tuberosity,

T. Gorbachova (✉)
Department of Radiology, Jefferson Einstein Hospital, Jefferson Health, Philadelphia, PA, USA

Sidney Kimmel Medical College at Thomas Jefferson University, Philadelphia, PA, USA
e-mail: Tetyana.Gorbachova@jefferson.edu

E. Llopis
Department of Radiology, Hospital IMSKE, Hospital de la Ribera, Valencia, Spain

J. Hodler et al. (eds.), *Musculoskeletal Diseases 2026-2029*, IDKD Springer Series,
https://doi.org/10.1007/978-3-032-17040-8_2

and thin-shaped lower portion attaches onto the surgical neck [1].

The supraspinatus and infraspinatus muscles are innervated by the suprascapular nerve; the teres minor is innervated by the axillary nerve [4]. Suprascapular artery supplies all three muscles while infraspinatus muscle also receives contribution from circumflex scapular artery and teres minor from the dorsal scapular artery.

The primary role of the supraspinatus is shoulder abduction, teres minor is responsible for external rotation and adduction, and infraspinatus function is critical to both abduction and external rotation.

The subscapularis is the largest muscle of the rotator cuff and has a multipennate structure. It originates broadly from the anterior surface of the scapula, the subscapular fossa, and has a complex insertion onto the humerus. Four distinct facets of insertion have been described from superior to inferior in a three-dimensional perspective; the first two facets represent approximately 60% of the entire subscapularis tendon [7, 8]. The superior 60% is the tendinous insertion onto the lesser tuberosity, forming a trapezoidal, comma-shaped footprint that is wider superiorly and narrower inferiorly. The inferior 40% consists of muscular fibers inserting directly into the bone [7, 9]. At the superolateral corner of the subscapularis, a discrete bundle of fibers connects with the anterior fibers of the supraspinatus [10]. The subscapularis is innervated by the upper and lower subscapular nerves of the brachial plexus. Its blood supply arises mainly from the subscapular artery, with contributions from the anterior humeral circumflex artery [10].

Functionally, the subscapularis is the primary internal rotator of the shoulder and contributes to elevation. In addition, it plays a critical role in stabilizing the anterior glenohumeral joint, preventing anterior dislocation [7].

Key Points

- Supraspinatus tendon has smaller insertional footprint compared to the infraspinatus.
- Both supraspinatus and infraspinatus tendons share insertions on the horizontal facet of greater tuberosity. This anatomic relation should be considered when describing the location of rotator cuff tears.
- Subscapularis has a complex insertion on the humerus.

2.2 Tendinopathy

Tendinopathy, or tendinosis, of the rotator cuff is characterized by tendon degeneration without discrete tears. On MRI, tendinopathy is diagnosed by combined findings of (1) increased signal intensity within the cuff that does not reach signal intensity of fluid and does not extend to either the articular and bursal surface and (2) abnormally increased thickness of the tendon (Fig. 2.1). Signal alterations without morphologic changes in the rotator cuff should be interpreted with caution, as tendon pathology may be mimicked by magic angle effect that is observed in the characteristic areas where tendon fibers change their orientation relative to the main magnetic field [11].

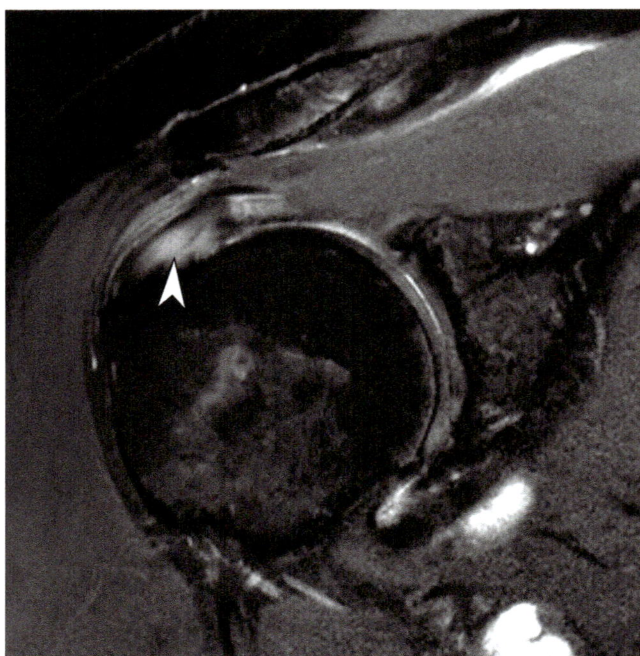

Fig. 2.1 Tendinopathy. Coronal fat-suppressed T2-weighted MR image demonstrates tendinopathy of the infraspinatus tendon (arrowhead) depicted by increased signal intensity within the tendon that does not reach signal intensity of fluid and abnormally increased thickness of the tendon

2.3 Rotator Cuff Tears

Rotator cuff tears are characterized by morphologic abnormalities, such as fiber discontinuity or thinning of the tendon, as well as a signal changes on fluid sensitive sequences that reach the signal intensity of fluid. Various classifications of the rotator cuff tears exist based on the tear morphology, location and extent of tendon disruption, and tendon retraction.

Full-thickness tears involve all the layers of the rotator cuff while partial-thickness tears can be classified into articular-sided, bursal-sided, and intrasubstance tears (also referred to as interstitial or intratendinous tears) (Fig. 2.2). Partial-thickness tears are diagnosed based on signal alterations on fluid sensitive sequences if the signal abnormality

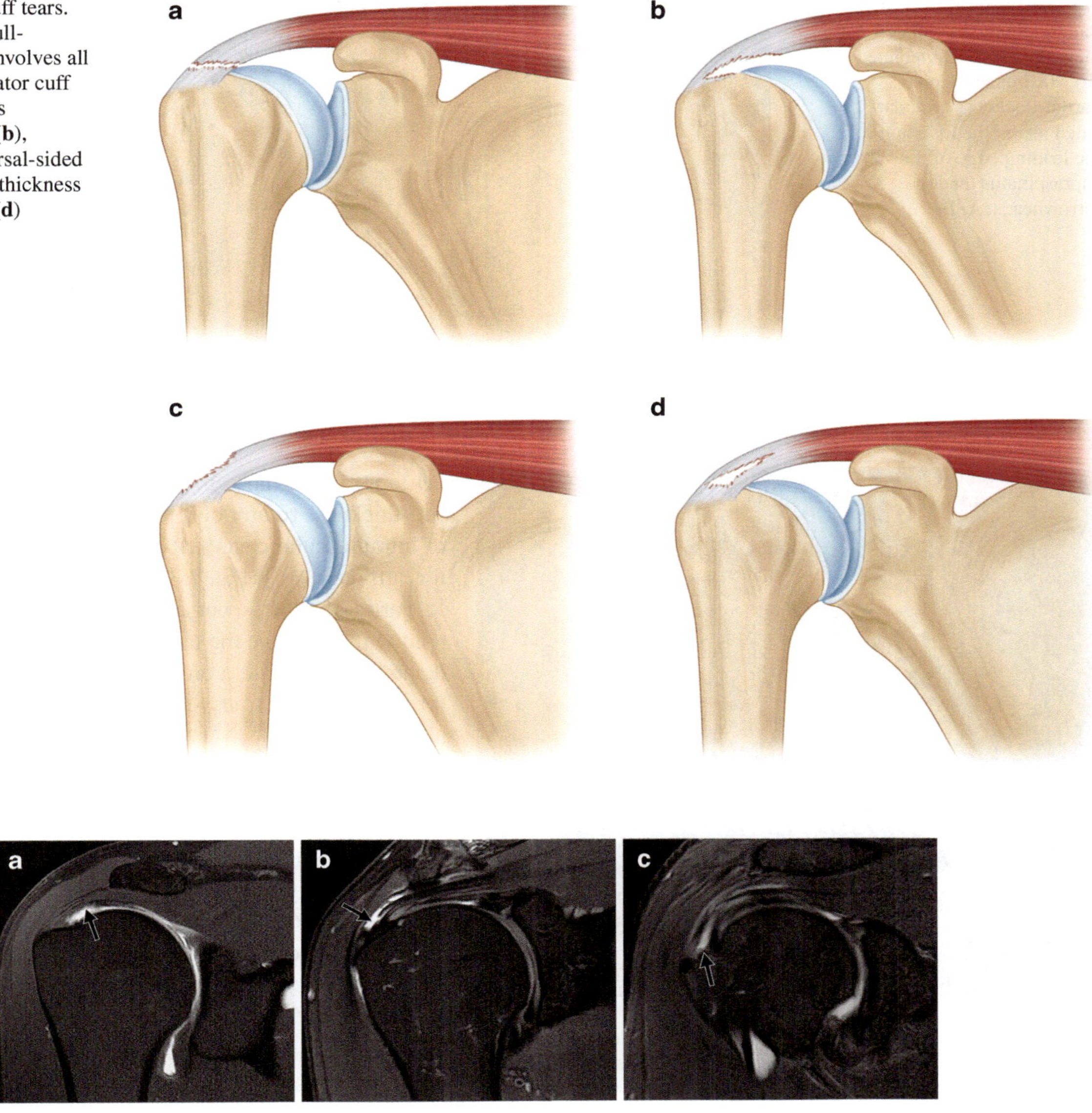

Fig. 2.2 Rotator cuff tears. Drawing showing full-thickness tear that involves all the layers of the rotator cuff (**a**), partial-thickness articular-sided tear (**b**), partial-thickness bursal-sided tear (**c**), and partial-thickness intrasubstance tear (**d**)

Fig. 2.3 Partial-thickness rotator cuff tears. Coronal fat-suppressed T1-weighted direct MR arthrography image (**a**) and fat-suppressed proton-density-weighted MR images (**b, c**) demonstrate partial-thickness articular-sided (arrow, A), bursal-sided (arrow, B), and intrasubstance (arrow, C) tears of the supraspinatus tendon

approaches the intensity of fluid and involves either articular or bursal surface of the tendon or resides within the tendon (Fig. 2.3). Additionally, alterations of normal tendon caliber may be present with either abrupt caliber changes or gradual tapering of the tendon in more chronic cases. Anatomic tendon footprints should be carefully examined as its incomplete coverage by the tendon indicates an insertional tear [1]. Partial-thickness articular-sided tears at the tendon insertion are sometimes referred as “rim-rent” tears (Fig. 2.4). Although rotator cable represents a normal anatomic structure, thickening along the rotator cable suggests the presence of the partial-thickness articular-sided tear and should prompt careful evaluation of the undersurface of the cuff [12].

Based on the assumption that an average normal cuff thickness is 10–12 mm, Ellman classification characterizes partial-thickness tears a low grade (grade 1, <3 mm deep), moderate grade (grade 2, 3–6 mm deep), or high grade (grade 3, >6 mm deep) [13]. Current classification by the International Society of Arthroscopy, Knee Surgery and Orthopaedic Sports Medicine (ISAKOS) recommends characterization of the partial-thickness rotator cuff tear as tendon tissue involvement greater or lesser than 50% of tendon thickness as tears involving less than 50% of tendon thickness are usually treated conservatively [14].

Full-thickness tendon tears vary in width, ranging from very focal, pinhole-sized tears to large tears that involve the entire tendon width, referred to as a full-thickness full-width

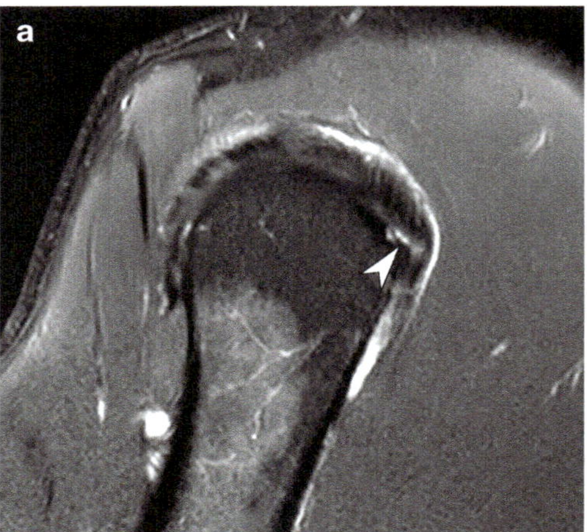

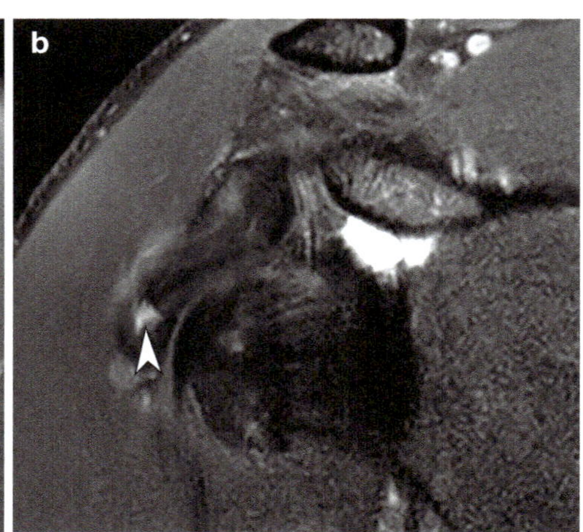

Fig. 2.4 "Rim-rent" tear. Sagittal STIR (**a**) and coronal fat-suppressed T2-weighted (**b**) MR images depict partial-thickness articular-sided tear at the insertion of the leading edge of the supraspinatus tendon (arrowheads, A, B)

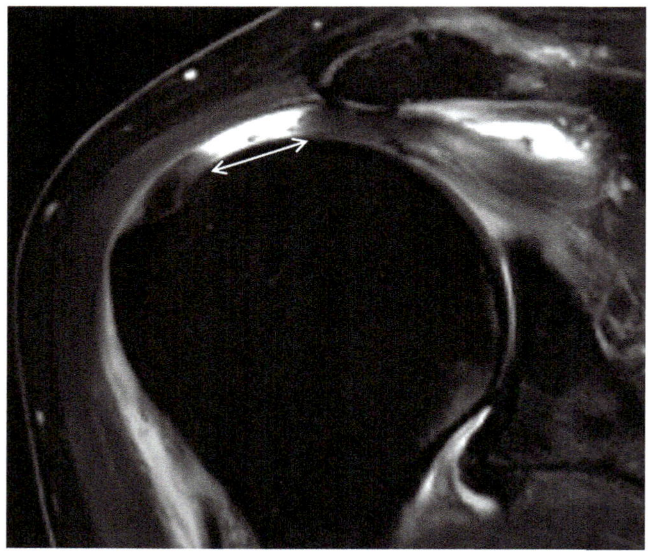

Fig. 2.5 Full-thickness tear of the supraspinatus tendon. Coronal fat-suppressed T2-weighted MR image shows full-thickness fiber discontinuity with 1.4 cm retraction (double-headed arrow) of the supraspinatus tendon

tendon tear. Full-thickness tears are classified based on the tear extension anterior to posterior, tendon retraction medial to lateral, and morphology (C-shaped, U-shaped, L-shaped, or reverse L-shaped) [14] (Fig. 2.5). Full-thickness tears that are equal or greater than 5 cm involve two or more rotator cuff tendons are referred to as massive tears.

Delaminated tear is defined as intratendinous horizontal splitting between the articular and bursal layers (Fig. 2.6). Delamination can be present with partial-thickness intrasubstance tears or represent an additional delaminating component of full-thickness tears (Fig. 2.7). Delamination should be described on imaging as it carries clinical implications: it can be missed during routine arthroscopy; its presence adversely affects a healing potential of the tendon and represents negative prognostic factor that requires different surgical approach. Intrasubstance delamination of partial or full-thickness rotator cuff tears may lead to the development of intramuscular cysts that are strongly associated with rotator cuff tears [15] (Fig. 2.8).

Partial-thickness bursal-sided tears of the infraspinatus tendon that involve the transverse head and accompanied by delamination create a unique tear pattern with avulsion and retraction of the transverse head from the oblique portion [16] (Fig. 2.9).

MRI is highly accurate for diagnosis of full-thickness cuff tears with 92% sensitivity and 93% specificity of standard MRI and 95% sensitivity and 99% specificity for MR arthrography. For partial-thickness tears, standard MRI demonstrate 64% sensitivity and 92% specificity, and MR arthrography demonstrate 86% sensitivity and 96% specificity [17]. Same meta-analysis demonstrated ultrasound to have 92% sensitivity and 94% specificity for full-thickness tears and 67% sensitivity and 94% specificity for partial-thickness tears [17].

Key Points

- Partial thickness tears involving less than 50% of tendon thickness are usually treated conservatively.
- The presence of delamination in both partial and full thickness tears may influence treatment decisions.
- Intramuscular cysts are strongly associated with the rotator cuff tendon tears.

In addition to the classifications above, tears of the supraspinatus and infraspinatus tendons may be referred to as posterior superior cuff tears while tears of the subscapularis are referred to as anterior cuff tears.

The subscapularis tears, or anterior cuff tears, are frequently underestimated by both arthroscopists and radiologists and often referred to as "hidden lesions." Subscapularis

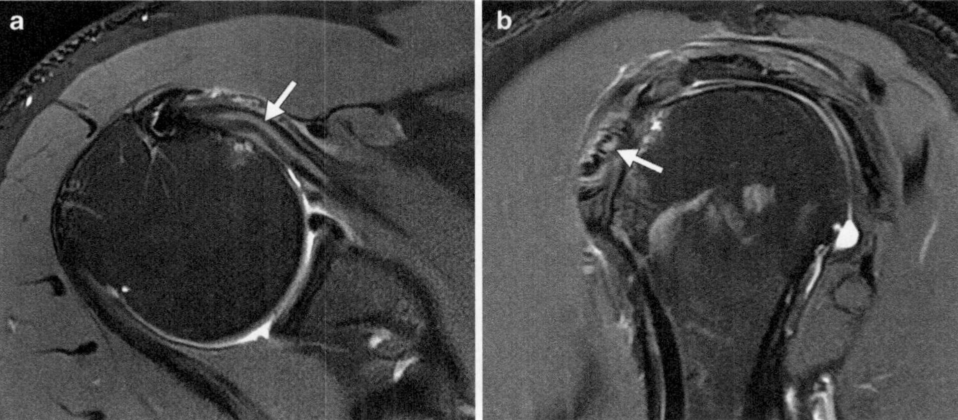

Fig. 2.6 Delaminated tear. Axial (**a**) and sagittal (**b**) fat-suppressed proton-density-weighted MR images demonstrate low-grade intrasubstance delaminated tear (arrows, A, B) of the subscapularis tendon

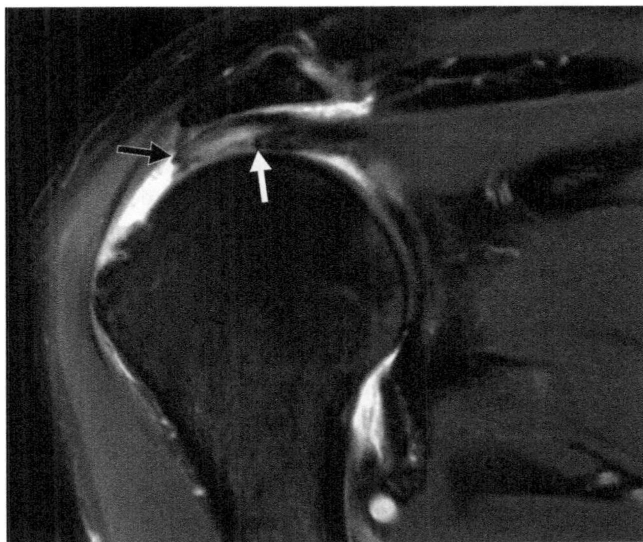

Fig. 2.7 Full-thickness delaminated tear. Coronal fat-suppressed T2-weighted MR image demonstrates full-thickness delaminated tear of the supraspinatus tendon with differential retraction of the bursal (black arrow) and articular (white arrow) fibers

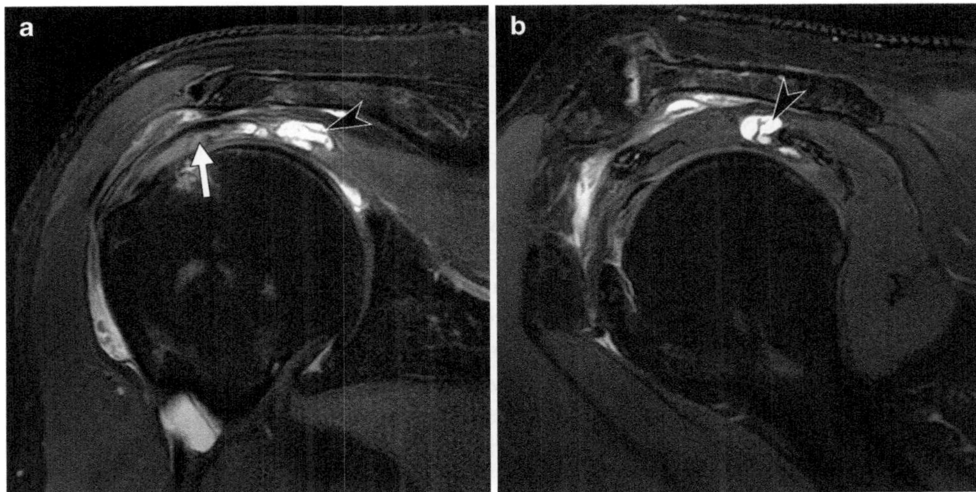

Fig. 2.8 Intramuscular cysts. Coronal (**a**) and sagittal (**b**) fat-suppressed proton-density-weighted MR images demonstrate delaminated tear (arrow, A) of the infraspinatus tendon with intramuscular cyst formation (arrowheads, A, B)

injuries are highly prevalent, being present in approximately 50% of patients undergoing shoulder arthroscopy. The reported sensitivity and specificity of different diagnostic studies vary widely, with accuracy decreasing particularly in small tears located in the upper third. This is partly due to the complex anatomy in this region, which involves the superior glenohumeral ligament, the coracohumeral ligament, and the anterior fascicle of the supraspinatus tendon.

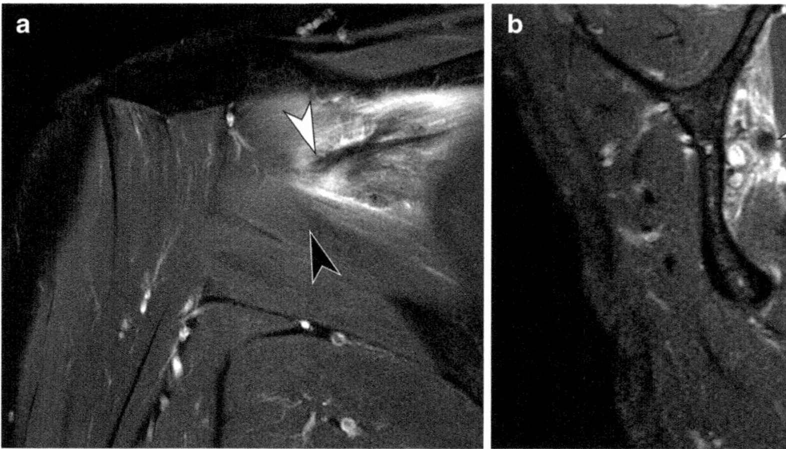

Fig. 2.9 "Novel lesion." Coronal fat-suppressed T2-weighted (**a**) and sagittal STIR (**b**) MR images depict delaminating infraspinatus tendon tear with retracted tear of the transverse portion (white arrowhead, A, B). The deeper fibers of the oblique portion are intact (black arrowhead, A, B) and can be traced to the greater tuberosity footprint (not shown)

To avoid missing these lesions, arthroscopists must perform a systematic and thorough evaluation during surgery. Similarly, imaging techniques should be optimized with high-resolution protocols. MRI and MR arthrography are considered more reliable than ultrasound for detecting subscapularis tears [9, 18]. Both axial and sagittal planes must be carefully assessed (Fig. 2.6). Some studies have also suggested that internal rotation of the shoulder during imaging may improve diagnostic accuracy [19]. Isolated subscapularis tears are uncommon and most often occur in association with other shoulder pathologies, particularly concomitant other rotator cuff tears. These tears typically originate in the superior third of the tendon and extend distally [9, 18]. Lesions involving the superior third frequently compromise the biceps pulley complex as well as the anterior articular fibers of the supraspinatus tendon (Fig. 2.10).

Several classification systems for subscapularis tears have been proposed, most of them based on the insertion site; however, none has been universally accepted. The Lafosse classification is one of the most widely used and has been adopted by ISAKOS. This system includes five grades, extending caudally from partial tear of the upper third, grade 1, to complete tear of the upper third, and grade 2, to complete lesion of the superior two-thirds in grade 3, and grades 4 and 5 are complete tear, being in grade 4 the humeral head centered and less than stage 3 fatty atrophy and grade 5 the humeral head is disbalanced and located eccentrically with fatty atrophy [9, 18, 20, 21] (Fig. 2.11). Yoo et al. [8] proposed a subdivision of the upper third tears involving the first facet, starting with fraying, grade 1, less than 50% of the attachment; in grade 2A and ig ,the detachment is greater than 50% but without complete disruption of the lateral hood attachment grade 2B. If there is a detachment from the complete first facet, it is grade 3 and grade 4 when it is the first and second facet, involving the entire tendinous attachment. If the muscle insertion is involved, it is grade 5[8]. Additionally, longitudinal tears of the subscapularis have been described,

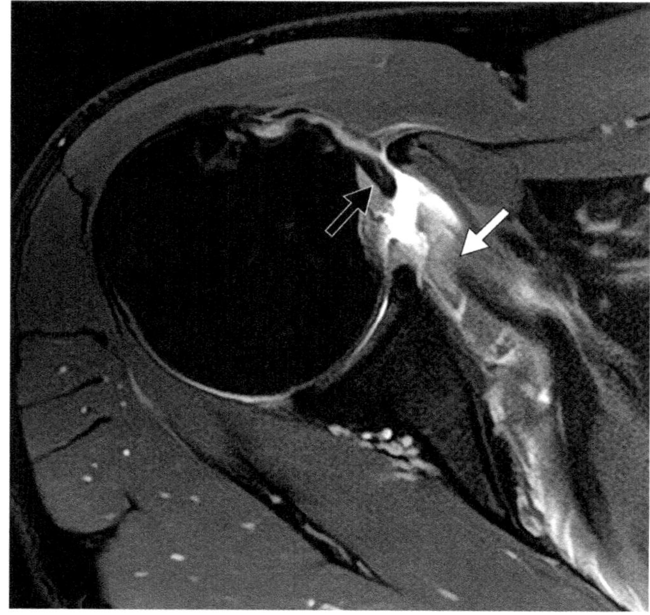

Fig. 2.10 Biceps pulley complex injury and subscapularis tendon tear. Axial fat-suppressed proton-density-weighted MR image demonstrates complete rupture of subscapularis tendon with retraction (white arrow) and biceps dislocation (black arrow)

occurring with or without disruption of the footprint insertion [22].

The superior retraction of the upper third of the subscapularis tendon was described by Burkhart as the "comma sign" on arthroscopic examination. This sign can be identified on MRI and has been also referred to as the "bridging sign." It appears as a soft tissue band bridging the subscapularis and supraspinatus tendons, located anteriorly and medially to the anterior labrum. This band is composed of the superior glenohumeral ligament, the coracohumeral ligament, and the residual subscapularis fascia (Fig. 2.12). Although the presence of this structure is frequently associated with supraspinatus tears, this is not always the case [23–25].

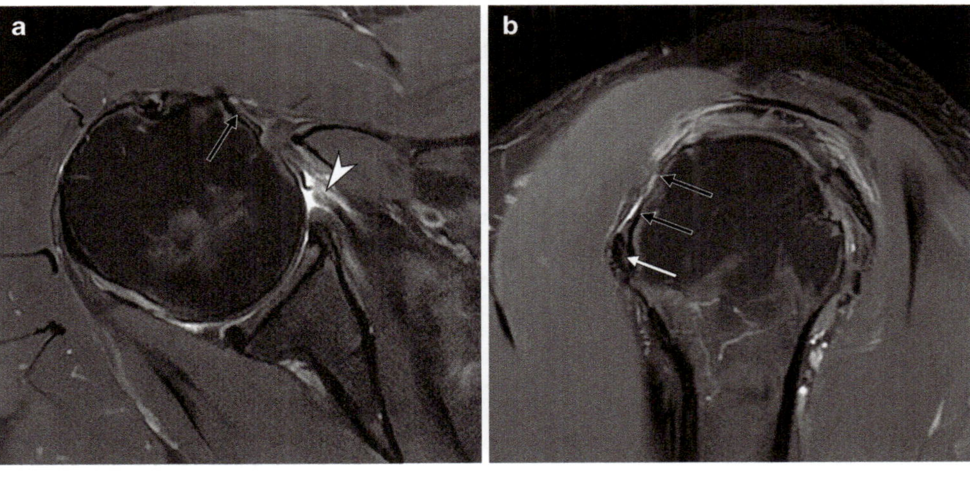

Fig. 2.11 Full-thickness subscapularis tendon tear. Axial (**a**) and sagittal (**b**) fat-suppressed proton-density-weighted MR images demonstrate a full-thickness tear of the upper and middle portions of the subscapularis tendon (black arrows, A, B) with tendon retraction (arrowhead) and intact lower third of the tendon (white arrow)

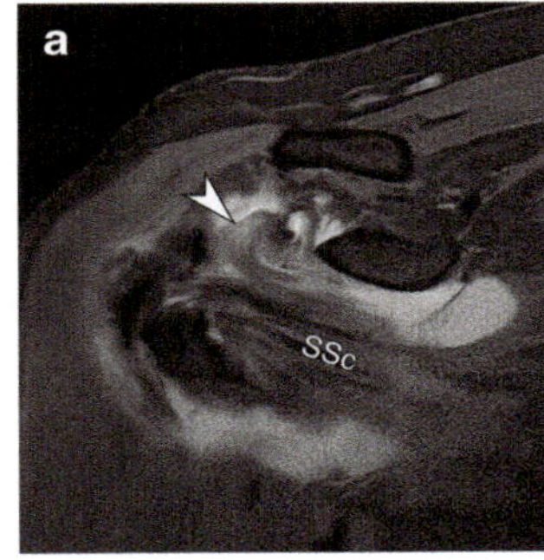

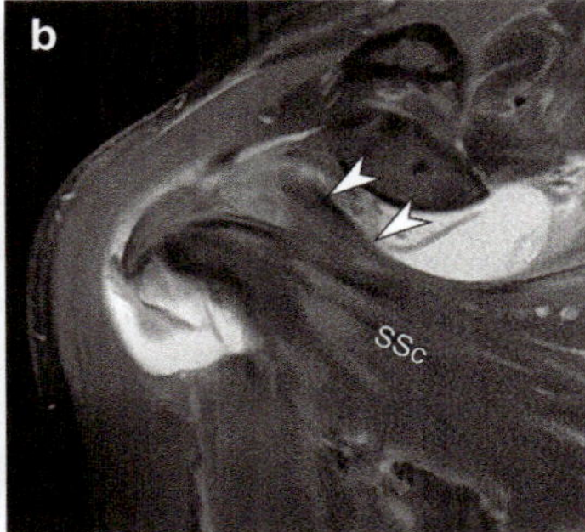

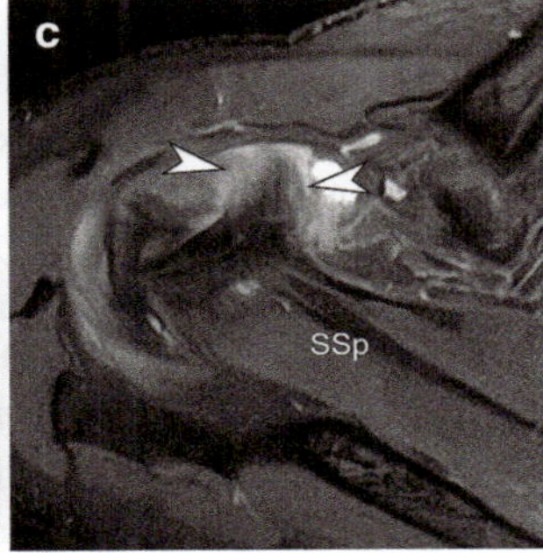

Fig. 2.12 "Comma sign" and "bridging sign" of subscapularis tendon tear in two patients. Coronal (Patient1, A, Patient 2, B) and axial (Patient 2, C) fat-suppressed proton-density-weighted MR images demonstrate full-thickness tear of the superior fibers of the subscapularis tendon (SSc, A, B) retracted superiorly and contiguous with a curved soft tissue band (arrowheads A, B, C) bridging the subscapularis and supraspinatus tendons (SSp)

Key Points

- Tears of subscapularis are often difficult to detect arthroscopically.
- MRI description of subscapularis tears should include their craniocaudal extent and thickness.
- "Comma sign" and "bridging sign" refer to a curved soft tissue band bridging the subscapularis and supraspinatus tendons representing retracted tissues in setting of full-thickness tears of the upper third of the subscapularis tendon.

2.4 Muscle Atrophy and Fatty Infiltration

Assessment of the rotator cuff musculature is an important part of MRI reporting, as it affects treatment decisions. Following the rotator cuff tendon tear, the cuff musculature undergoes atrophy and fatty infiltration which correlates with poor structural and functional outcomes of cuff repair. Various qualitative and quantitative methods have been introduced to access muscle degeneration on imaging. One of the most popular classification for assessment of fatty infiltration was introduced by Goutallier et al. using CT and subsequently adapted for MRI [26, 27]. Fatty infiltration can be classified as Stage 0, normal muscle; Stage 1, some fatty streaks; Stage 2, more muscle than fat; Stage 3, equal muscle and fat; and Stage 4, more fat than muscle [26]. Thomazeau et al. calculated the volume loss of the supraspinatus muscle belly by occupation ratio, defined as surface of the supraspinatus muscle divided by the surface of the supraspinatus fossa determined on the sagittal oblique plane where osseous borders of the supraspinatus fossa assume Y-shaped configuration, and categorized muscle volume loss as minimal, moderate, or severe [28]. A tangent sign, introduced by Zanetti et al., uses a reference line drawn through the superior borders of the scapular spine and the superior margin of the coracoid on the most lateral sagittal oblique MR image; it is considered abnormal, or positive, when the supraspinatus muscle does not cross the tangent [29]. Positive tangent sign is predictive of worse outcome after rotator cuff repair [30]. Feuerriegel et al. recently introduced the blackbird sign that describes development of concave contour of the superior posterior muscle belly as the asymmetric pattern of early supraspinatus atrophy on sagittal MRI [31].

Key Points
- Reporting of rotator cuff tears should include description of the tear location, pattern, size, retraction, shape, and presence of muscle atrophy and fatty infiltration.
- Muscle atrophy adversely affects treatment outcomes.

2.5 Myotendinous Junction Injury

Myotendinous junction injuries of the rotator cuff are uncommon but important for functional outcome. They are most common in infraspinatus and supraspinatus but may affect all muscles of the rotator cuff [32] (Fig. 2.13). Muscle strain represents most common injury pattern, followed by partial tears. Although myotendinous junction injury typically occurs without associated rotator cuff tendon tear, concomitant insertional tendon tears are reported with the supraspinatus myotendinous junction injuries [33]. At least a portion of the injuries of the infraspinatus tendon described in the spectrum of the "novel lesion" by Lunn et al. and originally characterized as myotendinous junction injury [34] may represent delaminated tears with differential retraction involving more superficial transverse portion of the layered infraspinatus tendon [16] (Fig. 2.9).

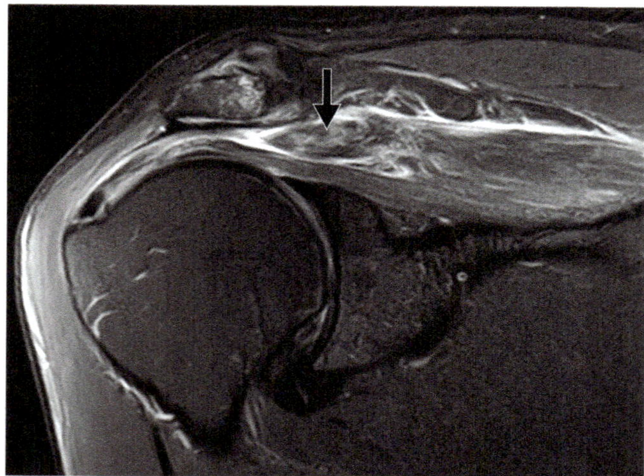

Fig. 2.13 Myotendinous junction injury. Coronal fat-suppressed proton-density-weighted MR image shows complete supraspinatus myotendinous tear (arrow)

2.6 Rotator Cuff Tear Mimickers

Several entities manifest with shoulder pain, weakness, or both and can mimic rotator cuff tears clinically. Additionally, imaging findings of some diseases overlap with appearance of a rotator cuff tear and may lead to diagnostic errors.

2.6.1 Calcific Tendinitis

Hydroxyapatite deposition disease (HADD) refers to a spectrum of musculoskeletal pathology, in which calcium hydroxyapatite crystals are deposited in the tendons, bursa, and other soft tissues and can migrate along the course of the tendon and into the bone. In the shoulder, manifestations of HADD include calcific tendinitis, calcific bursitis, and intraosseous loculation of the calcific deposits that may result in osteitis and osteolysis [35] (Fig. 2.14). On MRI imaging, calcific tendinitis is recognized by detecting calcific deposits of low-signal intensity on all pulse sequences and surrounding inflammation. When prominent, inflammation in the tendon may mimic rotator cuff tear and muscle strain. Small calcific deposits are often inconspicuous on MRI, and increased signal on fluid-sensitive sequences may be misinterpreted as a traumatic injury. Careful review of nonfat-suppressed sequences along with radiographs may be helpful in detecting calcifications, leading to accurate diagnosis of HADD.

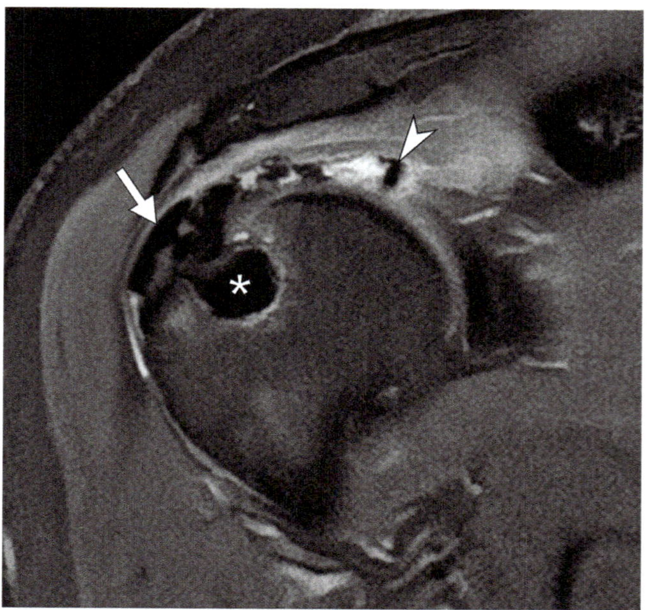

Fig. 2.14 Calcium hydroxyapatite deposition disease. Coronal fat-suppressed proton-density-weighted MR image depicts calcific tendinitis of the infraspinatus tendon with calcification in the tendon (white arrow) and within intramuscular cyst (arrowhead) as well as intraosseous loculation of the calcific deposits (asterisk)

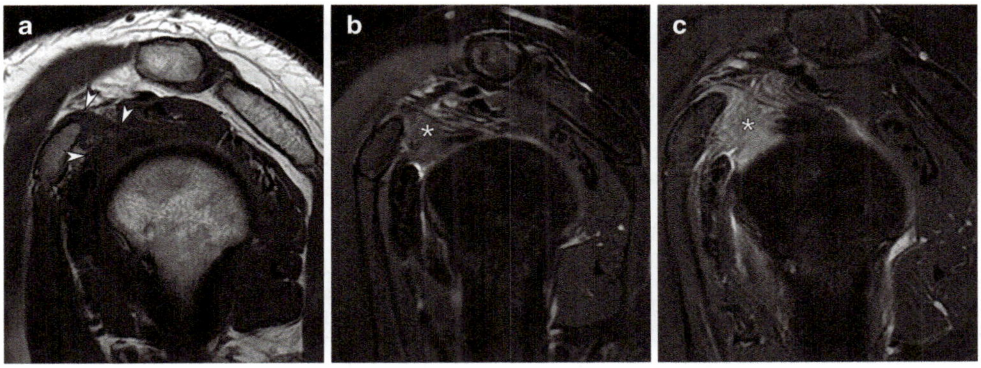

Fig. 2.15 Adhesive capsulitis. Sagittal T1-weighted (**a**), fat-suppressed proton-density-weighted (**b**) and contrast-enhanced fat-suppressed T1-weighted (**c**) MR images depict scarring of the rotator interval (arrowheads, A) and obliteration of the subcoracoid triangle of fat, edema of the rotator interval (asterisk, B) representing inflammatory changes with marked enhancement following administration of intravenous contrast (asterisk, C)

2.6.2 Adhesive Capsulitis

Adhesive capsulitis, a clinical condition referred to as a frozen shoulder, represents an idiopathic or secondary inflammatory process that affects the glenohumeral joint synovium, capsule, and glenohumeral ligaments, presents with pain, and results in capsular scarring and decreased passive and active range of motion. On MRI, adhesive capsulitis is diagnosed by detecting abnormalities of the signal and morphology that range from edema and thickening of the capsule and surrounding structures on fluid sensitive sequences due to inflammation to low-signal intensity on all pulse sequences due to scarring at the later phase of the process [36]. MRI abnormalities are best seen in the rotator interval and axillary pouch; however, they can also be observed along the posterior superior joint capsule. Typical changes in rotator interval include edema, thickening of the coracohumeral ligament, and obliteration of the subcoracoid triangle of fat [37] (Fig. 2.15). T2 hyperintensity of the inferior glenohumeral ligament demonstrated high sensitivity (85.3–88.2%) and high specificity (88.2%) for the diagnosis of adhesive capsulitis while the presence of a thin layer of signal hyperintensity adjacent to the external capsular surface of the inferior glenohumeral ligament on T2-weighted fat-saturated images is highly specific for the diagnosis of adhesive capsulitis (91.2–97%) [38]. Capsular scarring may result in altered distribution of the intraarticular fluid with disproportional distention of the biceps recess and subscapular recess compared to the glenohumeral joint [39]. Gadolinium-enhanced MRI might be useful as it increases the confidence in the diagnosis, showing inflammatory changes in earlier stages.

2.6.3 Muscle Denervation

Muscle denervation may present with weakness and may mimic rotator cuff tears clinically. Denervation in the shoulder may be caused by brachial plexopathy, acute trauma, or space-occupying lesions. Space-occupying lesions, commonly paralabral cysts, or trauma, such as glenohumeral dislocation typically affect single nerve territory while brachial plexopathy affects muscles in the multiple nerve distribution [40]. On MRI, denervation changes are characterized by uniform increased signal of muscles on fluid-sensitive sequences and absence of perifascial edema or inflammatory changes in the adjacent subcutaneous tissue. Initially the muscle bulk is preserved which later followed by atrophy and fatty infiltration.

2.7 Conclusion

Understanding the nuanced anatomy of the rotator cuff is important for analysis and reporting of clinical MR imaging. Current classifications and treatment implications of various injuries of the rotator cuff must be recognized for accurate communication between radiologists and surgeons. This review summarizes current anatomic concepts and accepted classifications of rotator cuff injuries as well as imaging pitfalls.

Take-Home Messages

- Knowledge of rotator cuff footprint anatomy and individual components of each muscle of the rotator cuff is essential for accurate reporting of the tear pattern and location.
- Various parameters of the cuff tear must be addressed utilizing accepted classifications.
- The presence of muscle atrophy and tendon delamination influences surgical decision-making.

Conflict of Interest Statement I/We declare no competing interests as defined by Springer Nature or other interests that might be perceived to influence results and/or discussion reported in this manuscript.

References

1. Chang EY, Chung CB. Current concepts on imaging diagnosis of rotator cuff disease. Semin Musculoskelet Radiol. 2014;18(4):412–24. https://doi.org/10.1055/s-0034-1384830.
2. Burkhart SS, Esch JC, Jolson RS. The rotator crescent and rotator cable: an anatomic description of the shoulder's "suspension bridge.". Arthroscopy. 1993;9:611.
3. Kim SY, Boynton EL, Ravichandiran K, Fung LY, Bleakney R, Agur AM. Three-dimensional study of the musculotendinous architecture of supraspinatus and its functional correlations. Clin Anat. 2007;20(6):648–55. https://doi.org/10.1002/ca.20469.
4. Kato A, Nimura A, Yamaguchi K, Mochizuki T, Sugaya H, Akita K. An anatomical study of the transverse part of the infraspinatus muscle that is closely related with the supraspinatus muscle. Surg Radiol Anat. 2012;34(3):257–65. https://doi.org/10.1007/s00276-011-0872-0.
5. Mochizuki T, Sugaya H, Uomizu M, et al. Humeral insertion of the supraspinatus and infraspinatus. J Bone Joint Surg. 2008;90(5):962–9. https://doi.org/10.2106/JBJS.G.00427.
6. Moser TP, Cardinal É, Bureau NJ, Guillin R, Lanneville P, Grabs D. The aponeurotic expansion of the supraspinatus tendon: anatomy and prevalence in a series of 150 shoulder MRIs. Skeletal Radiol. 2014;44(2):223–31. https://doi.org/10.1007/s00256-014-1993-4.
7. Kellam P, Kahn T, Tashjian RZ. Anatomy of the subscapularis: a review. J Shoulder Elb Arthroplast. 2019;3 https://doi.org/10.1177/2471549219849728.
8. Yoo JC, Rhee YG, Shin SJ, et al. Subscapularis tendon tear classification based on 3-dimensional anatomic footprint: a cadaveric and prospective clinical observational study. Arthroscopy. 2015;31(1):19–28. https://doi.org/10.1016/j.arthro.2014.08.015.
9. Yubran AP, Pesquera LC, Juan ELS, et al. Rotator cuff tear patterns: MRI appearance and its surgical relevance. Insights Imaging Springer. 2024; 15(1). https://doi.org/10.1186/s13244-024-01607-w.
10. Dhanaraj D, Parisien RL, McHale KJ, et al. The comma sign: the coracohumeral ligament and superior glenohumeral ligament exhibit similar quantitative characteristics with terminal confluence at the subscapularis insertion. Arthrosc Sports Med Rehabil. 2021;3(3):e645–9. https://doi.org/10.1016/j.asmr.2020.12.011.
11. Chang EY, Chung CB. Imaging diagnosis of rotator cuff pathology and impingement syndromes. In: The shoulder. Springer; 2019. p. 87–125. https://doi.org/10.1007/978-3-030-06240-8_5.
12. Sheah K, Bredella MA, Warner JJP, Halpern EF, Palmer WE. Transverse thickening along the articular surface of the rotator cuff consistent with the rotator cable: identification with MR arthrography and relevance in rotator cuff evaluation. Am J Roentgenol. 2009;193(3):679–86. https://doi.org/10.2214/AJR.08.2285.
13. Ellman H. Diagnosis and Treatment of Incomplete Rotator Cuff Tears.
14. Calvo E, Guardado CR, Morcillo D, Arce G. Rotator cuff tears: diagnosis and classification. In: Shoulder arthroscopy: principles and practice, Second Edition. Springer; 2023. p. 445–52. https://doi.org/10.1007/978-3-662-66868-9_33.
15. Kassarjian A, Torriani M, Ouellette H, Palmer W. Intramuscular rotator cuff cysts: association with tendon tears on MRI and arthroscopy. AJR Am J Roentgenol. 2005;185. https://doi.org/10.2214/ajr.185.1.01850160.
16. Huang BK, Chang EY. Delaminating infraspinatus tendon tears with differential retraction: imaging features and surgical relevance. Skeletal Radiol. 2017;46(1):41–50. https://doi.org/10.1007/s00256-016-2506-4.
17. De Jesus JO, Parker L, Frangos AJ, Nazarian LN. Accuracy of MRI, MR arthrography, and ultrasound in the diagnosis of rotator cuff tears: a meta-analysis. Am J Roentgenol. 2009;192(6):1701–7. https://doi.org/10.2214/AJR.08.1241.
18. Saremi H, seifrabiei M. Subscapularis tendon tear classification and diagnosis: a systemic review and meta-analysis. Front Surg Frontiers Media SA. 2023;10 https://doi.org/10.3389/fsurg.2023.916694.
19. Siriwanarangsun P, Pakdee W, Pisanuwongse A, Keyurapan E, Lektrakul N. Subscapularis tendon tear detection using axial internal rotation MRI: semiquantitative and quantitative analysis. Quant Imaging Med Surg. 2023;13(12):8274–89. https://doi.org/10.21037/qims-23-273.
20. Lafosse L, Jost B, Reiland Y, Audebert S, Toussaint B, Gobezie R. Structural integrity and clinical outcomes after arthroscopic repair of isolated subscapularis tears. J Bone Joint Surg. 2007;89(6):1184–93. https://doi.org/10.2106/JBJS.F.00007.
21. Willems J, Guttmann D, Arce G, Bain G. Arthroscopy and repair. In: Shoulder concepts 2013: consensus and concerns. Springer; 2013. p. 87–94. https://doi.org/10.1007/978-3-642-38097-6_11.
22. Dierckman BD, Shah NR, Larose CR, Gerbrandt S, Getelman MH. Non-insertional tendinopathy of the subscapularis. Int J Shoulder Surg. 2013;7(3):83–90. https://doi.org/10.4103/0973-6042.118876.
23. Jung JY, Yoon YC, Cha DI, Yoo JC, Jung JY. The "bridging sign": a MR finding for combined full-thickness tears of the subscapularis tendon and the supraspinatus tendon. Acta Radiol. 2013;54(1):83–8. https://doi.org/10.1258/ar.2012.120353.
24. Zappia M, Ascione F, Romano AM, et al. Comma sign of subscapularis tear: diagnostic performance and magnetic resonance imaging appearance. J Shoulder Elb Surg. 2021;30(5):1107–16. https://doi.org/10.1016/j.jse.2020.07.047.
25. Atinga A, Dwyer T, Theodoropoulos JS, Dekirmendjian K, Naraghi AM, White LM. Preoperative magnetic resonance imaging accurately detects the arthroscopic comma sign in subscapularis tears. Arthroscopy. 2021;37(10):3062–9. https://doi.org/10.1016/j.arthro.2021.04.040.
26. Goutallier D, Postel JM, Bernageau J, Lavau L, Voisin MC. Fatty muscle degeneration in cuff ruptures. pre- and postoperative evaluation by CT scan. Clin Orthop Relat Res. 1994;(304):78–83. http://www.ncbi.nlm.nih.gov/pubmed/8020238
27. Fuchs B, Weishaupt D, Zanetti M, Hodler J, Gerber C. Fatty degeneration of the muscles of the rotator cuff: assessment by computed tomography versus magnetic resonance imaging. J Shoulder Elb Surg. 1999;8(6):599–605. https://doi.org/10.1016/s1058-2746(99)90097-6.
28. Thomazeau H, Rolland Y, Lucas C, Duval JM, Langlais F. Atrophy of the supraspinatus belly: assessment by MRI in 55 patients with rotator cuff pathology. Acta Orthop Scand. 1996;67(3):264–8. https://doi.org/10.3109/17453679608994685.
29. Zanetti M, Gerber C, Hodler J. Quantitative assessment of the muscles of the rotator cuff with magnetic resonance imaging. Investig Radiol. 1998;33(3):163–70. https://doi.org/10.1097/00004424-199803000-00006.
30. Naimark M, Trinh T, Robbins C, et al. Effect of muscle quality on operative and nonoperative treatment of rotator cuff tears. Orthop J Sports Med. 2019;7(8) https://doi.org/10.1177/2325967119863010.
31. Feuerriegel GC, Marcus RP, Goller SS, et al. A visual marker for early atrophy of the supraspinatus muscle on conventional MRI: introduction of the blackbird sign. Eur Radiol. 2025;35(1):313–22. https://doi.org/10.1007/s00330-024-10946-7.
32. Taneja AK, Kattapuram SV, Chang CY, Simeone FJ, Bredella MA, Torriani M. MRI findings of rotator cuff myotendinous junction injury. Am J Roentgenol. 2014;203(2):406–11. https://doi.org/10.2214/AJR.13.11474.
33. Miranda MO, Bureau NJ. Supraspinatus myotendinous junction injuries: MRI findings and prevalence. Am J Roentgenol. 2019;212(1):W1–9. https://doi.org/10.2214/AJR.18.19776.

34. Lunn JV, Castellanos-Rosas J, Tavernier T, Barthélémy R, Walch G. A novel lesion of the infraspinatus characterized by musculotendinous disruption, edema, and late fatty infiltration. J Shoulder Elb Surg. 2008;17(4):546–53. https://doi.org/10.1016/j.jse.2007.11.016.
35. Porcellini G, Paladini P, Campi F, Pegreffi F. Osteolytic lesion of greater tuberosity in calcific tendinitis of the shoulder. J Shoulder Elb Surg. 2009;18(2):210–5. https://doi.org/10.1016/j.jse.2008.09.016.
36. Polster JM, Schickendantz MS. Shoulder MRI: what do we miss? Am J Roentgenol. 2010;195(3):577–84. https://doi.org/10.2214/AJR.10.4683.
37. Mengiardi B, Pfirrmann CWA, Gerber C, Hodler J, Zanetti M. Frozen shoulder: MR arthrographic findings. Radiology. 2004;233(2):486–92. https://doi.org/10.1148/radiol.2332031219.
38. Gondim Teixeira PA, Balaj C, Chanson A, Lecocq S, Louis M, Blum A. Adhesive capsulitis of the shoulder: value of inferior glenohumeral ligament signal changes on T2-weighted fat-saturated images. Am J Roentgenol. 2012;198(6) https://doi.org/10.2214/AJR.11.7453.
39. Barua R, Umans H, Wilde G, Tobin K, Perou P, Levy H. Conventional MRI evaluation of adhesive capsulitis: new perspectives. In: Conference: annual meeting of the American-roentgen-ray-society, vol. 198. Preprint posted online; 2012.
40. Yanny S, Toms AP. MR patterns of denervation around the shoulder. Am J Roentgenol. 2010;195(2):157–63. https://doi.org/10.2214/AJR.09.4127.

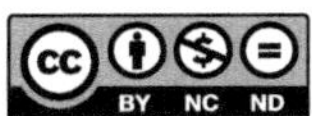

MRI of the Elbow

3

Kathryn J. Stevens and Mark Anderson

Learning Objectives

1. Describe the normal anatomy of the elbow and the soft tissue stabilizing structures.
2. Optimize imaging techniques and MR protocols for imaging the elbow.
3. Recognize examples of common osseous, ligamentous, tendinous synovial, and neural pathologies of the elbow.
4. Integrate clinical information with imaging findings for accurate diagnosis and optimal clinical management.

3.1 Introduction

The elbow is a complex joint comprising the humeroulnar, radiocapitellar, and proximal radioulnar articulations contained within a common synovial capsule. Together, these joints enable flexion and extension of the elbow, in conjunction with the distal radioulnar joint pronation and supination of the forearm. Stability of the elbow relies on the complex interplay of osseous geometry, ligaments, tendons, and muscles. Knowledge of normal anatomy is critical in the accurate interpretation of imaging studies, ultimately helping guide clinical management and treatment options.

K. J. Stevens (✉)
Department of Radiology, Stanford University Medical Center, Stanford, CA, USA
e-mail: kate.stevens@stanford.edu

M. Anderson
Department of Radiology, University of Virginia, Charlotteville, VA, USA
e-mail: mwa3a@virginia.edu

3.2 Imaging Modalities

Radiographs are usually performed first in a patient presenting with elbow pain and may demonstrate fracture, effusion, arthritis, soft tissue calcification, or joint bodies. Fat pad signs—anterior "sail sign" or visible posterior fat pad—indicate a joint effusion, and in the setting of trauma, this should raise concern for an underlying occult fracture [1].

Ultrasound is portable, low-cost, and excellent for superficial structures such as tendons, ligaments, and nerves and detection of calcification or foreign bodies [1, 2]. Ultrasound also enables dynamic evaluation of tissues, revealing abnormalities that may be occult on static imaging. Limitations include operator dependency, variable reproducibility, and reduced ability to evaluate deep osteochondral injuries.

CT provides high-resolution bony detail and is excellent for treatment planning in fractures. CT arthrography may be helpful in cases where MRI is contraindicated. Limitations include radiation exposure and inferior soft tissue contrast [1].

MRI is excellent for evaluating the complex anatomy of the elbow, particularly at 3T using a dedicated surface coil, which can improve signal-to-noise ratio and spatial resolution. Patients can be imaged supine with the arm resting at the side, which is comfortable and well tolerated, but the peripheral location of the elbow in the bore of the magnet may result in poor fat saturation. Imaging the patient prone in the "superman" position places the elbow in the center of the bore, but this position is less comfortable, and images are therefore prone to motion artifact.

A combination of fat-sensitive (T1 and PD) and fluid-sensitive (PD and T2 with fat saturation or STIR) images should be acquired in orthogonal scan planes [3]. Axial images should extend from the distal humeral diaphysis through the bicipital tuberosity of the radius. Coronal oblique images are obtained parallel to the humeral epicondylar axis. Sagittal oblique images should be perpendicular to the humeral epicondylar axis. More recently three-dimensional

J. Hodler et al. (eds.), *Musculoskeletal Diseases 2026-2029*, IDKD Springer Series,
https://doi.org/10.1007/978-3-032-17040-8_3

isotropic sequences have shown promise in imaging of the elbow, particularly for obliquely oriented structures and complex anatomical regions [4]. MR arthrography with dilute gadolinium contrast can improve detection of subtle osteochondral injuries, partial ligamentous tears, synovial plicae, and joint bodies, particularly in the absence of a joint effusion, and fat-saturated T1-weighted MR sequences should be included in the arthrography protocol [3, 5]. Limitations of MRI include cost, scan time, contraindications such as pacemakers and aneurysm clips, and relative contraindications such as claustrophobia.

3.3 Normal Anatomy of the Elbow

The humeroulnar joint is a hinge joint between the trochlea of the distal humerus and trochlear notch of the proximal ulna, providing osseous stability of the joint when the elbow is fully flexed or extended. The radial head articulates with the capitellum at the radiocapitellar joint, which allows both hinge and pivot motions. The proximal radioulnar joint is a pivot joint between the periphery of the radial head and sigmoid notch of the ulna, facilitating pronation and supination of the forearm in conjunction with the distal radioulnar joint [6].

The joint capsule envelops all three articulations, and supporting ligamentous structures are formed by capsular thickenings both medially and laterally (Figs. 3.1 and 3.2). On the medial side, the **ulnar collateral ligament** (UCL) is composed of three bundles [7]. The anterior bundle arises from the medial epicondyle and inserts into the ulnar sublime tubercle (Fig. 3.3). It is the most important bundle and provides the main constraint to valgus stress. The anterior bundle can be further subdivided into two bands: the anterior band which is taut in extension and the posterior band which tightens with flexion. The fan-shaped posterior bundle of the UCL is thinner and less robust. It courses from the medial humeral epicondyle to the trochlear notch and forms the floor of the cubital tunnel. The thin transverse bundle bridges the ulnar attachment of the other two bundles, is rarely seen on imaging, and plays no role in stability.

On the lateral side, there are also three ligaments (Fig. 3.3): the **radial collateral ligament** (RCL) extending from the lateral humeral epicondyle to insert into the annular ligament, the **annular ligament** attached to the radial sigmoid notch and encircling the radial head, and the **lateral ulnar collateral ligament** (LUCL) that extends from the lateral humeral epicondyle to the supinator crest of the ulna providing support for the radial head. It is also the main constraint to varus stress at the elbow [6].

Muscles and tendons provide dynamic stabilization of the joint (Fig. 3.4) [8]. Anteriorly the biceps and brachialis muscles are the main flexors of the elbow, and the biceps muscle also helps supinate the forearm. The long and short heads of

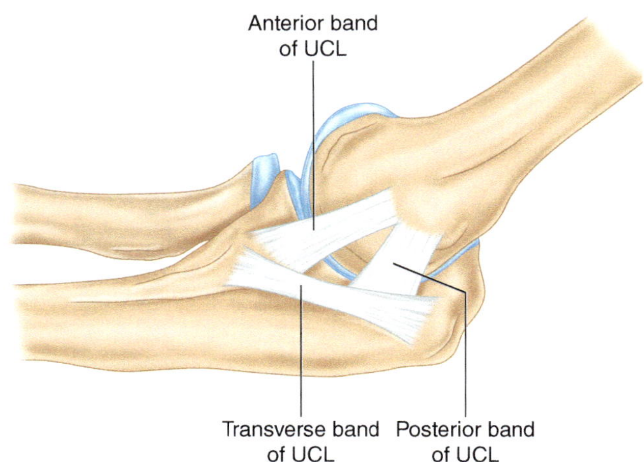

Fig. 3.1 Components of the ulnar collateral ligament (UCL)

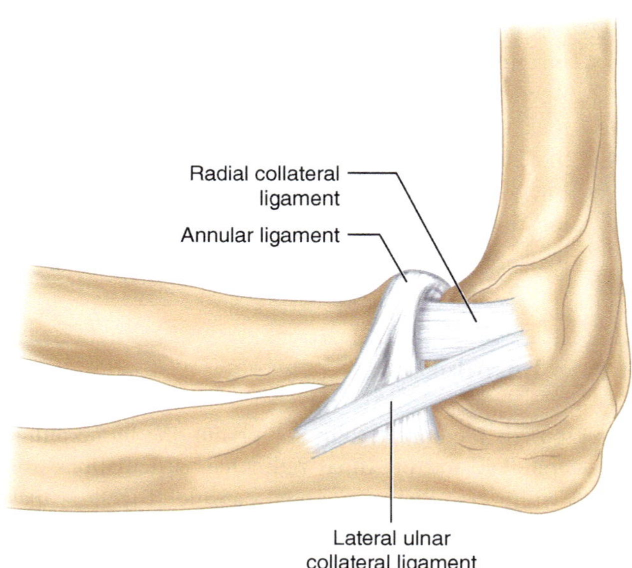

Fig. 3.2 Components of the lateral collateral ligament complex

biceps brachii typically unite to form a common tendon that passes through the antecubital fossa to insert into the bicipital tuberosity. Superficial fibers sweep across the antecubital fossa from the short head as a fascial extension known as the bicipital aponeurosis (lacertus fibrosis) that inserts into the superficial flexor pronator mass and helps to prevent tendon retraction in the case of a distal tendon rupture. Occasionally the tendons of the short and long heads remain divided throughout their length, and this can mimic a longitudinal split tear on axial MRI or result in an isolated rupture of one of the tendons [9]. The **brachialis** inserts into the ventral coronoid process or ulnar tuberosity and helps to stabilize the elbow joint during flexion and extension. In the posterior compartment, the **triceps brachii** has three heads: the long

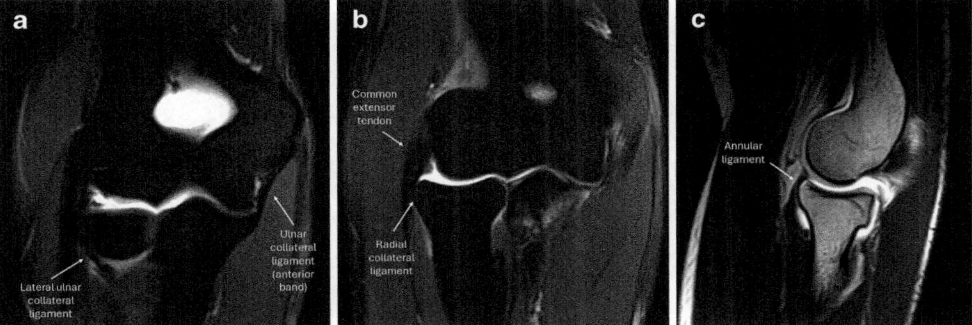

Fig. 3.3 Ligaments. (**a**) Coronal T1W fat-saturated (FS) arthrographic image demonstrates the anterior bundle of the UCL as well as the lateral ulnar collateral ligament. (**b**) Coronal T1W FS image at a slightly volar position compared with (**a**) shows the radial collateral ligament lying just deep to the common extensor tendon. (**c**) Sagittal T1W image displays the annular ligament in cross-section (arrow)

and lateral heads unite to form the superficial triceps tendon, and the medial head has a deeper more muscular insertion into the olecranon process. The anconeus muscle arises from the lateral epicondyle and inserts into the olecranon process. Medially, the flexor-pronator muscles arise from a **common flexor tendon** originating from the medial epicondyle of the humerus and include the pronator teres, flexor carpi radialis, palmaris longus, flexor digitorum superficialis, flexor carpi ulnaris, and flexor digitorum profundus. On the lateral aspect of the elbow, muscles can be divided into three layers: the superficial layer is formed by the brachioradialis and extensor carpi radialis longus (ECRL), arising from the lateral supracondylar ridge. The **common extensor tendon** arises from the lateral epicondyle, giving rise to the extensor carpi radialis brevis (ECRB), extensor digitorum, extensor digiti minimi, and extensor carpi ulnaris muscles. The supinator muscle forms the deepest layer.

The three major nerves around the elbow are the ulnar, median, and radial nerves (Fig. 3.4) [3, 8]. The **ulnar nerve** passes posterior to the medial humeral epicondyle to enter the cubital tunnel and is prone to compression in this location. The floor of the cubital tunnel is formed by the joint capsule and posterior bundle of the UCL, and the roof is formed proximally by the cubital tunnel retinaculum (Osborne ligament) and distally by the flexor carpi aponeurosis (arcuate ligament). Variants include a thickened cubital tunnel retinaculum, replacement of the retinaculum by an accessory anconeus epitrochlearis muscle, or an absent retinaculum which can predispose to friction neuropathy [9]. The **median nerve** lies adjacent to the brachial artery and vein, passing under the bicipital aponeurosis, between the two heads of pronator teres, and under a fibrous arch formed by the two heads of flexor digitorum superficialis, giving off an anterior interosseous branch 4 cm distal to the medial epicondyle which innervates the deep flexor muscles. The **radial nerve** courses between the biceps and brachialis, passing into the radial tunnel, bounded by the brachialis, brachioradialis, and ECRL, where it divides into superficial sensory and deep posterior interosseous branches.

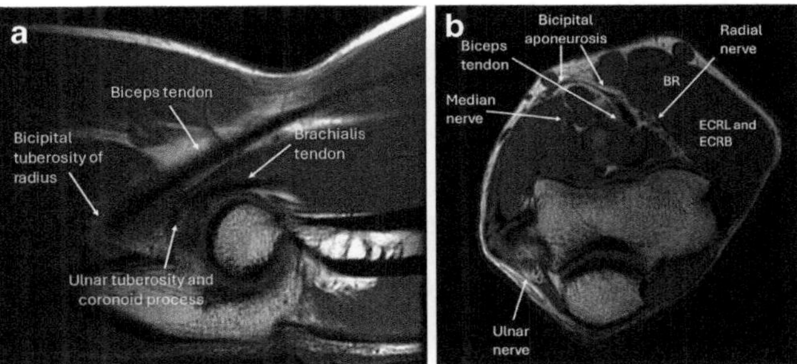

Fig. 3.4 Tendons/nerves. (**a**) Sagittal and (**b**) axial T1W images display the tendons and nerves of the elbow

3.4 Osteochondral Pathology

Radiographs are helpful in acute trauma to look for joint effusion and displaced fractures. However, in patients with a joint effusion on radiographs and a history of recent trauma, MRI may be needed to detect osseous contusions and/or occult fractures and identify any associated chondral or soft tissue injury (Fig. 3.5) [10].

MRI is also the imaging modality of choice if there is concern for a stress fracture. Stress fractures in the elbow most commonly occur in the olecranon process as a result of repetitive posteromedial shear forces in overhead throwing athletes in the setting of valgus extension overload [11, 12]. In adolescent athletes, this can result in olecranon apophysitis, manifesting as widening or delayed closure of the olecranon apophysis and periphyseal bone marrow edema (Fig. 3.6).

Osteochondral injuries are common in adolescent throwers and gymnasts due to repetitive impaction forces across the radiocapitellar joint and posterior humeroulnar joint,

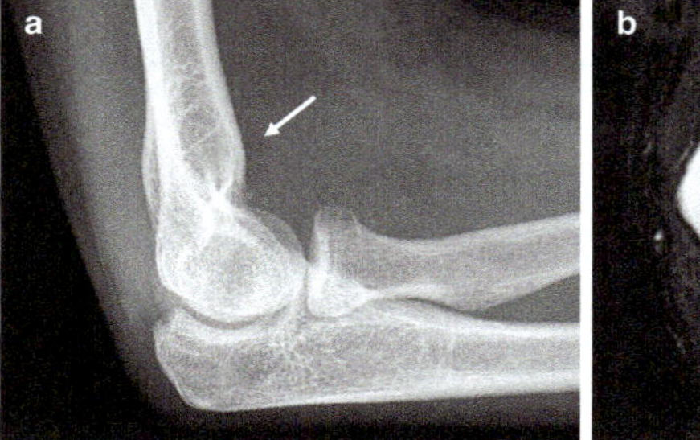
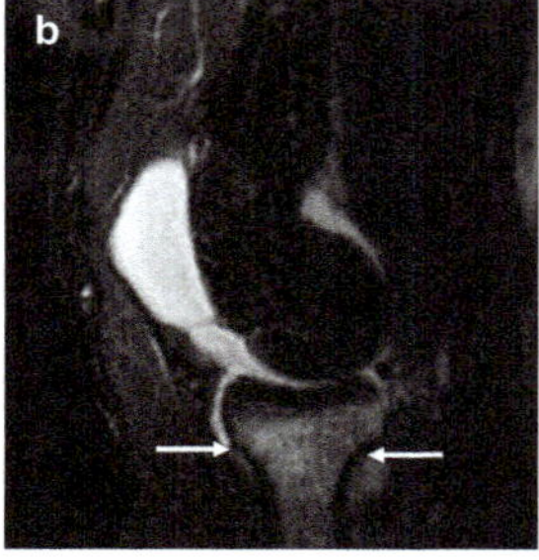

Fig. 3.5 A 20-year-old female with fall on outstretched hand. (**a**) Lateral radiograph demonstrates mild elevation of the anterior fat pad (arrow) ("sail sign") compatible with a small effusion. (**b**) Sagittal T2W FS image demonstrates a nondisplaced fracture of the radial neck with bone marrow edema (arrows)

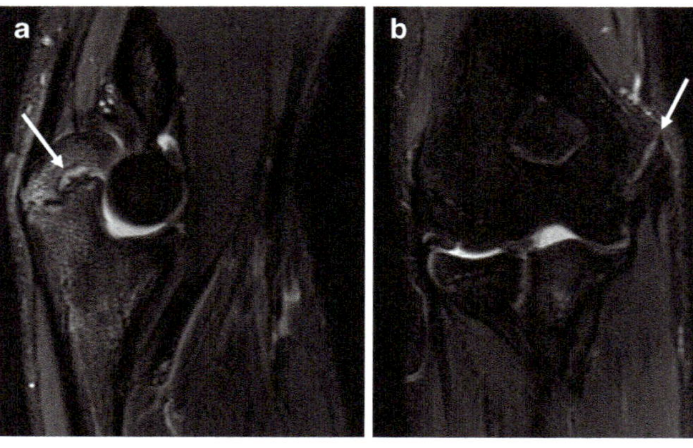

Fig. 3.6 A 15-year-old baseball pitcher with posteromedial elbow pain. (**a**) Sagittal T2W FS image shows widening and irregularity of the olecranon physis (arrow) and prominent periphyseal edema, compatible with olecranon apophysitis. (**b**) Coronal PD FS image also shows mild periphyseal edema along the medial apophysis (arrow), compatible with mild apophysitis

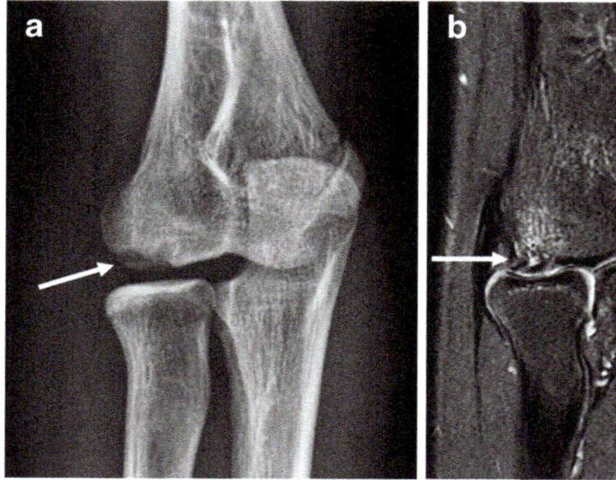
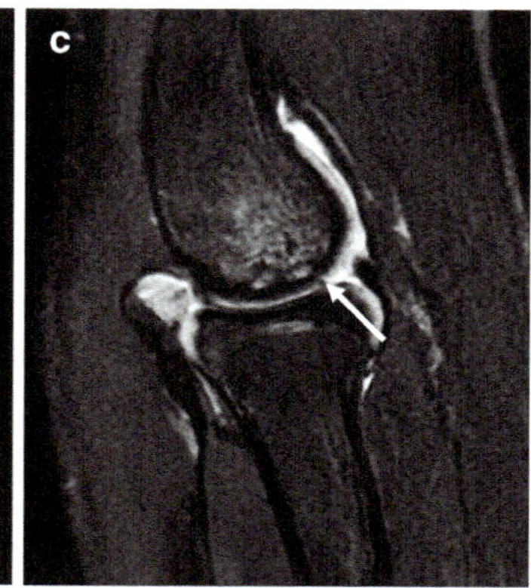

Fig. 3.7 A 12-year-old elite gymnast with elbow pain. (**a**) AP oblique radiograph shows cortical irregularity and subchondral lucency along the capitellum (arrow). (**b**) Coronal T2 FS image demonstrates irregularity of the capitellum with subchondral cystic change and bone marrow edema (arrow) compatible with osteochondritis dissecans ("osteochondral lesion"). (**c**) Sagittal T2 FS image demonstrates a subtle defect in the cartilage and subchondral bone plate along the anterior capitellum (arrow) with underlying cystic change and bone marrow edema

resulting in osteochondral lesions of the capitellum and trochlea, respectively (Figs. 3.7 and 3.8) [12–15]. MRI readily depicts articular cartilage and subchondral bone and is critical for detecting signs of instability, including undermining fluid, cystic change, or displacement. MR or CT arthrography can also be helpful in identifying an unstable osteochondral lesion. Repetitive posteromedial shear resulting from repetitive valgus extension overload also results in chondral thinning, subchondral sclerosis, and osteophytosis in the posterior humeroulnar joint, as well as fragmentation of the tip of the olecranon process and joint bodies [2, 16].

Key Point

Osteochondral injuries of the elbow most commonly involve the capitellum but may also be seen in the trochlea. These typically occur in young throwers or gymnasts secondary to repetitive activity-related impaction forces and are well demonstrated with MRI. If a subchondral fragment is present, the finding of underlying fluid or cystic changes suggests fragment instability which is usually an indication for surgical intervention.

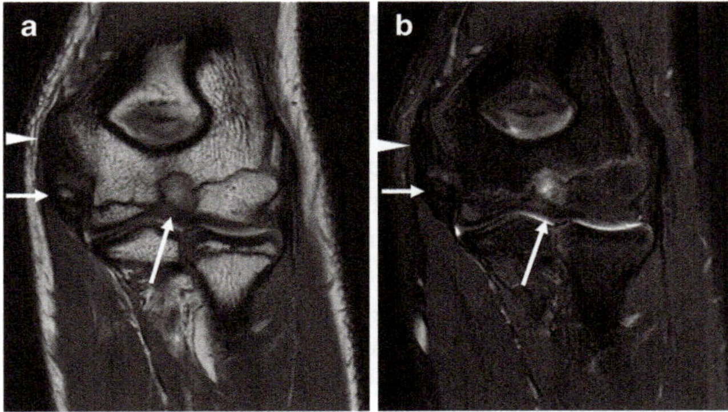

Fig. 3.8 A 14-year-old baseball pitcher with elbow pain. (**a**) Coronal T1W and (**b**) coronal T2W FS images demonstrate a nonacute avulsion injury of the medial condyle (short arrow). The overlying flexor tendon (arrowhead) is intact. There is also an osteochondral lesion of the trochlea with subchondral cystic change (long arrow) but no disruption of the articular surface

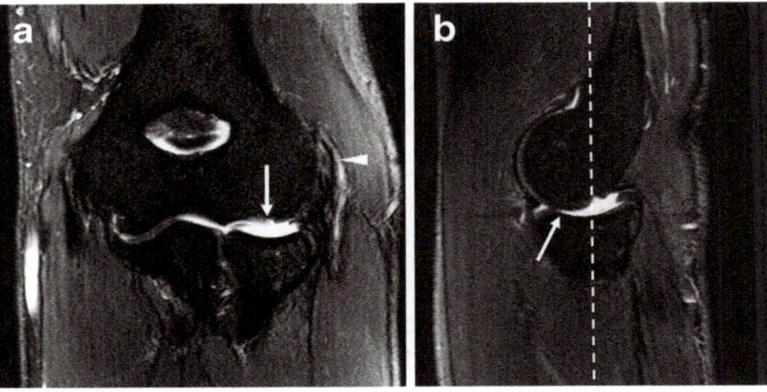

Fig. 3.9 Pseudodefect of the capitellum. (**a**) Coronal fat-saturated T2W image shows cortical irregularity of the capitellum (arrow), concerning for an osteochondral lesion. (**b**) Sagittal T2W FS image reveals that the plane of section of (**a**) (dotted line) lies just posterior to the articular surface of the capitellum (arrow)

Potential pitfalls include the "pseudodefect" of the capitellum which may mimic an osteochondral defect on coronal MR images, particularly when accompanied by subchondral cystic change [9, 10, 17]. However, cross referencing with sagittal images shows that this region corresponds to the normal transition from the smooth anterior articular surface of the capitellum to the roughened and irregular posterior nonarticular surface (Fig. 3.9). Other normal variants include the "pseudodefect "of the trochlear groove, a cartilage-free groove within the mid trochlea, and the transverse trochlear ridge, a bony ridge along the mid-trochlear groove, which can be mistaken for the sequela of a healed fracture on sagittal imaging or an intraarticular osteophyte [3, 9].

3.5 Ligamentous Injury

UCL injuries result from valgus stress, either as a result of acute injury or chronic repetitive valgus stress. MRI readily depicts complete and partial tears, although partial undersurface tears of the distal UCL can be subtle and may be better seen on MR arthrography (Fig. 3.10) [2, 3]. Ultrasound is a complementary tool for evaluation of the UCL, and dynamic examination during the application of valgus stress can be as effective as MRI in detecting UCL tears [2]. Chronic repetitive stress is common in overhead throwing athletes, particularly in baseball pitchers and javelin throwers due to valgus loading during the late cocking and acceleration phases of throwing. This may result in adaptive thickening of the UCL and heterotopic ossification [16]. Traction spurs and bone marrow edema may be seen along the sublime tubercle of the proximal ulna, and the spurs may become very large in elite athletes. The resultant valgus instability may in turn lead to lateral osteochondral injuries and posteromedial shear injuries in throwing athletes, termed **valgus extension overload** [16]. Professional throwing athletes may be imaged in the flexed elbow valgus external rotation (FEVER) position, which can increase conspicuity of UCL tears and result in abnormal gapping of the joint [18, 19]. In skeletally immature athletes, the apophysis is the weakest link at the medial elbow, and repetitive valgus stress may result in medial epicondylar apophysitis ("Little League elbow") (Fig. 3.11) and acute trauma can result in medial apophyseal avulsion [20, 21].

Key Point

Valgus extension overload syndrome is common in throwing athletes. Medial tension overload results in UCL thickening, UCL injury, heterotopic ossification, and ulnar traction spurs. In adolescent athletes, medial tensile forces may result in medial apophysitis or apophyseal avulsion. Lateral compressive forces result in osteochondral injuries of the radiocapitellar joint. Repetitive posteromedial shear leads to olecranon stress injuries, trochlear osteochondral lesions, degenerative changes in the posterior humeroulnar joint, and fragmentation of the olecranon tip and joint bodies.

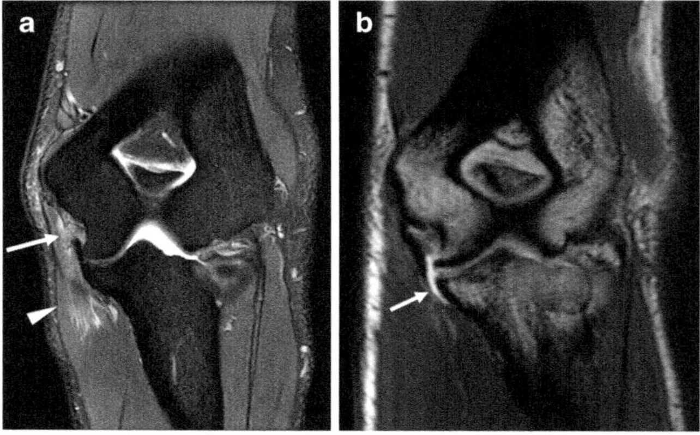

Fig. 3.10 Ulnar collateral ligament injuries. (**a**) Coronal proton density FS image in a 19-year-old baseball pitcher with acute valgus injury demonstrates a complete tear of the proximal to mid fibers of the UCL (arrow) with edema in the overlying flexor-pronator muscles (arrowhead) indicating associated muscle strain. (**b**) Coronal T1W MR arthrographic image in an 18-year-old baseball pitcher with medial elbow pain demonstrates a high-grade undersurface tear of distal UCL, with fluid tracking between the distal UCL and sublime tubercle (arrow) forming the "T-sign"

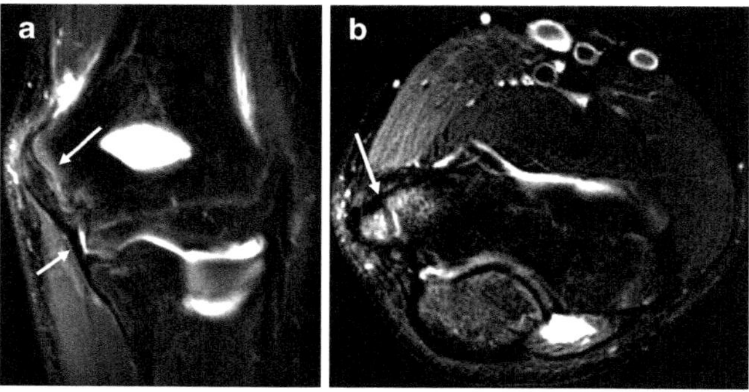

Fig. 3.11 (**a**) Coronal T2W FS arthrographic image in a 13-year-old baseball pitcher with medial elbow pain reveals prominent periphyseal edema along the medial epicondylar apophysis (long arrow) compatible with apophysitis ("little leaguer's elbow). Note the UCL is intact (short arrow). (**b**) Axial T2W FS image confirms the prominent periphyseal edema (arrow)

Lateral collateral ligament complex injuries often result from varus stress or posterior elbow dislocation and may result in posterolateral rotatory instability (PLRI), with posterior subluxation of the radial head [3, 8]. LUCL injuries may coexist with moderate to severe lateral epicondylosis and may require surgical repair or reconstruction [20, 22].

3.6 Tendon Pathology

Tendinous injuries around the elbow encompass a spectrum ranging from chronic overuse to acute traumatic injuries. MRI plays a pivotal role in characterizing the extent of pathology, differentiating partial from complete tears, identifying associated osseous, ligamentous, or bursal abnormalities, and guiding management decisions.

Lateral epicondylosis (tennis elbow) is the most common tendinopathy of the elbow, typically representing degenerative change in the common extensor tendon resulting from overuse of extensor muscles, particularly the extensor carpi radialis brevis. This is most commonly seen in patients between the ages of 40 and 60 years and presents with chronic lateral elbow pain. On MRI, this manifests as tendon thickening and increased signal (Fig. 3.12), often associated with underlying RCL or LUCL injury, which if untreated can destabilize the elbow and impair surgical outcomes [1, 20, 22]. Ultrasound may show thickening, areas of hypoechogenicity, calcifications, or abnormal Doppler flow in the common extensor tendon and can be used to guide therapeutic interventions such as platelet-rich plasma (PRP) injection [1, 2].

Medial epicondylosis (Golfer's elbow) is less common than its lateral counterpart but is seen most frequently as an overuse injury in athletes or workers subjected to repetitive valgus and wrist flexion forces. Patients present with chronic medial elbow pain. The differential diagnosis of medial elbow pain can be more challenging, so MRI is helpful for diagnosis, demonstrating tendon thickening, increased T2 signal, and possible underlying UCL injury [1, 20]. Ultrasound again aids diagnosis and can guide percutaneous therapy [1, 2]. The common flexor tendon can also be avulsed in elbow dislocations in association with underlying UCL disruption.

Biceps tendon injuries are predominantly seen in males between the ages of 40 and 60 years, usually resulting from a sudden eccentric load against a flexed elbow or forceful hyperextension against resistance. Risk factors include heavy lifting, anabolic steroid use, and smoking. Tears may be partial or complete, most commonly involving the distal insertion (Fig. 3.13). It is important to report both the extent and degree of retraction on imaging, as well as the integrity of the bicipital aponeurosis, as an intact aponeurosis may mask the diagnosis on clinical examination. Scanning the patient in

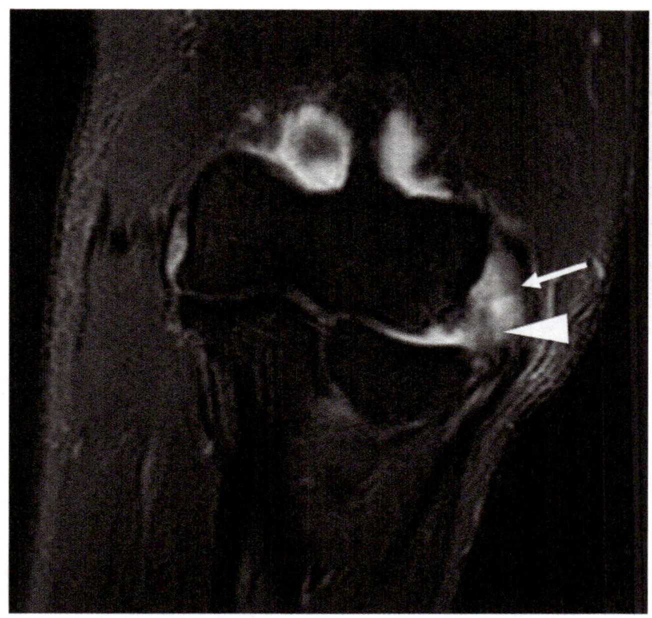

Fig. 3.12 A 56-year-old male with severe lateral epicondylosis. Coronal T2W FS image demonstrates high-grade undersurface tearing of the common extensor tendon (arrow) and a complete tear of the underlying proximal LUCL (arrowhead)

the flexed abduction and supinated (FABS) position may help differentiate high-grade from complete tears [1, 3, 20]. Ultrasound offers the added advantage of dynamic assessment [1, 23]. Repetitive traction forces may also result in biceps tendinopathy, bony hypertrophy of the bicipital tuberosity, and inflammation of the adjacent bicipitoradial and interosseous bursae, which can predispose to tendon tears (Fig. 3.14) [1, 24].

Key Point

Partial and complete tears of the distal biceps tendon typically result from an eccentric load applied to a flexed elbow. A complete tear can be missed on clinical examination if the bicipital aponeurosis is intact and restricts the degree of tendon retraction. Important MRI findings include differentiating partial from complete tears and measuring the degree of tendon retraction. Ultrasound may also be used in this setting and allows for real-time dynamic assessment of the tendon.

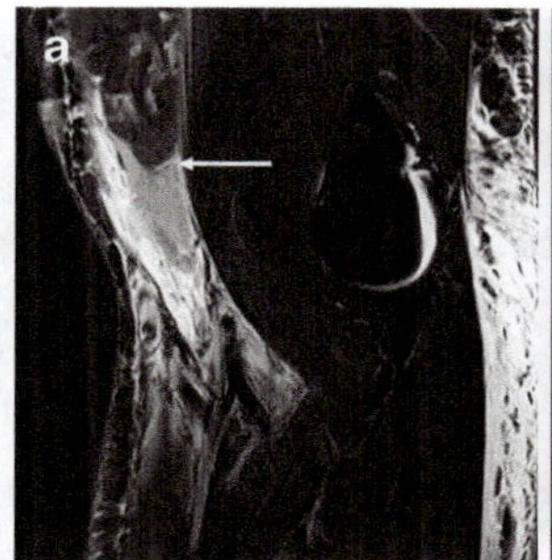

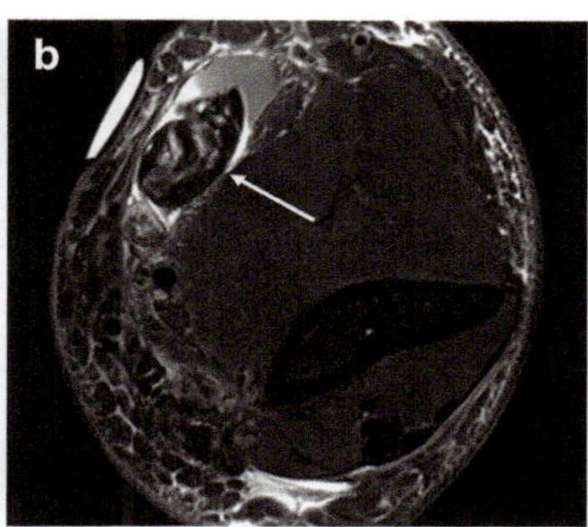

Fig. 3.13 A 49-year-old male with sudden onset of pain while lifting a kayak. (**a**) Sagittal and (**b**) axial T2W FS images demonstrate a complete tear of the distal biceps tendon with prominent retraction of the torn tendon end (arrows), with extensive surrounding fluid and soft tissue edema

Brachialis tendon tears are rare, typically following direct trauma or eccentric overload. **Triceps tendon tears** are uncommon, usually resulting from a fall on an outstretched hand, direct trauma, or forceful deceleration of an actively contracting triceps muscle. Risk factors include systemic diseases such as renal insufficiency, inflammatory arthropathies, olecranon bursitis, or anabolic steroid use [1]. The most common tear pattern involves the superficial tendon formed by the long and lateral heads, with varying involvement of the deep layer. Isolated tears of the deep layer are rare [25]. Triceps tendon avulsion from the olecranon may be accompanied by radial head fractures, which are sustained via a similar mechanism of injury. Radiographs are helpful in cases of suspected triceps tendon ruptures to look for a small flake fracture of the olecranon (Fig. 3.15). MRI and ultrasound are both able to differentiate between partial and complete tears, and the degree of retraction can be measured on both [1, 8]. Triceps tendinopathy can occur as a result of repetitive forceful or rapid extension, for example, in weightlifting, manifesting as tendon thickening and increased intrasubstance signal on MRI, often accompanied by enthesopathy along the olecranon process [1, 20].

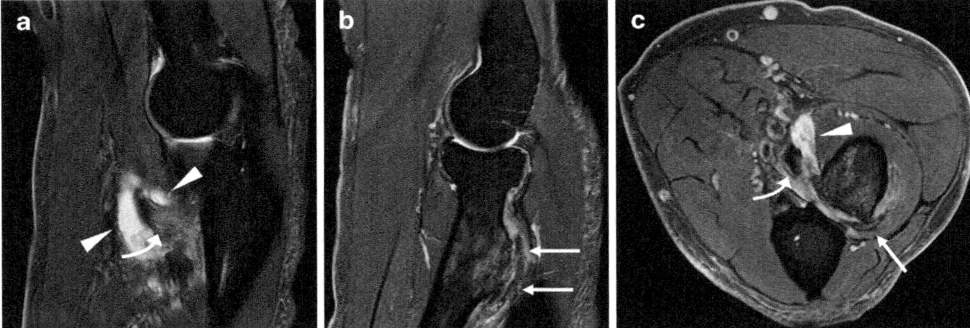

Fig. 3.14 A 46-year-old male with chronic elbow pain. (**a**, **b**) Sagittal T2W FS images demonstrate severe tendinopathy of the distal biceps tendon with thickening and increased signal (curved arrow) and surrounding fluid in the bicipitoradial bursa (arrowheads). Hypertrophic bone changes and bone marrow edema are seen along the radial tuberosity (arrows) with adjacent soft tissue edema. (**c**) Axial PD FS image shows tendinopathy and at least partial tearing of the distal biceps tendon (curved arrow), bicipitoradial bursitis (arrowhead), and hypertrophic bony reactive change (arrow) along the bicipital tuberosity

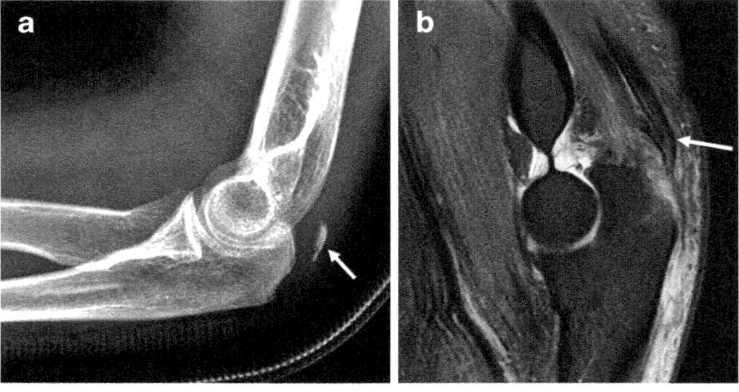

Fig. 3.15 A 34-year-old male with posterior elbow pain after falling off bike. (**a**) Lateral radiograph in splint shows a linear avulsed fracture fragment (arrow) adjacent to the olecranon process. (**b**) Sagittal T2W FS image demonstrates complete avulsion of the distal triceps tendon proper which is attached to the avulsed fragment (arrow) and edema within the surrounding soft tissues

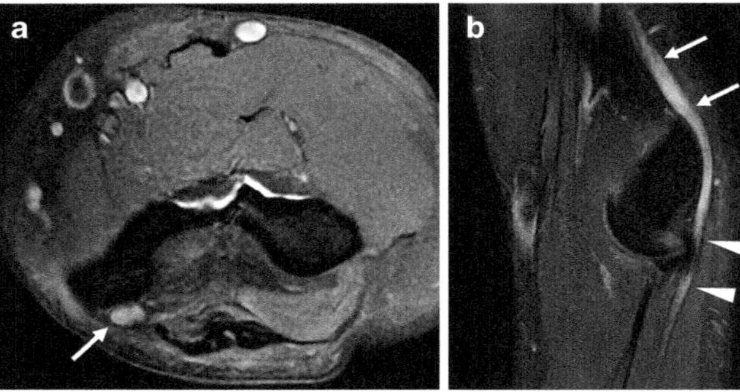

Fig. 3.16 A 38-year-old male with severe ulnar nerve symptoms. (**a**) Axial T2W FS image shows thickening of the ulnar nerve with increased T2 signal as it enters the cubital tunnel (arrow). (**b**) Sagittal T2 FS image shows marked thickening and increased signal within the ulnar nerve proximal to the cubital tunnel (arrows). The ulnar nerve returns to normal caliber and signal distal to the cubital tunnel (arrowheads)

3.7 Nerve Pathology

The ulnar, median, and radial nerves course in close proximity to osseous structures and through narrow fibromuscular or fibroosseous tunnels, making them vulnerable to injury from direct trauma, repetitive motion, or entrapment.

Ulnar neuropathy is the most common neuropathy at the elbow, most commonly due to compression in the cubital tunnel by osteophytes, an anomalous anconeus epitrochlearis muscle, and low-lying medial head of triceps or mass. Less common sites of entrapment include the arcade of Struthers, a fibrous band extending from the medial head of triceps to the medial intermuscular septum in the upper arm, compression between the two heads of flexor carpi ulnaris, or compression subjacent to the deep flexor-pronator aponeurosis. Patients typically present with medial elbow discomfort, paresthesia and numbness in the ulnar nerve distribution, and possible weakness of the intrinsic hand musculature. MRI shows nerve enlargement, fascicular prominence, and high T2 signal (Fig. 3.16) and may demonstrate anatomic variants or neural compressive lesions [3, 8]. However, it is important to correlate imaging findings with clinical symptoms, as increased T2 signal can be seen within the ulnar nerve in asymptomatic individuals [26]. Ultrasound is also widely used in the evaluation of ulnar nerve pathology at the elbow and has the advantage of dynamic assessment and identification of ulnar nerve subluxation [1, 27].

Median neuropathy may result from compression at various sites, including the ligament of Struthers (rare anatomic variant), thickened bicipital aponeurosis, flexor digitorum superficialis arch, or an accessory head of FPL (Gantzer muscle) [1, 9]. However, the most common site of compression is where the median nerve leaves the antecubital fossa by passing between the superficial and deep heads of the pro-

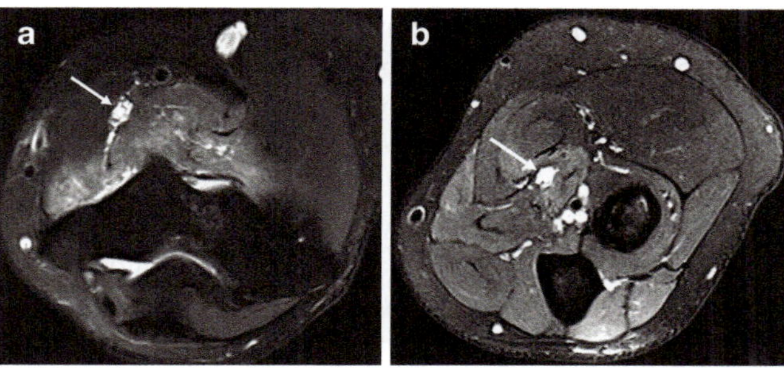

Fig. 3.17 A 31-year-old male with right-hand pain and numbness. (**a**, **b**) Axial and T2 FS images at the elbow (**a**) and proximal forearm (**b**) reveal marked thickening of the median nerve with asymmetrical internal fascicles (arrow) compatible with median neuropathy. Note also the edema-like signal with the flexor muscles at that level and in the proximal forearm

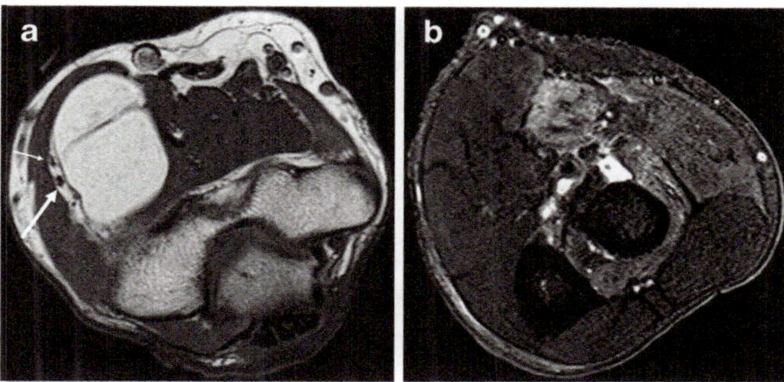

Fig. 3.18 A 61-year-old male with intermittent numbness and weakness in the arm and hand. (**a**) Axial T1W image demonstrates a large lipomatous mass in the region of the radial tunnel displacing the superficial (small arrow) and deep (large arrow) branches of the radial nerve. (**b**) Axial T2W FS image at the proximal forearm reveals diffuse edema within the extensor and supinator muscles compatible with subacute denervation changes

nator teres muscle, where fibrous bands can occur and cause selective compression of the anterior interosseous branch, just as it diverges from the median nerve. Compression of the median nerve is more common in manual laborers, athletes, and weightlifters and can cause pronator syndrome, presenting with deep volar forearm pain and sensory changes in the median nerve distribution. Selective compression of the anterior interosseous branch causes Kiloh-Nevin syndrome resulting in motor weakness in the flexor pollicis longus, flexor digitorum profundus, and pronator quadratus. MRI may demonstrate the cause of impingement as well as denervation changes within the forearm flexor muscles (Fig. 3.17) [1, 3]. In acute or subacute denervation, there is increased T2 signal within the affected muscles, whereas chronic denervation results in fatty infiltration and atrophy, best seen on fat-sensitive sequences.

Radial neuropathy at the elbow can result from compression in the radial tunnel or at the arcade of Frohse, a tendinous or fibrous arch formed by the supinator muscle in the proximal forearm [1, 3]. Distension of the bicipitoradial bursitis can also result in compression of the radial nerve. Radial tunnel syndrome can present with vague dorsal forearm pain exacerbated by repetitive forearm rotation, and symptoms may mimic lateral epicondylosis. Selective involvement of the posterior interosseous nerve produces finger and wrist extensor weakness without sensory loss. MRI may show the cause of compression as well as denervation changes in the forearm extensor muscles (Fig. 3.18) [1, 3].

> **Key Point**
> The most common neuropathy at the elbow involves the ulnar nerve and often results from nerve compression within the cubital tunnel. Other less common sites include the arcade of Struthers, between the two heads of the flexor carpi ulnaris or along the deep flexor aponeurosis. MRI findings of neuritis include nerve enlargement, asymmetric fascicle size, and increased T2 signal intensity although the latter can be seen in asymptomatic patients, especially if it is the only imaging finding.

3.8 Synovial Pathology

Synovial processes can affect the elbow including rheumatoid arthritis, gout, CPPD, synovial osteochondromatosis, and tenosynovial giant cell tumor, manifesting as joint effusion, synovial hypertrophy and enhancement, and periarticular erosions. Septic arthritis can present with a similar appearance.

Synovial folds are common in the elbow, and the posterior radiocapitellar plica can become thickened and result in mechanical symptoms [28].

Several bursae are located around the elbow, and the most clinically relevant include the olecranon and bicipitoradial bursae. The **olecranon bursa** is located superficial to the olecranon process and distal triceps tendon and can become inflamed in chronic repetitive stress, trauma, inflammatory arthropathies, and sepsis [8, 29]. MRI and ultrasound show a well-defined fluid collection dorsal to the olecranon, often with associated synovial thickening (Fig. 3.19). Intravenous gadolinium should be considered if there is concern for sepsis and can essentially be excluded if there is no bursal or soft tissue enhancement. The **bicipitoradial bursa** is located between the distal biceps tendon and bicipital tuberosity and can become inflamed with distal biceps tendinopathy, inflammatory arthropathy, or sepsis [8, 30]. Significant distension of the bursa can result in compression of the radial nerve.

Key Point

Inflammation of the olecranon or bicipitoradial bursae may result from a variety of etiologies. The olecranon bursa overlies the dorsal margin of the olecranon and distal triceps tendon. The radiobicipital bursa is found along the distal biceps tendon, and given that there is no distal biceps tendon sheath, any fluid collection in this region is most likely related to bursal inflammation. At either site, MRI and ultrasound will demonstrate a distended fluid-filled structure with associated synovial thickening and enhancement/hypervascularity.

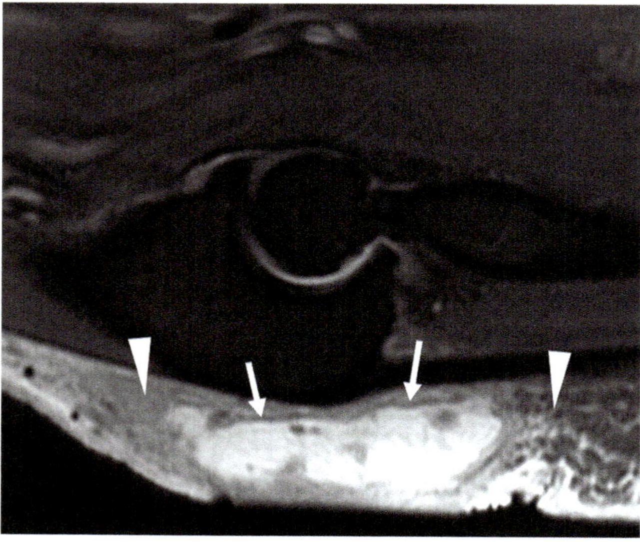

Fig. 3.19 Sagittal T2W FS image in an 80-year-old male with septic olecranon bursitis. There is complex fluid within the olecranon bursa (arrows) with extensive edema in the surrounding soft tissues (arrowheads). Of note there is no abnormal signal in the olecranon process, and the triceps tendon is intact

In conclusion, MRI is integral in the evaluation of patients with elbow pain, offering unparalleled visualization of the intricate interplay between bone, cartilage, ligaments, tendons, nerves, and bursae. The high spatial resolution and multiplanar capabilities of MRI allow detection of subtle injuries that may be clinically occult and can differentiate between acute and chronic pathologies. It is important to integrate the MRI findings with the patient's history, physical examination, and adjunct imaging studies, in order to tailor management strategies to the individual and improve clinical outcome. Ultrasound is also a valuable tool in the evaluation of soft tissue pathology around the elbow and has the advantages of dynamic visualization of structures as well as guiding therapeutic interventions.

Take-Home Messages

1. It is important to understand the complex anatomy of the elbow and some of the normal variants that can be encountered in order to prevent misdiagnosis.
2. MRI is an invaluable tool in the evaluation of patients with elbow pain, particularly when pain is poorly localized.
3. Imaging findings should be interpreted in conjunction with clinical history and mechanism of injury.

Conflict of Interest Statement I/We declare no competing interests as defined by Springer Nature or other interests that might be perceived to influence results and/or discussion reported in this manuscript.

References

1. Stevens KJ, McNally EG. Magnetic resonance imaging of the elbow in athletes. Clin Sports Med. 2010;29(4):521–53.
2. Gustas CN, Lee KS. Multimodality imaging of the painful elbow: current imaging concepts and image-guided treatments for the injured thrower's elbow. Radiol Clin North Am. 2016;54(5):817–39.
3. Acosta Batlle J, Cerezal L, Márquez MV, López Parra MD, Soteras C, Resano S, et al. MRI of the normal elbow and common pathologic conditions. Radiographics. 2020;40(2):468–9.
4. Mogharrabi B, Cabrera A, Chhabra A. 3D isotropic spine echo MR imaging of elbow: how it helps surgical decisions. Eur J Radiol Open. 2022;9:100410.
5. Magee T. Accuracy of 3-T MR arthrography versus conventional 3-T MRI of elbow tendons and ligaments compared with surgery. AJR Am J Roentgenol. 2015;204(1):W70–5.
6. Alcid JG, Ahmad CS, Lee TQ. Elbow anatomy and structural biomechanics. Clin Sports Med. 2004;23(4):503–17. vii
7. Lynch JR, Waitayawinyu T, Hanel DP, Trumble TE. Medial collateral ligament injury in the overhand-throwing athlete. J Hand Surg Am. 2008;33(3):430–7.
8. Stevens KJ. Magnetic resonance imaging of the elbow. J Magn Reson Imaging. 2010;31(5):1036–53.

9. Antil N, Stevens KJ, Lutz AM. Elbow imaging: variants and asymptomatic findings. Semin Musculoskelet Radiol. 2021;25(4):546–57.
10. Porrino J, Wang A, Taljanovic M, Stevens KJ. Comprehensive update of elbow magnetic resonance imaging. Curr Probl Diagn Radiol. 2021;50(2):211–28.
11. Furushima K, Itoh Y, Iwabu S, Yamamoto Y, Koga R, Shimizu M. Classification of olecranon stress fractures in baseball players. Am J Sports Med. 2014;42(6):1343–51.
12. Helm JM, Myers NL, Conway JE. Non-medial ulnar collateral ligament elbow pathology in the thrower: valgus extension overload, osteochondritis dissecans, olecranon stress fracture, and ulnar nerve. Clin Sports Med. 2025;44(2):195–214.
13. Nguyen JC, Degnan AJ, Barrera CA, Hee TP, Ganley TJ, Kijowski R. Osteochondritis dissecans of the elbow in children: MRI findings of instability. AJR Am J Roentgenol. 2019;213(5):1145–51.
14. Marshall KW, Marshall DL, Busch MT, Williams JP. Osteochondral lesions of the humeral trochlea in the young athlete. Skeletal Radiol. 2009;38(5):479–91.
15. Wang KK, Bixby SD, Bae DS. Osteochondritis dissecans of the humeral trochlea: characterization of a rare disorder based on 28 cases. Am J Sports Med. 2019;47(9):2167–73.
16. Stevens KJ, Chaudhari AS, Kuhn KJ. Differences in anatomic adaptation and injury patterns related to valgus extension overload in overhead throwing athletes. Diagnostics (Basel). 2024;14(2):217.
17. Rosenberg ZS, Beltran J, Cheung YY. Pseudodefect of the capitellum: potential MR imaging pitfall. Radiology. 1994;191(3):821–3.
18. Lund P, Waslewski GL, Crenshaw K, Schenk M, Munday G, Knoblauch T, et al. FEVER: the flexed elbow valgus external rotation view for MRI evaluation of the ulnar collateral ligament in throwing athletes-a pilot study in major league baseball pitchers. AJR Am J Roentgenol. 2021;217(5):1176–83.
19. Patel M, Schenk M, Rangan P, Crenshaw K, Caplinger R, Raasch W, et al. Correlation of joint space widening on valgus stress magnetic resonance imaging with level of play and innings pitched in professional pitchers. Orthop J Sports Med. 2023;11(11) https://doi.org/10.1177/23259671231209704.
20. Kheterpal AB, Bredella MA. Overuse injuries of the elbow. Radiol Clin North Am. 2019;57(5):931–42.
21. Tariq SM, Patel V, Gendler L, Shah AS, Ganley TJ, Zoga AC, et al. Pediatric thrower's elbow: maturation-dependent MRI findings in symptomatic baseball players. Pediatr Radiol. 2024;54(1):105–16.
22. Bredella MA, Tirman PF, Fritz RC, Feller JF, Wischer TK, Genant HK. MR imaging findings of lateral ulnar collateral ligament abnormalities in patients with lateral epicondylitis. AJR Am J Roentgenol. 1999;173(5):1379–82.
23. Al-Ani Z, Lauder J. Ultrasound assessment in distal biceps tendon injuries: techniques, pearls and pitfalls. Clin Imaging. 2021;75:46–54.
24. Stevens K, Kwak A, Poplawski S. The biceps muscle from shoulder to elbow. Semin Musculoskelet Radiol. 2012;16(4):296–315.
25. Vicentini JRT, Hilgersom NFJ, Martinez-Salazar EL, Simeone FJ, Bredella MA, Palmer WE, et al. Distal triceps tendon tears: magnetic resonance imaging patterns using a systematic classification. J Comput Assist Tomogr. 2022;46(2):224–30.
26. Husarik DB, Saupe N, Pfirrmann CW, Jost B, Hodler J, Zanetti M. Elbow nerves: MR findings in 60 asymptomatic subjects--normal anatomy, variants, and pitfalls. Radiology. 2009;252(1):148–56.
27. Becciolini M, Pivec C, Raspanti A, Riegler G. Ultrasound of the ulnar nerve: a pictorial review: part 2: pathological ultrasound findings. J Ultrasound Med. 2024;43(6):1153–73.
28. Lee HI, Koh KH, Kim JP, Jaegal M, Kim Y, Park MJ. Prominent synovial plicae in radiocapitellar joints as a potential cause of lateral elbow pain: clinico-radiologic correlation. J Shoulder Elb Surg. 2018;27(8):1349–56.
29. Floemer F, Morrison WB, Bongartz G, Ledermann HP. MRI characteristics of olecranon bursitis. AJR Am J Roentgenol. 2004;183(1):29–34.
30. Yap SH, Griffith JF, Lee RKL. Imaging bicipitoradial bursitis: a pictorial essay. Skeletal Radiol. 2019;48(1):5–10.

4 Wrist and Hand

Anna Hirschmann and Michael J. Tuite

Learning Objectives

- Review common fractures affecting the hand and wrist.
- Describe common injuries to ligamentous, tendinous, and capsular structures of the hand and wrist.
- Discuss the approach to MR and ultrasound imaging of injuries to the hand and wrist.

4.1 Introduction

Wrist and hand imaging requires an integrated understanding of the complex anatomy of tendons, pulleys, ligaments, joints, and bones, along with the relative strengths and weaknesses of imaging methods, especially MRI and ultrasound. This chapter is divided into two main parts: wrist imaging and hand imaging. The wrist section addresses the most common fracture types, scaphoid avascular necrosis, carpal dislocations, and instability patterns, along with associated ligament injuries. Conditions contributing to ulnar-sided wrist pain, including triangular fibrocartilage complex (TFCC) tears, distal radioulnar joint pathology, and extensor carpi ulnaris tendon abnormalities, are also reviewed. Other topics include tendon pathologies and median nerve disorders. The second part of the chapter focuses on hand imaging, covering extensor and flexor tendon systems, the thumb's carpometacarpal (TMC) and metacarpophalangeal (MCP) joints, and common fracture patterns of the hand. For each anatomical region, we highlight relevant trauma, degenerative disease, and instability, while presenting characteristic imaging findings on radiographs, CT, MRI, and ultrasound. Special emphasis is placed on selecting the most appropriate imaging modality for accurate diagnosis and effective treatment planning.

4.2 Wrist Anatomy

The wrist is made up of eight carpal bones, four in the proximal row and four in the distal row, held together by many ligaments but with only a few tendon attachments [1]. The pisiform is unique because it only articulates with one bone, the triquetrum, and is a sesamoid for the flexor carpi ulnaris tendon.

Imaging of the wrist usually begins with radiographs, from two views (e.g., posterior-anterior (PA) and lateral views to follow-up a Colle's fracture) up to four or more projections (e.g., including oblique and scaphoid views after wrist trauma). On the PA view, the proximal and distal carpal rows form a series of three arcs which should each form a smooth curve (Fig. 4.1) [2]. The two proximal arcs are along the edge of three of the proximal-row bones, the scaphoid, lunate, and triquetrum. The middle arc also extends along the trapezoid's capitellum-facet in the distal row. The distal arc is along the two distal row bones, the hamate and capitellum. A disruption in one of more of the arcs should lead one to search for a fracture or dislocation injury.

A. Hirschmann (✉)
Imamed Radiology Nordwest, University of Basel, Basel, Switzerland
e-mail: Anna.hirschmann@unibas.ch

M. J. Tuite
Department of Radiology, University of Wisconsin School of Medicine and Public Health, Madison, USA
e-mail: mjtuite@wisc.edu

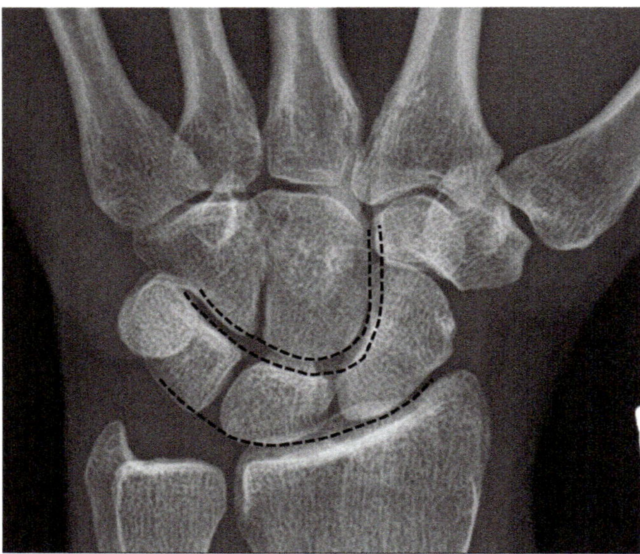

Fig. 4.1 Posterior-anterior view of a normal wrist radiograph shows the three smooth arcs. Disruption of the arcs indicates a subluxation or dislocation abnormality

4.3 Wrist Fractures

Radiographs of the wrist demonstrate almost all distal radius fractures but are less sensitive for scaphoid fractures. The scaphoid is the most fractured carpal bone, and radiographs have about an 80% sensitivity for scaphoid fractures [3]. If radiographs are negative and there is high clinical suspicion (e.g., focal snuff box tenderness), then MR is the best advanced imaging modality with a sensitivity of 94% and a specificity of 98%. CT and US are less accurate with a sensitivity of 82%, and a specificity of 96% and 77%, respectively. The second most common carpal bone fracture is the triquetrum and is usually a dorsal avulsion fracture at the insertion of the dorsal radiocarpal ligament. These triquetral fractures are seen best on a lateral radiograph.

The next most common carpal bones to fracture are the hamate and trapezium. A common location for a hamate fracture is the hook of the hamate, which can occur after a fall or in sports where a stick is held in the hand as in baseball, golf, or hockey. These often require a carpal tunnel radiographic view or CT or MR scan to diagnose. Trapezium fractures are also often missed on radiographs. These fractures commonly occur along with fractures of the base of the first metacarpal, the Bennett and Rolando fractures [4]. Isolated fractures often involve the tubercle, also called the volar or palmar ridge of the trapezium. Trapezium tubercle fractures are frequently only detected at CT or MR imaging.

4.4 Scaphoid Avascular Necrosis

Although chronic advanced scaphoid avascular necrosis (AVN) can be seen on radiographs, MRI is much more sensitive for detecting early AVN. The most common cause of scaphoid AVN is a proximal pole fracture with nonunion, but AVN can also be seen in scaphoid waist and/or healed fractures. Scaphoid AVN in some cases is not related to trauma and is termed Preiser's disease. The MRI appearance of scaphoid AVN is variable but usually appears as low signal on T1 and high signal on T2-weighted images in the proximal pole of the scaphoid (Fig. 4.2). Confluent low signal in the proximal pole on T1-weighted images has a 79% accuracy for AVN in patients with scaphoid nonunion but can be seen in some healing fractures [5]. T2 high signal in the proximal pole can be seen in both viable and osteonecrotic proximal poles and therefore is less helpful. There is debate in the literature if contrast-enhanced images or dynamic post gadolinium images significantly improve the accuracy for scaphoid AVN; some have reported that it does [6], while others have reported that it does not [5, 7] because contrast enhancement can be seen in 50% of nonviable scaphoid proximal poles.

Key Point

- Scaphoid AVN on MRI is usually confluent low signal on T1-weighted images involving the proximal pole.

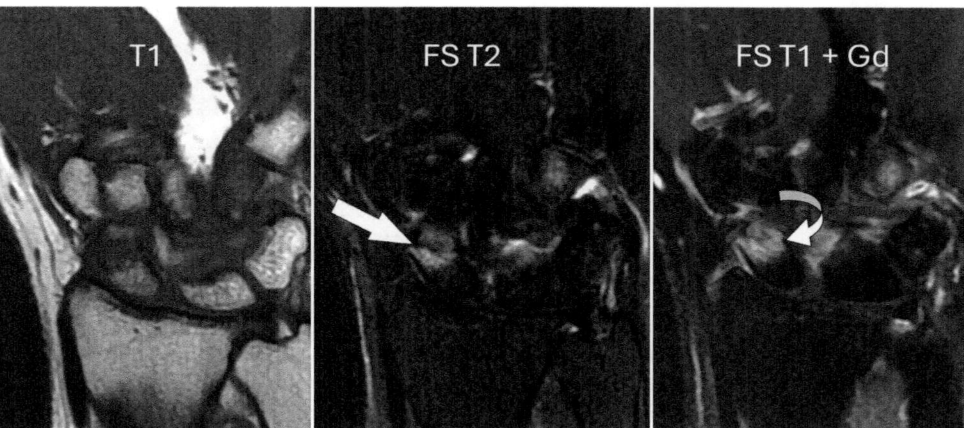

Fig. 4.2 Patient with progressive angulation of a nonhealing scaphoid fracture, so an MRI was obtained to assess viability of the proximal pole prior to surgery. The fracture (arrow) has adjacent bone marrow edema-like signal and enhancement (curved arrow) but normal marrow signal with no AVN in the proximal pole

4.5 Wrist Dislocation

A common pattern of wrist dislocations are the "perilunate injuries" which typically occur with axial loading and dorsiflexion, often combined with ulnar deviation and supination [8]. These dislocation injuries have been described as having progressive stages with increasing force. Stage I is scapholunate dissociation. Stage II is a perilunate dislocation where the lunate remains articulating with the radius, but the remainder of the carpal bones dislocate dorsally. Stage III is a midcarpal dislocation where there is partial reduction of the distal carpal bones with respect to the radius while the lunate subluxes volar, and Stage IV is where the lunate dislocates volar and the triquetrum and distal carpal row align with the radius. The higher-grade perilunate dislocation injuries are commonly associated with fractures of the scaphoid waist but can also involve other carpal bones. Another classification system divides the instability into four different groups mainly depending on whether the dislocation is within a single row (dissociative) or between the proximal carpal row and either the radius or distal row (nondissociative) [9].

4.6 Wrist Instability

Instability of the wrist can occur after an acute injury where the ligaments fail to heal or from repetitive trauma. A common static instability in the wrist is scapholunate dissociation from a large scapholunate ligament tear resulting in a wide scapholunate interval. Scapholunate dissociation can progress to scapholunate advanced collapse (SLAC wrist), particularly in patients with chronic arthritis.

Other common instability patterns are dorsal intercalated segment instability (DISI) and volar intercalated segment instability (VISI). The three bones of the proximal carpal row, the scaphoid, lunate, and triquetrum, form an intercalated segment, which means they do not have tendon attachments and can therefore rotate volar or dorsal independent of the radius or distal carpal row. The fourth proximal carpal bone, the pisiform, does have tendon attachments from the flexor carpi ulnaris and abductor digiti minimi tendons.

DISI and VISI instability are diagnosed best on neutral lateral radiographs. In DISI there is scapholunate dissociation, and the lunate is dorsi flexed >10 degrees and the scapholunate angle is >70 degrees [10]. In VISI, there is typically lunotriquetral ligament injury, and on a lateral view, the lunate is volar flexed >15 degrees relative to the longitudinal axis of the radius and capitate, and the scapholunate angle is <30 degrees.

4.7 Carpal Ligaments

The carpal ligaments are classified as either intrinsic (only attached to carpal bones) or extrinsic (where at least one attachment is to a structure other than a carpal bone). The scapholunate (SL) and lunotriquetral (LT) ligaments are intrinsic ligaments that are subclassified as intraarticular ligaments, while most of the dorsal and palmar intrinsic and extrinsic ligaments are considered intracapsular ligaments. The SL and LT ligaments are important because when injured they can cause chronic pain. These ligament tears can occur without radiographically visible dissociation and are best imaged with MRI. Both ligaments are U-shaped with dorsal, central, and volar components. For the SL ligament, the dorsal component is the thickest and strongest portion. Small tears within the interosseous and volar components can be seen in asymptomatic patients, while dorsal tears are frequently symptomatic and can extend to involve the adjacent portions. Complete tears of the SL ligament can lead to dissociation, SLAC wrist, or DISI. Conversely, the volar component of the LT ligament is the thickest portion, and isolated tears of the volar portion can extend to involve the remainder

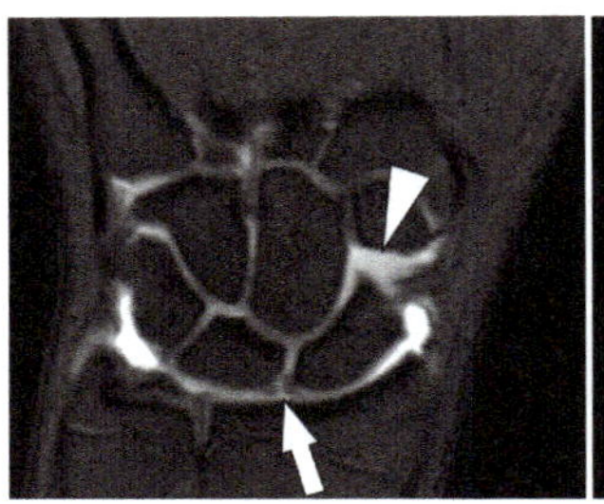
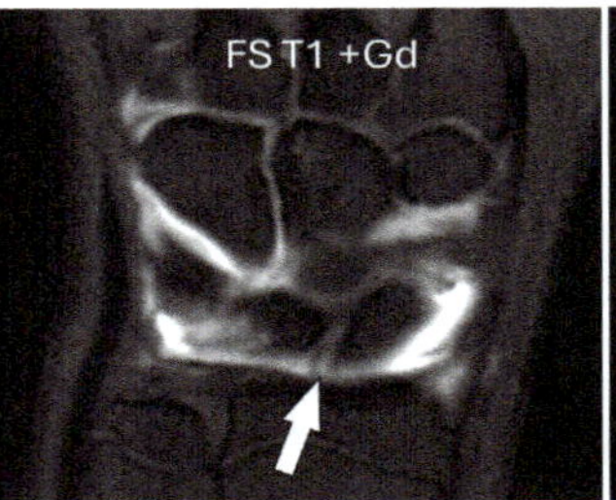

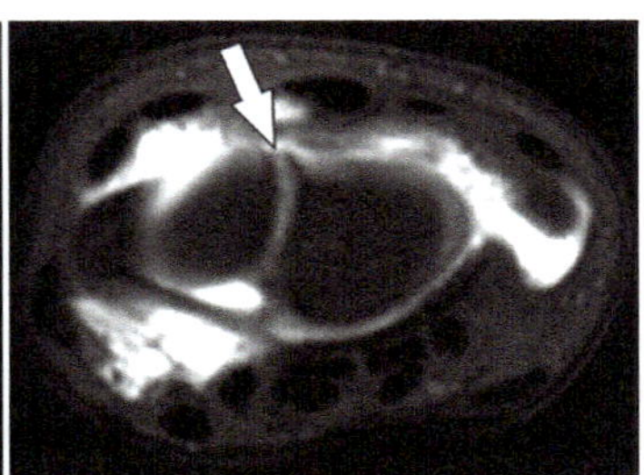

Fig. 4.3 Fat-suppressed T1 MR arthrogram images show a scapholunate ligament tear (arrows) in the central (left) and dorsal portions (middle and right images) of the ligament, with gadolinium extending into the midcarpal joint (arrowhead)

of the ligament. The volar component also blends with the ulnocarpal ligaments to form part of the triangular fibrocartilage complex (TFCC). Complete tears of the LT ligament can result in palmar rotation of the lunate and VISI.

When imaging the SL and LT ligaments with MRI, it is important to use a small field-of-view (8–10 cm) and thin sections. Many centers recommend a fat-suppressed fluid-sensitive thin section three-dimensional isotropic volume acquisition not only to minimize partial averaging but also to allow reformatted images. SL and LT tears appear as absence of or linear fluid signal extending across the ligament (Fig. 4.3).

Key Point

- The dorsal portion of the SL ligament is thickest, but tears in this region are more likely to progress to a complete tear and be symptomatic.

The two main dorsal ligaments, the dorsal intercarpal and dorsal radiocarpal ligaments, are also commonly injured, particularly after a fall on an outstretched hand. Patients present with dorsal wrist soft tissue swelling, and on MRI, there will typically be T2 high-signal edema surrounding one or both ligaments.

4.8 Triangular Fibrocartilage Complex (TFCC) and Ulnar Impaction Syndrome

The TFCC is composed of a central triangular fibrocartilage (TFC) disk surrounded by multiple attached supporting ligaments [11]. The attachment of the TFC to the radius occurs between the radius articular surface and the sigmoid notch (Fig. 4.4). There are two attachments of the TFC to the ulna: a proximal lamina which inserts into the fovea and a distal lamina which connects to the ulnar styloid. The fibers between the proximal and distal lamina make up the ligamentum subcruentum.

There are also dorsal and palmar ligamentous attachments to the TFC that are important stabilizers of the TFCC. The volar and dorsal radioulnar ligaments are attached along the anterior and posterior margins of the TFC and are often considered part of the TFC disk proper.

The meniscus homologue lies distal to the distal lamina and blends with the dorsal radioulnar ligament. The distal lamina also has fibers that extend peripherally to join the ulnar collateral ligament and extensor carpi ulnaris (ECU) subsheath before attaching to the triquetrum.

TFCC tears can be classified using the Palmer classification [12]. This classification divides TFCC tears into Class I Traumatic and Class II degenerative. The Class II degenerative tears are graded IIA up to IIE with progressive TFCC wear or perforation. The Class I traumatic injuries are categorized based on location of the tear. The most common location for an acute TFCC tear is a central perforation of the TFC disc, and this is categorized as IA. Traumatic tears involving the proximal and/or distal lamina are IB, distal avulsion from the carpus with tearing of the ulnocarpal ligaments is IC, and radial-side avulsion is ID.

The distal ulna is often slightly longer or shorter than the radius by 1 or 2 mm in normal asymptomatic individuals and when longer is termed +'ve ulnar variance. The length of the ulna relative to the radius changes with positioning and can become an additional 1–2 mm longer with wrist pronation or a firm grip.

Ulnar impaction syndrome, or ulnar abutment syndrome, is defined as ulnar-side wrist pain due to +'ve ulnar variance (typically >2 mm) with the ulna impacting on the TFCC [13]. Because wrist pronation or a firm grip can increase positive ulnar variance, ulnar impaction syndrome can be seen in patients with zero ulnar variance at neutral positioning who develop symptoms with pronation, firm grip, or ulnar deviation. Patients with ulnar impaction syndrome may develop a tear of the TFCC.

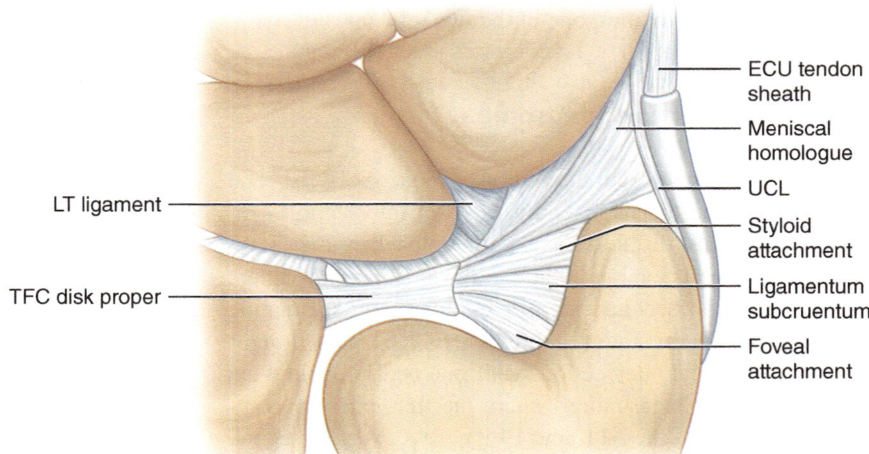

Fig. 4.4 Drawing of the triangular fibrocartilage complex showing the TFC disk proper and its two attachments to the ulna, one to the ulnar styloid and the other to the fovea of the ulna

4.9 Ulnar Impingement Syndrome and Negative Ulnar Variance

Ulnar impingement syndrome is different than ulnar impaction/abutment syndrome and is seen in patients where the ulna is short relative to the radius, that is, −'ve ulnar variance, and thus the opposite of what is seen in ulnar impaction syndrome. Ulnar impingement syndrome occurs with an ulna that is so short that the distal ulna lies proximal to the sigmoid notch and erodes into the side of the radius. It is often painful and causes bone remodeling, osteophytes, and focal bone marrow edema.

Negative ulnar variance, particularly when shorter by more than 2 mm, is also associated with Kienbock's osteonecrosis of the lunate [14]. Radiographs may show sclerosis or flattening of the lunate, but MRI is more sensitive for showing the bone marrow changes of early AVN. The symptoms are often relieved with an ulnar lengthening or radial shortening surgical procedure.

4.10 Wrist Tendons

4.10.1 Extensor Carpi Ulnaris

The ECU is the most common tendon to develop pathology and become symptomatic in the wrist. ECU tendon pathology includes tendinosis, tenosynovitis, tears, and subluxation or dislocation (Fig. 4.5). Tendinosis should not be confused with the common pseudolesion central increased signal within the tendon on T1- and T2-weighed images that can be seen with asymptomatic mucoid change. Displacement of the tendon partly out of the ulnar groove with supination, flexion, or ulnar deviation can also be seen in asymptomatic wrists where the displacement can measure up to 50% of the tendon diameter or up to 5 mm [15].

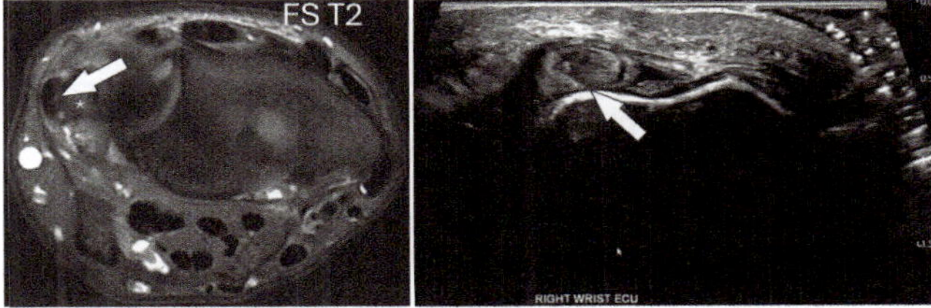

Fig. 4.5 Patient with ulnar-side wrist pain shows a partial tear of the extensor carpi ulnaris tendon (arrow) on a fat-suppressed T2 MR image (left) and ultrasound (right). On the MRI, the * is on the palmar aspect of the ulnar styloid; the ultrasound image is more proximal at level of the ulnar groove

4.10.2 Abductor Pollicis Longus and Extensor Pollicis Brevis

The APL and EPB are the tendons in the first extensor compartment and may become painful due to tenosynovitis. Stenosing tenosynovitis of the first extensor compartment is called de Quervain disease and occurs with overuse, pregnancy, and postpartum particularly in breastfeeding mothers. It can also result from abnormal thickening of the overlying extensor retinaculum. The MRI findings are typically thickening of the APL and EPB tendons and a first compartment tendon sheath effusion. There are several normal variants of the first extensor compartment including multiple slips of the APL or a septum that divides the compartment into two separate compartments. These variants are associated with an increased incidence of de Quervain disease, and identifying the two separate compartments on ultrasound is important when performing a therapeutic tendon sheath steroid injection to avoid only treating one of the two tendons.

4.10.3 Intersection Syndrome

There are two intersection syndromes near the wrist, and both involve the extensor tendons. Distal intersection syndrome occurs just distal to Lister's tubercle where the extensor pollicis longus tendon in the third extensor compartment crosses over the second extensor compartment containing the extensor carpi radialis brevis (ECRB) and longus (ECRL). Proximal intersection syndrome occurs about 4 cm proximal to the distal radius where the first extensor compartment tendons (the APL and EPB) cross over the second extensor compartment tendons ECRB and ECRL. Patients with intersection syndrome often have tendinosis and tenosynovitis of the deeper tendons.

4.11 Median Nerve

The most common entrapment neuropathy in the body is to the median nerve and is called carpal tunnel syndrome. Carpal tunnel syndrome is usually diagnosed with a combination of clinical findings and nerve conduction studies. The use of ultrasound and MRI in the initial diagnosis of carpal tunnel syndrome is controversial, although several imaging findings are utilized such as palmar bowing of the transverse carpal ligament (TCL), increased cross-sectional area of the median nerve, increased swelling ratio of the median nerve at the distal radius compared to at the level of the pisiform (proximal end of the transverse carpal ligament), and a flattening ratio greater than 2.0 [16]. Some institutions use ultrasound or MR only in patients with prior carpal tunnel release with continued or recurrent symptoms. Ultrasound is particularly helpful in postoperative cases because it can both assess for findings of incomplete retinaculum release or reassociation of the TCL and for imaging guidance of a perineural steroid injection.

4.12 Ganglion Cyst

Although studies often report that most wrist ganglion cysts are not painful, in some patients, the cyst can be painful enough to interfere with normal daily activities [17]. Wrist ganglion cysts may not be palpable, so imaging is useful to look for these occult ganglion cysts.

Around 70–80% of wrist ganglion cysts occur on the dorsal side of the wrist. A common location for dorsal ganglion cysts is arising from the scapholunate joint, typically between the dorsal radiocarpal and intercarpal ligaments, and felt to be due to a capsular tear at the attachment of the dorsal capsular scapholunate septum. Ganglion cysts are well seen on both MRI and ultrasound, with ultrasound also able to guide cyst fenestration and steroid injection for treatment.

4.13 Metacarpal and Phalangeal Fractures

Fractures of the metacarpals and phalanges are among the most common hand injuries, arising from falls, crush injuries, sports, or direct impact. Accurate imaging is essential for assessing fracture location, displacement, intraarticular extension, angulation, comminution, and associated soft tissue injuries. Among metacarpal fractures, the *neck fracture* of the fifth metacarpal (Boxer's fracture) is most commonly affected [18]. Phalangeal fractures may present with transverse, oblique, or intraarticular configurations. They may also be associated with small avulsion fragments involving tendon insertions or collateral ligament attachments. Intraarticular base fractures of the phalanges can involve the joint cartilage and require accurate mapping. Radiographs remain the cornerstone of fracture diagnosis: standard views (e.g., posteroanterior, oblique, lateral) typically visualize the fracture line, displacement, angulation, and alignment. CT facilitates detection of small articular fragments, subtle comminution, and planning for surgical fixation in complex and displaced fractures.

4.14 Thumb Including TMC Joint

The first carpometacarpal (TMC) joint is highly susceptible to both degenerative disease and traumatic instability, reflecting its saddle-shaped anatomy and its essential role in thumb opposition and pinch grip. Stabilized is provided by a complex ligamentous network including the anterior oblique ligament (beak ligament), the posterior oblique ligament, the dorsoradial ligament, and the intermetacarpal ligament [19]. The most frequent degenerative disorder of the hand is *thumb TMC osteoarthritis*, caused by chronic ligamentous insufficiency and progressive wear of the joint surfaces. Standard posteroanterior and lateral views typically suffice, though specialized stress views may be obtained in suspected instability. Several classification systems, such as the Eaton-Littler grading system, rely on plain radiographs to stage disease severity. Traumatic injuries to the TMC joint include intraarticular fractures of the metacarpal base, most commonly the Bennett fracture, an oblique intraarticular fracture with dislocation tendency, and the Rolando fractures, a comminuted intraarticular fracture, essentially a Bennett fracture with an additional dorsal or radial fragment [20]. CT is invaluable for acute assessment, offering precise characterization of fracture morphology, comminution, and subtle joint incongruity for surgical planning.

The thumb metacarpophalangeal (MCP) joint is supported by the ulnar and radial collateral ligaments, volar ligaments (including the Checkrein ligaments, the phalangoglenoid ligaments, and the volar plate), and the dorsal capsule [21]. Among these, the ulnar collateral ligament (UCL) is most frequently injured. In complete UCL tears, the ligament may retract proximally and become trapped above the adductor aponeurosis, forming the characteristic Stener lesion (Fig. 4.6) [22]. On ultrasound and MRI, this may appear as a "yoyo-on-a string" configuration. A displaced UCL prevents anatomic healing and mandates surgical repair. Both MRI (100%) and ultrasound (91%) have high specificities in diagnosing UCL tears; however MRI (92%) is more specific differentiating nondisplaced from displaced UCL tears than ultrasound (72%) [23]. Radiographs may demonstrate small avulsion fragments (Fig. 4.7) but usually provide only indirect information, such as MCP joint widening. Volar ligament injuries, although less common in the thumb than in the fingers, frequently (>92%) occur in association with UCL injuries and should be actively assessed on MRI and ultrasound (Fig. 4.8) [22].

Key Point

- A Stener lesion represents a proximally displaced and entrapped UCL of the first MCP joint. Both ultrasound and MRI reliably depict UCL tears and associated injuries of the thumb MCP joint.

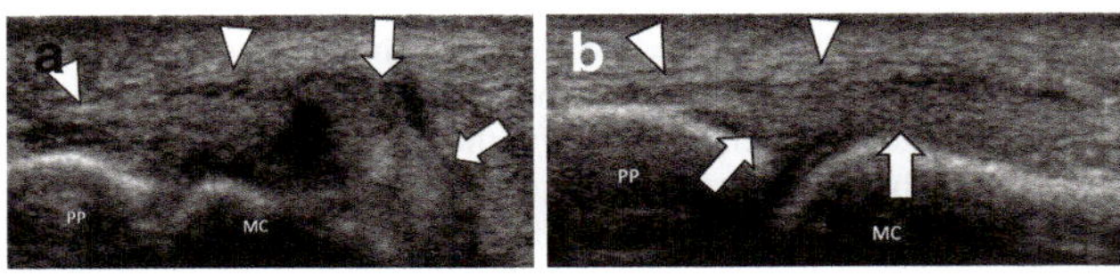

Fig. 4.6 Long-axis ultrasound of the metacarpophalangeal joint. (**a**) The ulnar collateral ligament (UCL) is proximally displaced and flipped superficial to the adductor aponeurosis (arrowheads), consistent with a Stener lesion. (**b**) The contralateral uninjured side demonstrates an intact UCL (arrows) lying deep to the adductor aponeurosis (arrowheads)

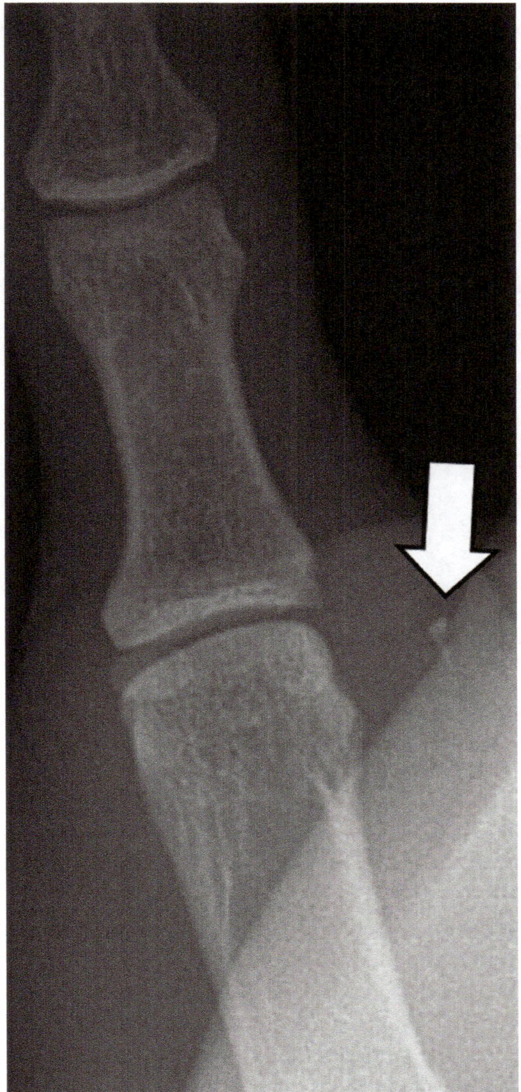

Fig. 4.7 Dorsopalmar radiograph of the thumb demonstrates a markedly displaced avulsion fracture (arrow) at the insertion of the ulnar collateral ligament of the metacarpophalangeal joint, with a small cortical defect along the ulnar base of the proximal phalanx, findings suspicious for a Stener lesion

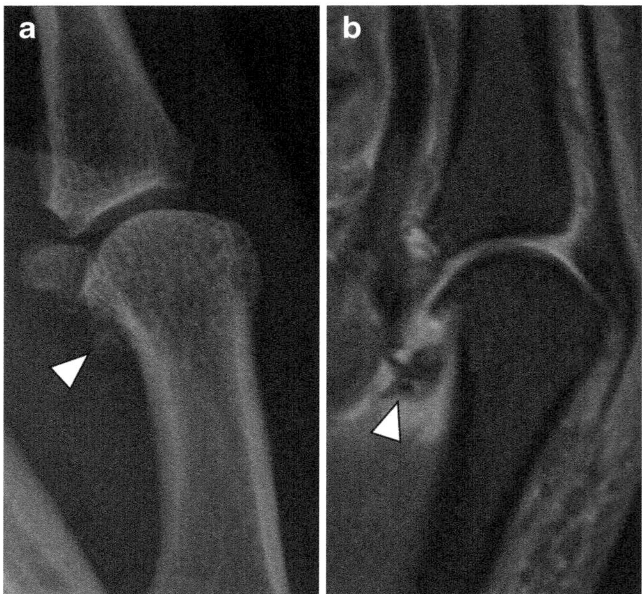

Fig. 4.8 (**a**) Lateral radiograph of the first metacarpophalangeal (MCP) joint demonstrates ossifications anterior to the metacarpal head (arrowhead) and mild osteoarthritic changes. (**b**) Sagittal proton density-weighted fat-suppressed MR image confirms avulsion of the volar capsuloligamentous structures (checkrein ligament, arrowhead) in association with an unshown UCL tear

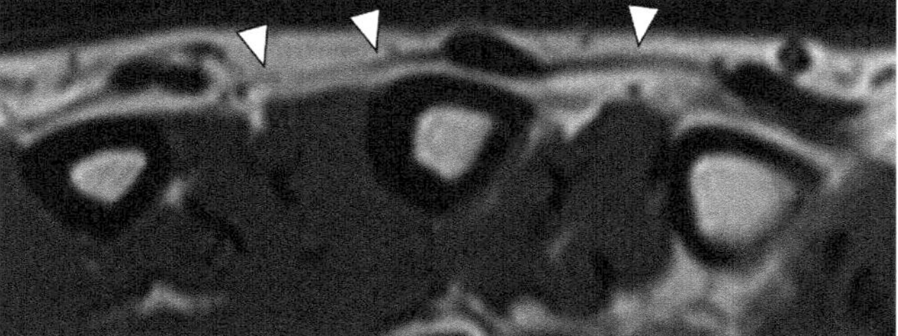

Fig. 4.9 Axial T1-weighted MR image demonstrates the connexus intertendinous between the extensor digitorum tendons of digits 2–4. These intertendinous bands stabilize the extensor tendons and distribute force during finger extension

4.15 Extensor Tendons and Sagittal Bands

The extensor apparatus of the fingers comprises the extensor digitorum communis (EDC) tendon, which extends into the extensor hood, lateral bands, and terminal tendon [24]. Anatomical variants are common, with double slips frequently seen at the fourth and fifth digits [24]. The connexus intertendinous are fibrous connections between the EDC tendons, most prominent between the index, middle, and ring fingers [24]. These intertendinous junctures stabilize the extensor tendons across the dorsum of the hand, distribute extensor force, and limit independent finger motion, explaining the frequent coupling of extension in central digits. On ultrasound, they appear as hyperechoic bands linking adjacent tendons; on MRI, they are seen as low-signal bands between tendons (Fig. 4.9). Although rarely injured in isolation, scarring or disruption may contribute to extensor lag or reduced finger independence after trauma or surgery.

At the level of the metacarpophalangeal (MCP) joint, the extensor tendon is stabilized by the radial and ulnar sagittal bands, which originate from the volar plate, deep transverse metacarpal ligament, and adjacent soft tissues. These structures envelop the tendon and maintain its central position over the metacarpal head (Fig. 4.10) [24, 25]. The sagittal bands resist ulnar or radial deviation of the tendon during MCP motion, preventing subluxation or dislocation. The extensor hood further divides into a central slip inserting on the middle phalanx and two lateral slips converging to form the terminal tendon at the distal phalanx [24]. The classic injury is a *sagittal band rupture,* historically termed boxer's knuckle. Injury to one or both sagittal bands allows the extensor tendon to sublux or dislocate. Patients typically present with painful snapping or loss of active extension at the MCP joint. The radial sagittal band is more often affected, especially in the middle finger, due to anatomical predisposition. Chronic instability may result in persistent extensor lag and reduced function. Ultrasound is excellent for evaluating sagittal band pathology. During a clenched fist maneuver, the subluxing or dislocating tendon can be visualized in real

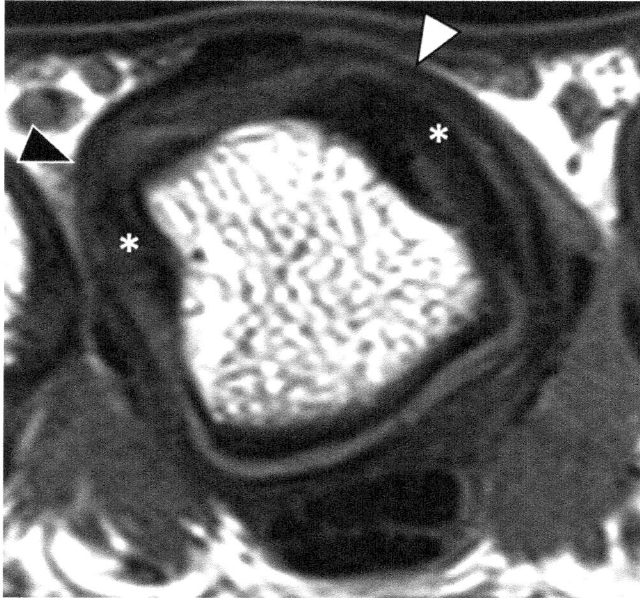

Fig. 4.10 Axial T2-weighted MR image shows the radial (white arrowhead) and the ulnar (black arrowhead) sagittal bands, which center and stabilize the extensor tendon at the metacarpophalangeal joint. Both sagittal bands course volarly, crossing the collateral ligaments (asterisks), and insert into the volar plate and deep transversal metacarpal ligament

time. Sagittal band tears appear as hypoechoic gaps or thinning in the fibrillar band structure (Fig. 4.11). Doppler signal may reveal associated hyperemia. MRI provides complementary static detail, showing displacement of the extensor tendon relative to the metacarpal head and fluid signal at the site of the torn sagittal band. On axial sequences, the normally centered tendon appears eccentrically positioned, though this may be obscured when the finger is imaged in extension.

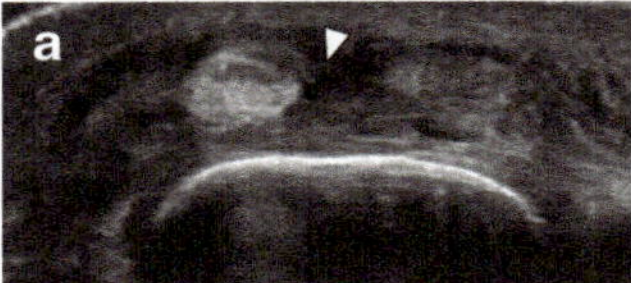

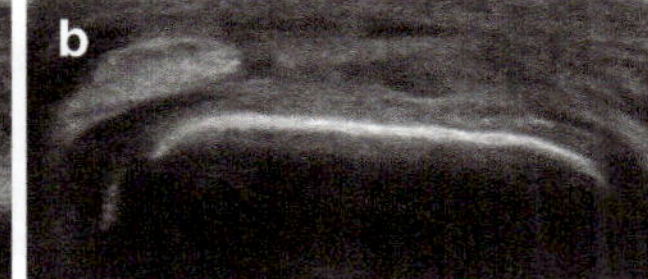

Fig. 4.11 (**a**) Ultrasound image demonstrates a tear of the radial sagittal band (arrowhead) of the middle finger. (**b**) Dynamic ultrasound during a clenched fist maneuver shows ulnar displacement of the extensor tendon

In combined sagittal band and collateral ligament injuries, the displaced collateral ligament may interpose with the extensor hood, producing a Stener-like lesion (Fig. 4.12) [26]. Radial collateral ligament injuries of the MCP joints more often affect the fourth and fifth digits, whereas ulnar collateral ligament injuries occur more often in the index finger, which lacks stabilizing support from adjacent interosseous muscles [26]. Other extensor tendon injuries include partial or full-thickness tears more distally, such as central or lateral slip tears from trauma or attrition. Mallet finger, another frequent injury, results from avulsion of the terminal extensor tendon at the base of the distal phalanx during forced flexion of an extended DIP joint [20]. Mallet injuries may occur with or without a bony fragment, with pure tendon injuries being more common [19]. In case of bony avulsion, description of the fragment size, degree of dislocation, and the percentage of articular surface involvement is essential.

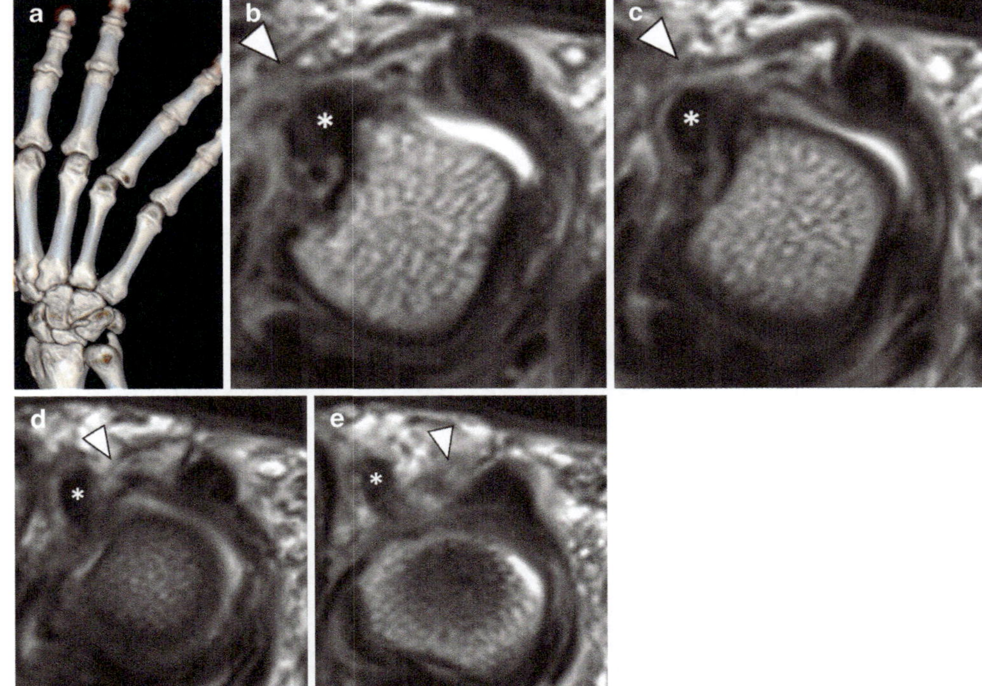

Fig. 4.12 (**a**) CT volume-rendered reconstruction of the right hand shows ulnar dislocation of the fourth MCP joint. (**b–e**) Axial T2-weighted MR images reveal a full-thickness tear of the radial sagittal band (arrowhead) and an associated displaced tear of the radial collateral ligament (RCL; asterisk). The RCL is interposed within the sagittal band defect and displaced superficially, representing a Stener-like lesion

4.16 Flexor Tendons and the Pulley System

The flexor tendons of the fingers consists of the flexor digitorum profundus (FDP) and flexor digitorum superficialis (FDS) tendons, which glide within a fibroosseous tunnel along the volar aspect of each finger. This tunnel is reinforced by a series of annular (A1–A5) and cruciform (C1–C3) pulleys. The A2 and A4 pulleys are most biomechanically important, preventing tendon bowstringing during finger flexion by maintaining the tendons in close apposition to the phalanges [18, 27, 28]. The A2 pulley is most commonly injured, particularly in rock climbers, followed by the A4 pulley (Fig. 4.13). Bowstringing of the flexor tendon is visualized as an increased distance between the tendon and the phalangeal cortex during active flexion—typically exceeding 1 mm at the level of the pulley [29, 30]. In forced flexion, a distance of ≥3 mm is indicative of a complete A2 pulley tear and of ≥5 mm suspicious of a combined A2/A3 pulley rupture [29, 30]. A distance ≥2.5 mm is indicative for an A4 pulley tear [29].

The A1 pulley resides at the metacarpal neck level and is frequently involved in stenosing tenosynovitis (trigger finger). *Trigger finger* is due to chronic overuse; the flexor tendon catches at the site of the A1 pulley due to thickening of the synovium or pulley itself. The most clinically urgent lesion is *Jersey finger*, a rupture of the FDP tendon at its distal insertion, typically in forced extension of a flexed DIP joint [20]. Tendon retraction into the palm may occur. The fourth finger is most commonly involved. Volar plate avulsions occur commonly at the weaker distal insertion and may be a result of joint dislocation; it mainly affects the proximal interphalangeal joint [20].

Tendon lacerations may occur, more frequently affecting the extensor tendons due to their superficial position. Lacerated flexor tendons have a higher tendency of retraction as they lack of a sufficient network of stabilizing surrounding fibers. MRI or ultrasound allow a precise detection of the degree of superficial and deep tendon involvement (Fig. 4.14). Description of the degree of tendon retraction, the quality of the tendon margins, and bony abnormalities which may be the cause of tendon laceration is crucial for the surgeon [18, 28].

Key Point

- On dynamic ultrasound, a tendon-to-bone distance greater than 3 mm (A2 pulley) or greater than 5 mm (A2 and A3 pulley) is diagnostic of pulley rupture with bowstringing.

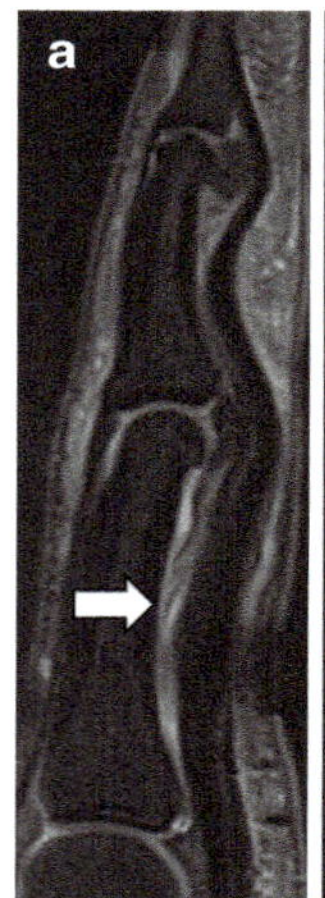

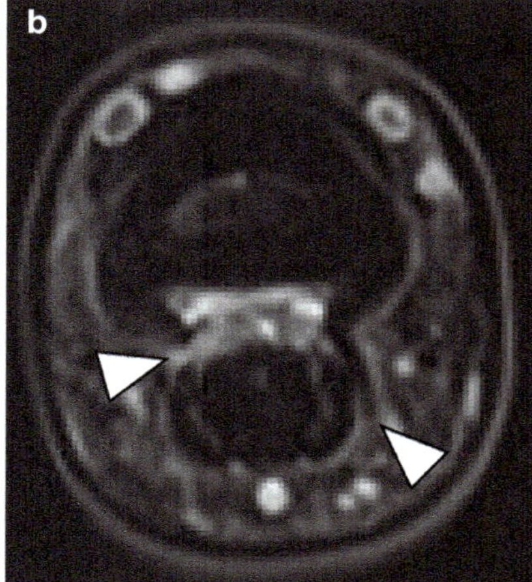

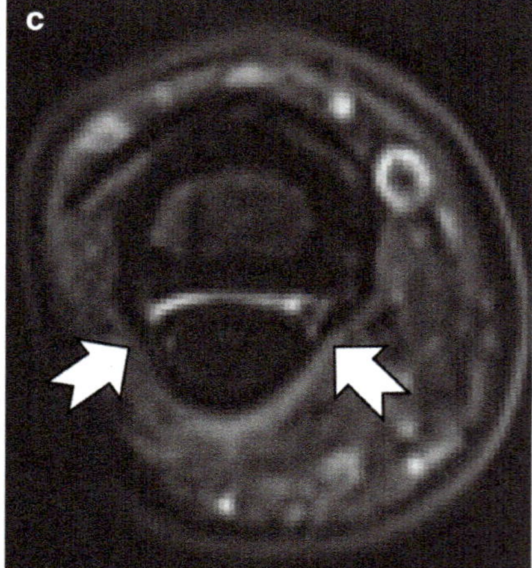

Fig. 4.13 (**a**) Sagittal proton density-weighted fat-saturated MR image demonstrates bowstringing of the flexor tendon (arrow) secondary to an A2 pulley tear. (**b**) Axial proton density-weighted fat-saturated MR image confirms discontinuity of the A2 pulley (arrowheads). (**c**) An adjacent intact A2 pulley for comparison (open arrows)

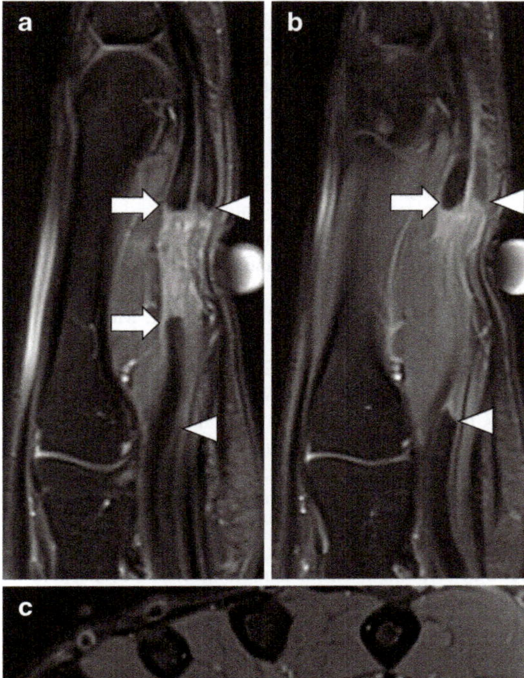

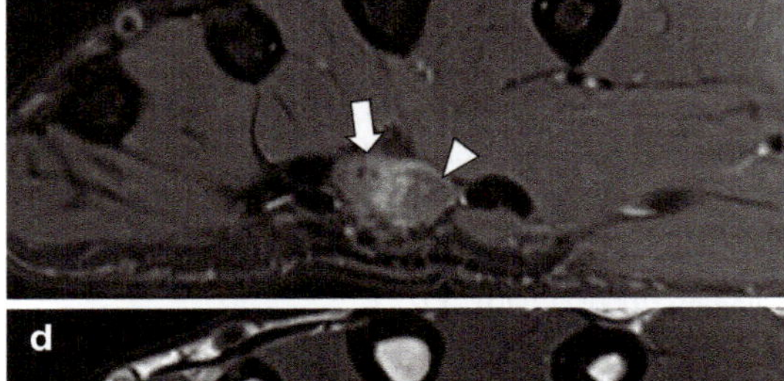

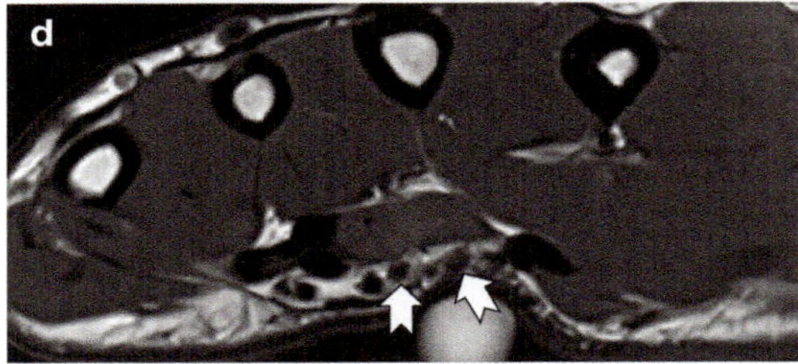

Fig. 4.14 (**a**) and (**b**) Sagittal proton density-weighted fat-saturated MR images demonstrate a full-thickness tear and retraction of the flexor digitorum profundus (FDP; arrows) and flexor digitorum superficialis tendons (FDS; arrowheads) tendons of the third digit. (**c**) Axial T2-weighted fat-saturated image depicts the torn FDP (arrow) and FDS (arrowhead). (**d**) Axial T1-weighted MR image shows the terminal branch of the median nerve (open arrows) adjacent to the torn tendons

4.17 Concluding Remarks

Imaging of the wrist and hand requires not only technical knowledge of available modalities but also a detailed understanding of anatomy and injury mechanisms. Radiographs continue to provide the essential first step in evaluation. Ultrasound, with its dynamic capability, is invaluable for assessing tendon and pulley integrity. MRI remains the gold standard for detecting subtle ligament tears, tendon disruptions, and cartilage or marrow pathology, while CT offers superior evaluation of complex intraarticular and comminuted fractures. Optimal patient care is achieved through a multimodality, problem-oriented approach that tailors imaging to the clinical question.

Take-Home Messages

- Radiographs are indispensable as the first-line tool for fractures and joint degenerative disease of the hand and wrist.
- Ultrasound is highly effective for the hands when evaluating tendon, pulley, and ligament integrity in real time, especially with dynamic maneuvers.
- MRI with dedicated coils is the modality of choice when detailed soft tissue characterization, surgical planning, or confirmation of subtle injuries is required, particularly in the TFC, extensor, flexor, or thumb and carpal ligamentous domains.

Conflict of Interest Statement I/We declare no competing interests as defined by Springer Nature or other interests that might be perceived to influence results and/or discussion reported in this manuscript.

References

1. Chang AL, Yu HJ, von Borstel D, Nozaki T, Horiuchi S, Terada Y, Yoshioka H. Advanced imaging techniques of the wrist. AJR Am J Roentgenol. 2017;209(3):497–510.
2. Loredo R, Sorge D, Garcia G. Radiographic evaluation of the wrist: a vanishing art. Semin Roentgenol. 2005;40(3):248–89.
3. Bäcker HC, Wu CH, Strauch RJ. Systematic review of diagnosis of clinically suspected scaphoid fractures. J Wrist Surg. 2020;9(1):81–9.
4. Beekhuizen SR, Quispel CR, Jasper J, Deijkers RLM. The uncommon trapezium fracture: a case series. J Wrist Surg. 2020;9(1):63–70.
5. Fox MG, Gaskin CM, Chhabra AB, Anderson MW. Assessment of scaphoid viability with MRI: a reassessment of findings on unenhanced MR images. AJR Am J Roentgenol. 2010;195(4):281–6.
6. Cerezal L, Abascal F, Canga A, Garcfa-Valtuille R, Bustamante M, del Pinal F. Usefulness of gadolinium- enhanced MR imaging in the evaluation of the vascularity of scaphoid nonunions. AJR Am J Roentgenol. 2000;174:141–9.
7. Murthy NS. The role of magnetic resonance imaging in scaphoid fractures. J Hand Surg Am. 2013;38(10):2047–54.
8. Mayfield JK, Johnson RP, Kilcoyne RK. Carpal dislocations: pathomechanics and progressive perilunar instability. J Hand Surg Am. 1980;5(3):226–41.
9. Wright TW, Dobyns JH, Linscheid RL, Macksoud W, Siegert J. Carpal instability non-dissociative. J Hand Surg Br. 1994;19(6):763–73.
10. Braun NS, Berger RA, Wolfe SW. Defining DISI and VISI. J Hand Surg Eur. 2021;46(5):566–8.
11. van der Post AS, Jens S, Smithuis FF, Obdeijn MC, Oostra RJ, Maas M. The triangular fibrocartilage complex on high-resolution

3 T MRI in healthy adolescents: the thin line between asymptomatic findings and pathology. Skeletal Radiol. 2021;50(11):2195–204.
12. Doarn MC, Wysocki RW. Acute TFCC injury. Oper Tech Sports Med. 2016:24:123–5.
13. Cerezal L, del Piñal F, Abascal F, García-Valtuille R, Pereda T, Canga A. Imaging findings in ulnar-sided wrist impaction syndromes. Radiographics. 2002;22(1):105–21.
14. Chen W. Kienböck disease and negative ulnar variance. J Bone Joint Surg Am. 2000;82(1):143–4.
15. Lee KS, Ablove RH, Singh S, De Smet AA, Haaland B, Fine JP. Ultrasound imaging of normal displacement of the extensor carpi ulnaris tendon within the ulnar groove in 12 forearm-wrist positions. AJR Am J Roentgenol. 2009;193(3):651–5.
16. Huang YT, Chen CJ, Wang YW, Horng YS. Comparing the carpal tunnel area and carpal boundaries in patients with carpal tunnel syndrome and healthy volunteers: a magnetic resonance imaging study. Diagnostics (Basel). 2025;15(10):1205.
17. Gude W, Morelli V. Ganglion cysts of the wrist: pathophysiology, clinical picture, and management. Curr Rev Musculoskelet Med. 2008;1(3–4):205–11.
18. Wieschhoff GG, Sheehan SE, Wortman JR, Dyer GSM, Sodickson AD, Patel KI, Khurana B. Traumatic finger injuries: what the orthopedic surgeon wants to know. Radiographics. 2016;36:1106–28.
19. Weintraub MD, Hansford BG, Stilwill SE, Allen H, Leake RL, Hanrahan CJ, Chan BY, Soltanolkotabi M, Kobes P, Mills MK. Avulsion injuries of the hand and wrist. Radiographics. 2020;40:163–80.
20. Smith TA, Bueno B, Phelan JV, Andand D, Kirschenbaum D, Katt BM. Stener-like lesions in the hand: a qualitative review. Hand. 2024;19(7):1097–101.
21. Hirschmann A, Sutter R, Schweizer A, Pfirrmann CWA. The carpometacarpal joint of the thumb: MR appearance in asymptomatic volunteers. Skeletal Radiol. 2013;42:1105–12.
22. Hirschmann A, Sutter R, Schweizer A, Pfirrmann CWA. MRI of the thumb: anatomy and spectrum of findings in asymptomatic volunteers. AJR Am J Roentgenol. 2014;202(4):819–27.
23. Manneck S, Del Grande F, Hirschmann A. Ulnar collateral ligament injuries of the first metacarpophalangeal joint: prevalence of associated injuries on radiographs and MRI. Skeletal Radiol. 2021;50:505–13.
24. Rashidi A, Haj-Mirzaian A, Dalili D, Fritz B, Fritz J. Evidence-based use of clinical examination, ultrasonography, and MRI for diagnosing ulnar collateral ligament tears of the metacarpophalangeal joint of the thumb: systematic review and meta-analysis. Eur Radiol. 2021;31:5699–712.
25. Clavero J, Golano P, Farinas O, Alomar X, Monill JM, Esplugas M. Extensor mechanism of the fingers: MR imaging-anatomic correlation. Radiographics. 2003;23:593–611.
26. Theumann NH, Pfirmmann CWA, Drapé JL, Trudell DJ, Resnick D. MR imaging of the metacarpophalangeal joints of the fingers. Part I. Conventional MR imaging and MR arthrographic findings in cadavers. Radiology. 2002;222:437–45.
27. McCarthy C. Ultrasound of normal and injured ligaments and retinacula of the hand. Semin Musculoskeletal Radiol. 2020;24:83–100.
28. Lapegue F, Andre A, Brun C, Bakouche S, Chiavassa H, Sans N, Faruch M. Traumatic flexor tendon injuries. Diagn Interv Imaging. 2015;96:1279–92.
29. Klauser A, Frauscher F, Bodner G, Halpern EJ, Schocke MF, Springer P, Gabl M, Judmaier W, zur Nedden D. Finger pulley injuries in extreme rock climbers: depiction with dynamic US. Radiology. 2002;222:755–61.
30. Hauger O, Chung CB, Lektrakul N, Botte MJ, Trudell D, Boutin RD, Resnick D. Pulley system in the fingers: normal anatomy and simulated lesions in cadavers at MR imaging, CT, and US with and without contrast material distention of the tendon sheath. Radiology. 2000;217:201–12.

The Current State of Hip Imaging

5

Reto Sutter and Donna G. Blankenbaker

Learning Objectives

- Recognize the key imaging features of common hip disorders—including fractures, avascular necrosis of the femoral head, osteoarthritis, femoroacetabular impingement, extraarticular hip impingement, and developmental hip dysplasia—and understand which imaging modality is indicated for which clinical situation.
- Apply imaging-based criteria that alter management, such as MRI signs of femoral neck stress fractures, subchondral fracture in avascular necrosis, MRI arthrography detection of cartilage delamination in FAI, and coverage/torsion metrics in FAI and developmental hip dysplasia.

5.1 Fractures

Stress fractures are due to a mismatch between native bone strength and chronic mechanical load applied on bone over time [1]. It is important to identify these injuries early as they can progress to complete fracture and lead to prolonged recovery and further complications. Stress fractures most often present in endurance athletes, such as runners and military recruits, but are also seen in recreational athletes with a rapid increase in activity [2, 3]. Stress fractures are categorized as fatigue fractures, caused by normal bone being subjected to abnormal repetitive forces, and insufficiency fractures, because of normal stress placed on abnormal bone [1]. The repetitive overloading leads to increased osteoclastic activity that exceeds the rate of osteoblastic new bone formation; this results in bone weakening and microtrabecular fractures (stress injury) and eventually may lead to cortical break (fracture) [3]. These injuries commonly occur along the medial femoral neck, where compressive forces are pronounced, but can develop along the outer aspect, where tensile forces predominate [1]. Clinical history and characteristic radiographic findings of focal periosteal reaction, cortex disruption, and trabecular sclerosis are classic for this injury. However, femoral neck stress fractures are frequently occult on radiographs. Typical MRI features include poorly defined focal or diffuse high T2 bone marrow signal because of microtrabecular fractures and edema, with or without corresponding low T1 signal and/or periosteal edema. When these features are present, carefully assess for a hypointense band in the marrow or focal cortical abnormality, indicating a stress fracture with a need for a prolonged period of nonweight-bearing or for rest from sports (Fig. 5.1).

Key Point

- MRI is the most sensitive test for femoral neck stress injury; look for marrow edema plus a hypointense band/cortical irregularity.

Subchondral insufficiency fracture (SIF) of the femoral head is a relatively uncommon entity and can be a cause of mechanical hip pain and typically occurs in elderly individuals with osteoporosis [4]. SIF is considered an important contributing factor of rapidly progressive osteoarthritis of the hip and an uncommon cause of acute hip pain in healthy adults. It was previously thought that this disease was mainly affected by osteoporosis in the elderly, but current evidence suggests that SIF can occur in adults of all ages and at different activity levels [4, 5] These fractures can progress to

R. Sutter (✉)
Department of Radiology, Balgrist University Hospital, University of Zurich, Zurich, Switzerland
e-mail: reto.sutter@balgrist.ch

D. G. Blankenbaker
Musculoskeletal Imaging & Intervention, University of Wisconsin School of Medicine and Public Health, Madison, WI, USA
e-mail: dblankenbaker@uwhealth.org

J. Hodler et al. (eds.), *Musculoskeletal Diseases 2026-2029*, IDKD Springer Series,
https://doi.org/10.1007/978-3-032-17040-8_5

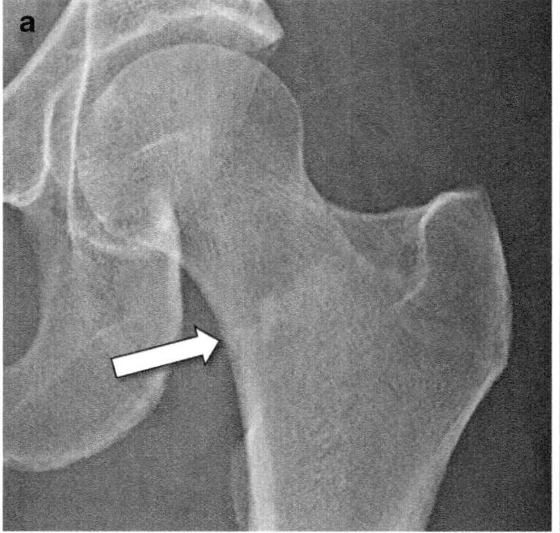

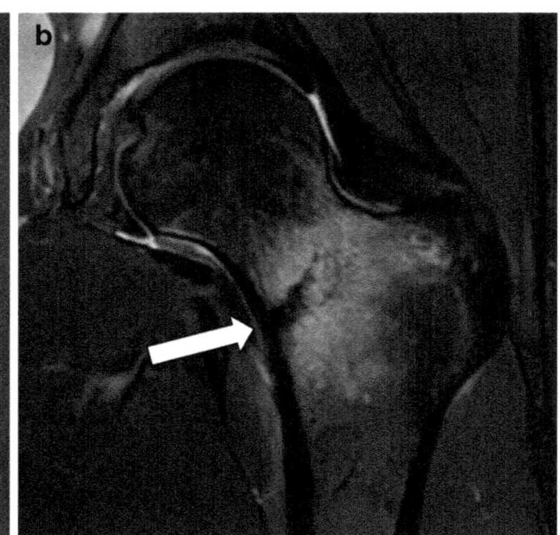

Fig. 5.1 Anteroposterior radiograph of the left hip (**a**) in a 36-year-old female runner shows a subtle band of sclerosis (arrow) along the medial femoral neck. Coronal T2-weighted fat-suppressed MR image (**b**) in the same patient shows a low-signal intensity line along the medial femoral neck (arrow) and extensive surrounding bone marrow edema

advanced collapse and it is therefore crucial to recognize them on imaging [6]. Distinguishing SIF from osteonecrosis is important not only for the determination of the appropriate initial treatment but also for planning an effective pre- and postoperative management. Characteristic MRI findings are that of a low-signal subchondral line that parallels the articular surface and extensive bone marrow edema (BME) of the femoral head and/or neck. Contrast-enhanced MRI can be helpful to distinguish SIF from osteonecrosis: hips with SIF will enhance on the articular side of the low-signal intensity band in the femoral head, whereas necrotic segments in osteonecrosis do not enhance [7].

Complete femoral head fractures are rare and most often accompany posterior hip dislocation after high-energy trauma [8]. Multiple classification systems for proximal femur fracture-dislocations have been used, but the Pipkin classification system is still in use due to its simplicity [8]. Pipkin 1 fractures are confined to the femoral head caudal to the fovea, type 2 fractures extend cranial to the fovea, type 3 is a type 1 or 2 femoral head fracture combined with a femoral neck fracture, and type 4 combine a type 1 or 2 femoral head fracture with an acetabular fracture. Osteochondral femoral head impaction fractures are commonly seen following both posterior and anterior hip dislocations. These injuries may be subtle or occult on radiographs, where only a slight contour flattening or a focal impaction defect of the femoral head may be seen. CT or MRI improves detection of these subtle lesions. Femoral neck fractures are classified as subcapital, transcervical, or basicervical and as displaced or nondisplaced. In older adults, low-energy trauma more commonly produces transverse subcapital femoral neck fractures or intertrochanteric fractures [8]. The Garden classification is most commonly used for elderly patients. This system describes four categories: stage 1, incomplete or valgus impacted; stage 2, complete but nondisplaced; stage 3, complete and partially displaced; and stage 4, complete and fully displaced [8]. Most femoral neck fractures are usually well characterized on anteroposterior and lateral radiographs; MRI is used for equivocal cases for definite detection especially in osteoporotic patients.

5.2 Avascular Necrosis of the Hip

Avascular necrosis (AVN) of the femoral head is an ischemic osteonecrosis characterized by death of trabecular bone and marrow with a high risk of subchondral collapse and secondary osteoarthritis. Nontraumatic AVN is commonly linked to corticosteroids, alcohol misuse, hemoglobinopathies, chemotherapy, and transplantation (Fig. 5.2). Early disease is frequently oligosymptomatic; once collapse occurs, pain and functional limitation accelerate. Contemporary staging uses the 2019 revised ARCO system, where at stage 1 radiographs are normal, but MRI or bone scans are positive. At stage 2 radiographic abnormalities are present without fracture or flattening of the femoral head, and at stage 3 a fracture is seen in the subchondral or necrotic zone (either with femoral head depression $\leq$2 mm [IIIA] or > 2 mm [IIIB]). When secondary osteoarthritis is present, this is classified as stage 4. Treatment decisions are driven primarily by lesion size and location and by the presence of subchondral collapse [9].

Standard radiographs are insensitive in early disease but depict late sclerosis, subchondral crescent sign (impending collapse), segmental flattening of the femoral head, and secondary osteoarthritis (OA). MRI is the modality of choice for early detection and mapping of necrotic extent. The hallmark is the low-signal intensity band on T1-weighted images circumscribing the necrotic segment; on fluid-sensitive sequences, a double-line sign is typical. Bone marrow edema (BME) may be reactive or reflect superimposed subchondral fracture, which indicates an impending collapse [10]. Involvement of the superior weight-bearing portions of the femoral head and a subchondral fracture are the most powerful imaging predictors of poor outcome and the need for total

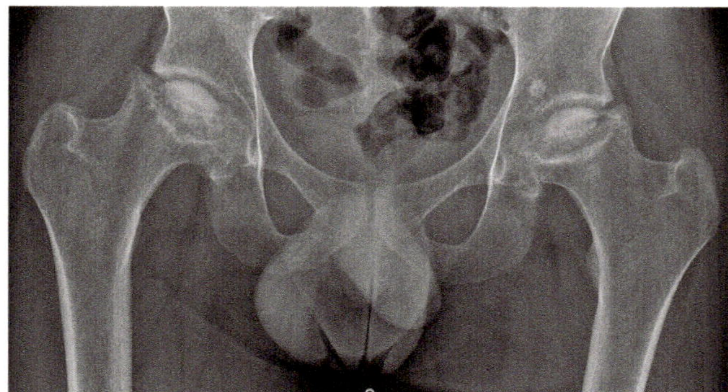

Fig. 5.2 Anteroposterior radiograph of the pelvis in an 18-year-old male with bilateral avascular necrosis of the femoral head after chemotherapy for leukemia, showing bilateral sclerosis of the necrotic femoral head with fracture, fragmentation, and collapse. Note that the joint space is preserved in both hips

hip arthroplasty; small, medial lesions without fracture are candidates for joint-preserving interventions [10].

There are two main differentials for AVN: transient osteoporosis (bone-marrow-edema syndrome) shows diffuse femoral head/neck BME without a circumscribing T1 low-signal band and typically resolves over time. Subchondral insufficiency fractures show a low-signal line parallel to the articular surface of the femoral head with surrounding edema in osteopenic patients. When it comes to treatment, early-stage disease with small or medium lesions may be managed with core decompression, sometimes in combination with biologic adjuncts that enhance revascularization and osteogenesis. In the presence of a femoral head collapse (ARCO III), larger subchondral fractures, extensive superolateral involvement, or substantial cartilage delamination, usually total hip arthroplasty will be performed [9].

Key Point

Use MRI to quantify the size and location of hip AVN (percent head involvement, relation to the superior weight-bearing dome); larger, superolateral lesions predict collapse and steer management away from joint preservation toward total hip arthroplasty.

5.3 Osteoarthritis of the Hip

Hip OA is common and age-related, with the incidence rising substantially after 50–60 years and a lifetime risk of symptomatic hip OA of roughly one in four adults; it remains a leading indication for total hip arthroplasty and a major contributor to disability. Radiographs remain the first-line test for suspected OA because they are accessible and inexpensive and correlate with structural severity (Fig. 5.3). MRI may be used in unclear cases, for example, when clinical signs of inflammation are present, and to rule out differential diagnoses, and readily depicts cartilage defects, labral tears and paralabral cysts, bone marrow edema, joint effusion, and synovitis, as well as subchondral insufficiency fractures [11]. In addition, MRI is useful for assessing disorders of the insertion of the hip abductor tendons at the greater trochanter, which are commonly present in elderly patients and can be a cause of pain and substantial morbidity. CT is not indicated for primary OA diagnosis, but it aids in preoperative templating and detecting occult subchondral fractures when MRI is contraindicated.

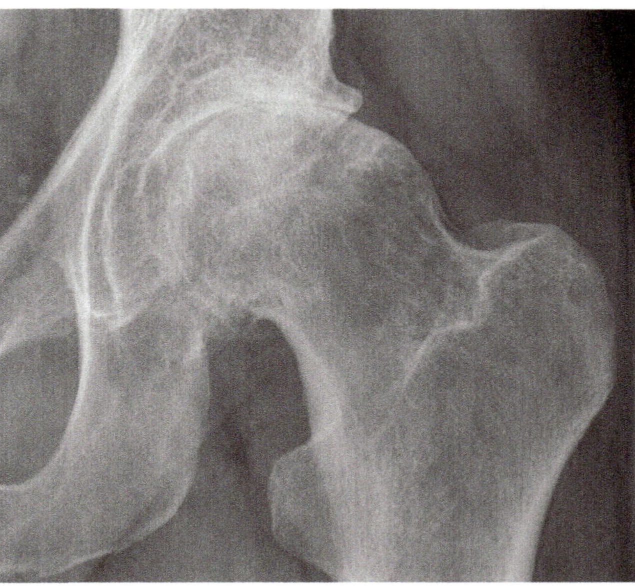

Fig. 5.3 Anteroposterior radiograph shows advanced osteoarthritis of the left hip in a 51-year-old patient with known femoroacetabular impingement. The typical radiographic features of osteoarthritis are present, with large osteophytes, marked joint space narrowing, pronounced subchondral sclerosis of the articular surfaces, deformity of the femoral head contour, and large subchondral cysts of the femoral head

OA of the hip most commonly affects the superior-lateral compartment. Femoroacetabular impingement (FAI)-related OA often demonstrates labral ossification, rim osteophytes, and anterosuperior chondrolabral damage; dysplasia-related OA shows lateral uncovering of the femoral head with a hypertrophic and severely degenerated labrum. Increased femoral antetorsion is associated with more severe OA, even in cases without hip dysplasia [12]. Differential diagnoses for hip OA include subchondral insufficiency fractures of the femoral head and AVN. And importantly, hip pain may originate from other locations, such as the peritrochanteric region (e.g., with abductor tendon tears and trochanteric bursitis), or from the spine or SI joints. When diagnosing hip OA, care should be taken not to overcall the presence of osteophytes, since to some degree small osseous spurs can be seen at some locations of the hip joint (e.g., at the rim of the fovea of the femoral head) also in asymptomatic individuals [13].

Key Point

Radiographs stage structural severity of hip OA; MRI can distinguish atypical/inflammatory presentations of hip diseases from OA, detects occult subchondral fractures, and is good for assessing pathologies of the periarticular muscles and tendons, such as the abductor tendons.

5.4 Femoroacetabular Impingement

FAI is a symptomatic hip disorder in young- and middle-aged individuals caused by an abnormal morphology of the femoral head-neck junction (cam-type morphology), the acetabulum (pincer-type morphology), and/or an abnormal femoral antetorsion, resulting in repetitive mechanical conflict and chondrolabral injury [14]. Male individuals are more commonly affected than female individuals, and athletes are affected most, probably due to a too high mechanical load on the hip joint during early adolescence, when the growth plate of the proximal femur is most susceptible. As with other hip disorders, standard radiographs are the first modality that is used for assessing the hip joint, usually consisting of an anteroposterior pelvic radiograph and a cross-table lateral or Dunn lateral radiograph of the affected side [16]. Crucially, a correct and consistent radiographic technique has to be applied, in order to allow a valid assessment of the osseous structures of the hip joint.

Radiographs are especially useful to assess the acetabular morphology (Fig. 5.4), where pincer-type impingement presents either with a global overcoverage of the hip joint (i.e., coxa profunda or acetabular protrusion) or with a focal acetabular retroversion (i.e., a relative anterior overcoverage of the hip joint). Coxa profunda is defined as the crossing of the floor of the acetabular fossa with the ilioischial line on the anteroposterior pelvic radiograph, while acetabular retroversion can be assessed on pelvic radiographs with the presence of one or more of the following signs: the crossover sign, posterior wall sign, or ischial spine sign. Cam-type deformities are best assessed on radial MRI images over the femoral head-neck junction, making it possible to assess the osseous morphology circumferentially around the femoral head. Alternatively, CT can be used to assess cam-type deformities, but generally MRI is preferred, because it allows the assessment of FAI morphology without using radiation. Care must be taken though when looking for cam-type impingement that some extent of an aspherical femoral head-neck junction can also be seen in asymptomatic volunteers, and similarly, a number of asymptomatic volunteers show coxa profunda. The presence of a moderate cam-type deformity or moderate coxa profunda is not sufficient to diagnose FAI, as the diagnosis of FAI is always made by combining the clinical signs and symptoms as well as the radiological findings [14]. If both cam- and pincer-type deformities are present, this is called mixed-type impingement.

Femoral antetorsion is a normal anatomical feature of the femur and is defined as the angle between the femoral neck axis (at the level of the proximal femur) and the tangent of

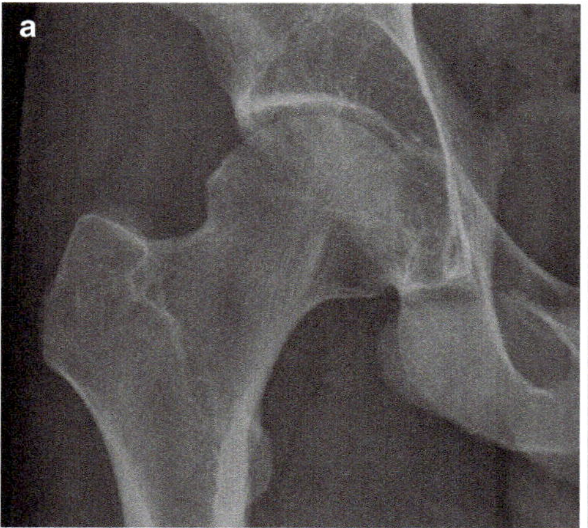

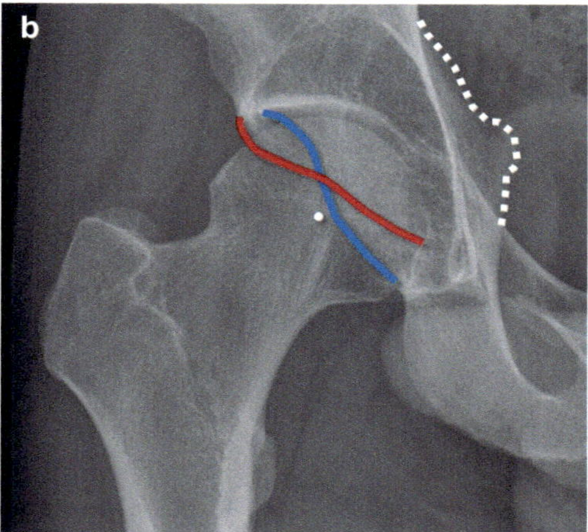

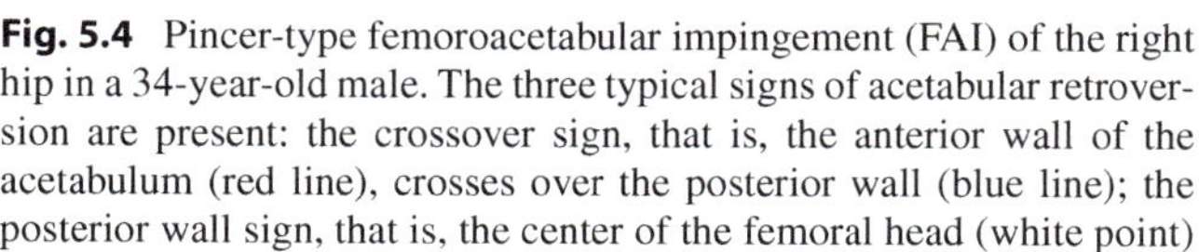

Fig. 5.4 Pincer-type femoroacetabular impingement (FAI) of the right hip in a 34-year-old male. The three typical signs of acetabular retroversion are present: the crossover sign, that is, the anterior wall of the acetabulum (red line), crosses over the posterior wall (blue line); the posterior wall sign, that is, the center of the femoral head (white point) is lateral to the posterior acetabular wall; the ischial spine sign, that is, the ischial spine is visible on the medial side of the pelvis (dotted line). The image shown is an enlarged portion of an anteroposterior pelvic radiograph and is shown twice for didactic purposes

the femoral condyles (at the level of the knee) (Fig. 5.5). Normal femoral antetorsion is usually around 12–13°, although with a substantial standard deviation of about 10° [15]. Both abnormally increased and decreased femoral torsions contribute to the development of FAI, with the typical case involving a cam-type FAI with a reduced femoral torsion, thereby creating an increased repetitive mechanical impaction between the femoral head and the labrum during flexion, internal rotation, and adduction of the hip joint. While initially only cam- and pincer-type morphologies were described as a cause of FAI, abnormal femoral antetorsion is now recognized as the third major osseous contributor to FAI, making it necessary to assess femoral torsion in all patients with suspected FAI. Femoral antetorsion can easily be measured on strictly axial images over the proximal and the distal part of the femur by using fast MRI sequences that can be integrated in the standard MRI protocol of the hip.

MRI arthrography is the best modality to assess the internal derangement of the hip joint in patients with FAI, readily depicting labrum tears (which are most commonly found in the anterosuperior quadrant of the hip joint), injury to the acetabular and femoral cartilage, abnormalities of the teres ligament, or the presence of joint bodies and synovitis (Fig. 5.6). Traction MRI arthrography increases the sensitivity of detecting articular cartilage delamination, which is an important information for both stratification of patient out-

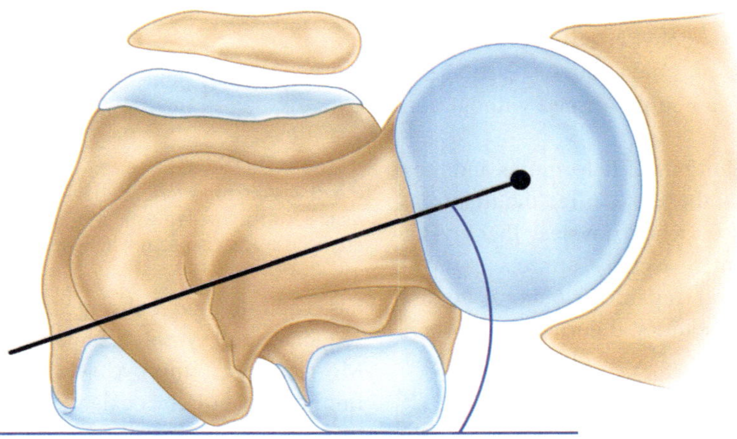

Fig. 5.5 Schematic drawing of the femoral antetorsion, showing the angle between the longitudinal axis along the femoral neck (thick straight line) and the tangent at the femoral condyles (thin straight line) at the level of the knee. Normal femoral antetorsion is around 12–13° ± 10°. Reduced femoral antetorsion results in increased mechanical impaction at the anterior part of the hip joint during internal rotation, while increased femoral antetorsion results in increased mechanical impaction at the posterior part of the hip during external rotation

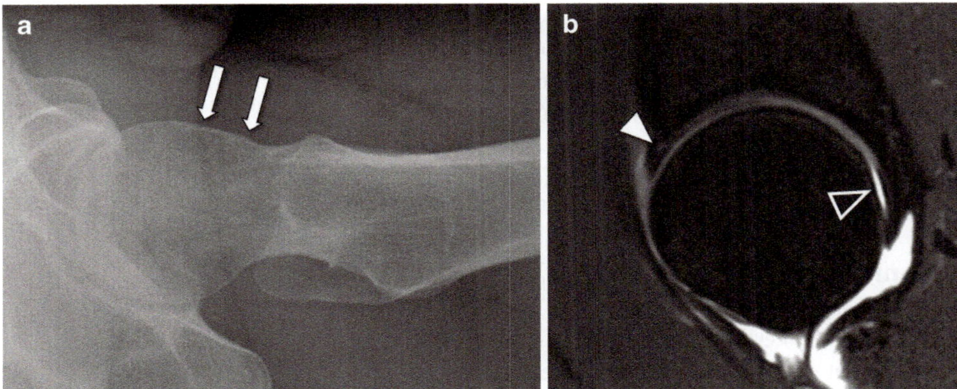

Fig. 5.6 Femoroacetabular impingement (FAI) of the left hip in a 32-year-old male with pain in the left hip. (**a**) Cross-table lateral radiograph of the left hip shows a cam deformity (arrows) at the femoral head-neck junction. (**b**) Sagittal proton-density fat-suppressed MRI arthrography image shows a tear of the anterosuperior labrum (white arrowhead), involving both the base and the substance of the labrum. Additionally, a deep cartilage defect at the posterior femoral head is present (outline arrowhead)

Key Point

Start the evaluation for FAI with radiographs, where pincer-type morphology is visible; radial MRI images are best for assessing cam-type morphology; femoral torsion can be measured on strictly axial MRI images over the hip and knee; traction MRI arthrography best reveals delamination of the articular cartilage.

come and surgical planning [17]. The actual impingement can be visualized with real-time assessment of the femoroacetabular motion on MRI, and recent developments with AI-accelerated MRI sequences have allowed obtaining images at a higher spatial resolution, which has started a discussion whether MRI arthrography is still necessary for detecting injuries to the labrum and articular cartilage or whether these examinations can be performed without contrast [18].

In patients with isolated cam/pincer deformities and focal chondrolabral injury, physical therapy is often the first treatment. In more severe cases or when physical therapy has failed, the surgical treatment is usually arthroscopy with osteochondroplasty and labral repair. If femoral torsion abnormalities are present, an additional derotational osteotomy of the femoral shaft may be considered. If there is already extensive cartilage loss present, the benefits of arthroscopy are quite limited, so these patients often first receive conservative therapy (physical therapy or corticosteroid injections for pain relief), and at a later stage, a total hip arthroplasty will be performed.

5.5 Extraarticular Impingement

Extraarticular impingement disorders are distinct in mechanism from the classic cam- and pincer-type impingement. Patients with extraarticular disorders are typically younger and present with hip, groin, or buttock pain and limited function [19]. Diagnosing extraarticular impingement guides appropriate treatment and patient outcomes.

5.5.1 Anterior Impingement

There are two discrete types of anterior impingement by etiology: subspine impingement related to the anterior-inferior iliac spine and iliopsoas impingement attributable to the iliopsoas tendon. Before apophyseal closure at the anterior inferior iliac spine (AIIS), avulsion can occur in adolescents engaged in high-load sports, from either a single traumatic event or repetitive traction [20]. An enlarged, prominent AIIS is typical, with an impingement between the AIIS and the proximal femur during hip flexion; therefore this disorder has been termed subspine impingement (Fig. 5.7). The sequelae and symptoms may persist into adulthood [21]. Most patients improve with conservative care. Subspine impingement often coexists with FAI, likely reflecting shared exposure to high-level sports during adolescence as the physes close [22]. In adolescents, imaging may show a widened, irregular AIIS apophysis with adjacent marrow edema. In chronic cases, a distal anterior femoral neck bump and superior capsular edema may be present; a more distal anterior cam lesion independently increases the risk of symptomatic subspine impingement [21].

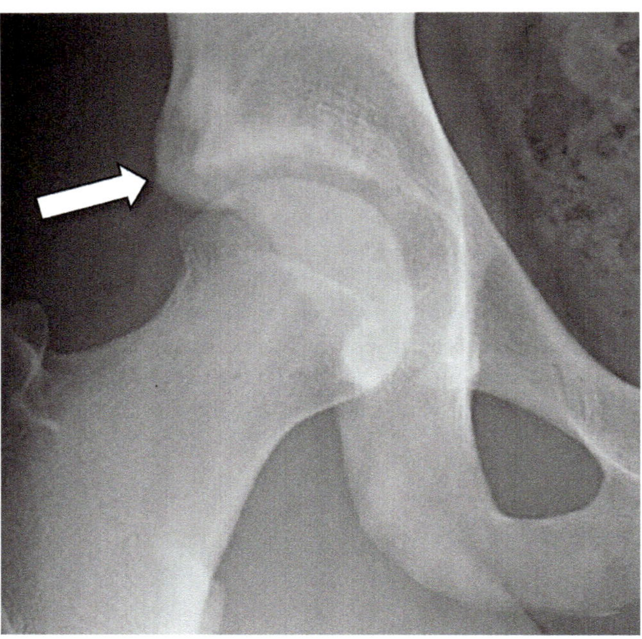

Fig. 5.7 Anteroposterior radiograph of the hip in a 17-year-old athletic male shows a low-lying anterior inferior iliac spine (arrow) which can predispose to subspine impingement

Iliopsoas impingement is less common and involves repetitive contact of the iliopsoas tendon against the anterior labrum. The chronic friction of the iliopsoas tendon against the anterior hip can result in labrum tears at this location. This tends to be inferior to the anterosuperior labral tears typical of FAI [19]. Several factors can predispose to psoas impingement including scar formation, prominent muscle or tendon bulk, or regional morphological variations in muscle anatomy more commonly seen in women. Iliopsoas impingement is also found in 3–5% of patients following total hip arthroplasty. In the past, labrum repair and tenotomy were performed; however, tenotomy has fallen out of favor as more recent concern about subsequent anterior hip instability has emerged [19].

5.5.2 Posterior Impingement

Posterior extraarticular impingement involves either the ischiofemoral interval or the deep gluteal space.

Ischiofemoral impingement refers to pain from entrapment of the quadratus femoris between the lesser trochanter and the ischial tuberosity/hamstring complex and is more commonly seen in women [23, 24]. Narrowing of the ischiofemoral space may be positional, acquired, or congenital [25], is often bilateral, and may be incidental and asymptomatic. Studies have shown that provocation depends on hip position—internal/external rotation, adduction/abduction, and flexion/extension can all influence symptoms [24]. Studies have shown significant reduction of the ischiofemoral space and quadratus femoris space when comparing patients with abnormal quadratus femoris muscle MRI signal with control groups [23]. Narrowing of this space can be congenital, or it can be seen secondary to prior fractures, surgical procedures (such as total hip arthroplasty or femoral osteotomy), the presence of an osteochondroma, ischial enthesopathy, or conditions leading to superomedial femoral migration [25]. Patients typically report nonspecific hip, groin, or lower buttock pain. Radiation to the thigh or knee can occur, and proximity to the sciatic nerve may produce radicular-type symptoms [19]. Pain symptoms in patients with ischiofemoral impingement can often be reproduced by a combination of extension, adduction, and external rotation of the hip [25].

> **Key Point**
> Ischiofemoral impingement: look for quadratus femoris edema and/or fatty replacement of the quadratus femoris muscle on MRI, as well as narrowing of the ischiofemoral and quadratus femoris space.

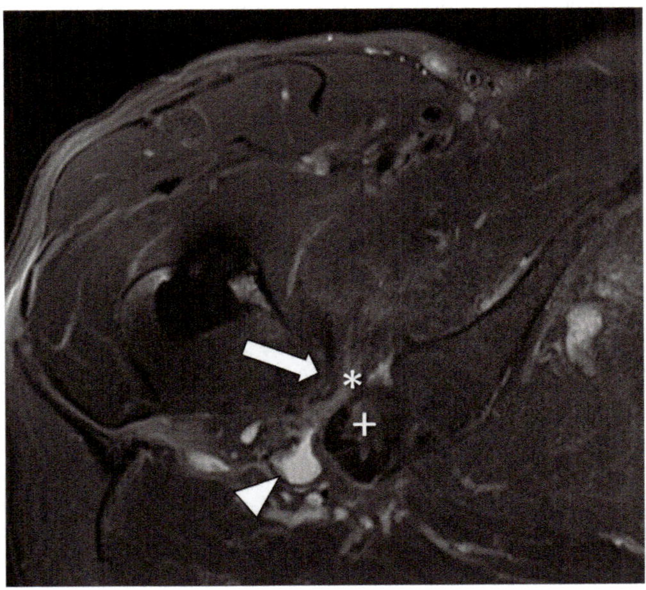

Fig. 5.8 Ischiofemoral impingement of the right hip in a 73-year-old woman after total hip arthroplasty. The quadratus femoris space is severely narrowed between the femoral lesser trochanter (arrow) and the markedly degenerated hamstring tendon origin (plus sign). The quadratus femoris muscle is compressed, demonstrating pronounced edema (asterisk) and associated neo-bursa formation (white arrowhead). These findings are shown on a transverse short-tau inversion recovery (STIR) MRI sequence with metal artifact reduction

There is no clear consensus about what constitutes a normal ischiofemoral or quadratus femoris space, and if measurements are used at imaging, there should be a reproducible positioning of the patient in the scanner. The classic morphologic signs on MRI are edema and fatty replacement of the quadratus femoris muscle on MRI (Fig. 5.8). Differential diagnosis of quadratus femoris muscle edema includes muscle strains or tearing of the muscle, which should be considered in cases without narrowing of the ischiofemoral or quadratus femoris space.

Currently, there is no consensus on how to treat patients with ischiofemoral impingement. Most commonly, conservative treatment is preferred, with rest, activity restriction, anti-inflammatory nonsteroidal medications, and physical therapy. Image-guided injections into the quadratus femoris muscle or next to the muscle have shown good results [19].

The deep gluteal space is anatomically confined by the gluteus maximus muscle, the posterior acetabular column, the proximal femur and hip joint, the linea aspera and greater trochanter, and the sacrotuberous ligament. This space is dynamically deformed with hip motion, and it contains the sciatic and smaller regional nerves, muscles, the hamstring tendons, and fibrous bands containing blood vessels [26]. Deep gluteal syndrome is commonly a diagnosis of exclusion; lumbar and intraarticular hip sources should be ruled out first. MRI of the pelvis is the most comprehensive imaging test to exclude alternative causes of sciatic nerve impingement and may reveal edema or neuritis of the sciatic nerve within the deep gluteal space. Other causes such as hamstring tendinosis, tear or peritendinous bursal inflammation, piriformis muscle anatomy and signal, integrity of regional and small nerves, or masses can also be assessed. Initial management is typically conservative with an emphasis on physical therapy or injections [26].

5.5.3 Lateral Impingement

Trochanteric-pelvic impingement denotes symptomatic contact between the greater trochanter and the ilium during hip abduction and extension [19, 27]. It most often follows proximal femoral deformity after Perthes disease but may also occur with congenital dislocation and other Perthes-like deformities [19]. These abnormalities alter hip biomechanics by shortening the abductor lever arm and reducing the trochanter-ilium distance, predisposing to abutment. Treatment begins conservatively, and if unsuccessful, a proximal femoral osteotomy may be considered [19].

> **Key Point**
> Developmental hip dysplasia can coexist with cam morphology and may precipitate secondary FAI if unrecognized.

5.6 Developmental Hip Dysplasia

Developmental dysplasia of the hip (DDH) encompasses a spectrum of abnormal development of the acetabulum and femoral head and is associated with hip pain, instability, and early-onset osteoarthritis. Dysplasia anatomically refers to a shallow acetabulum, and there are different variants with a different extent and location of the acetabular undercoverage. For the diagnosis of DDH, it is crucial to integrate symptoms, physical examination, and imaging [28]. Although historically applied to infants, DDH is increasingly recognized also in adolescents and adults as acetabular undercoverage [29]. Undercoverage reduces the load-bearing surface area, which results in cartilage injury and ultimately in osteoarthritis.

Preoperative imaging, including radiographs, CT, MRI, and ultrasound, is used to diagnose hip dysplasia, with ultrasound being pivotal in infants. Accurate, standardized imaging and careful interpretation are crucial for effective treatment planning. The lateral center-edge angle (LCEA) is the most widely used parameter to characterize acetabular coverage on the anteroposterior pelvic view, but it should not be used in isolation. The normal range of LCEA is 25–39°. The LCEA for borderline dysplasia is between 20° and 25° and < 20° is considered acetabular dysplasia. Acetabular version can also be assessed on CT or MRI. MRI has immense value in the evaluation of the labrum, cartilage, capsule, ligamentum teres, and surrounding supporting soft tissue structures of the hip. The typical findings on imaging include acetabular undercoverage together with a large, hypertrophied labrum that shows substantial degeneration (Fig. 5.9).

Acetabular dysplasia and FAI are known to coexist, with cam morphology most commonly found in these cases. In one study, 47% of patients being treated for FAI also had findings of acetabular dysplasia [30]. Pincer FAI is not frequently seen in DDH. Dysplastic hips can have retroversion, with a crossover sign and prominent ischial spine, but typically it is due to posterior acetabular deficiency and not due to anterior overcoverage. It is important to recognize coexisting femoral head asphericity to prevent secondary FAI after acetabular correction. When symptoms persist despite non-operative care, hip preservation surgery is indicated in young patients—surgery is performed arthroscopically, as open surgery (e.g., periacetabular and/or proximal femoral osteotomy), or combined [28].

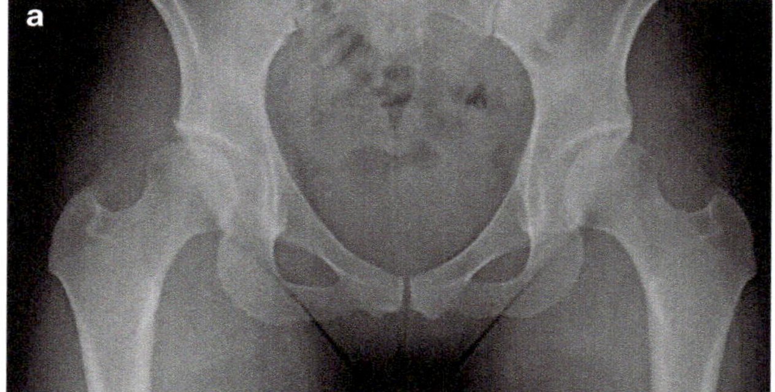

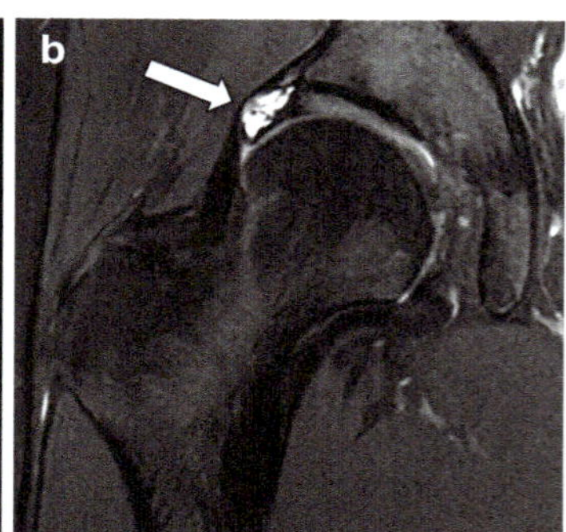

Fig. 5.9 Anteroposterior radiograph (**a**) of both hips in a 33-year-old active woman shows bilateral acetabular dysplasia with uncovering of the femoral heads. Coronal T2-weighted fat-suppressed MR image (**b**) in the same patient shows an enlarged labrum (arrow) with intrasubstance cysts

5.7 Concluding Remarks

A variety of imaging techniques are essential for the comprehensive evaluation of the hip joint. Radiographs are good for structural assessment; MRI detects early stress injury, subchondral insufficiency fractures, and avascular necrosis while also giving a good assessment of chondrolabral injuries and soft tissue pathologies; and CT contributes precise osseous detail for preoperative planning. Accurate recognition of osseous conflict—caused by cam and pincer morphology as well as abnormal femoral antetorsion—and of extraarticular impingement is essential to explain patient symptoms and in establishing the correct diagnosis.

Take-Home Messages

- Imaging plays a central role in evaluating the osseous architecture of the hip joint, detecting stress injuries and avascular necrosis, and identifying morphological abnormalities that contribute to femoroacetabular conflict.
- Abnormal femoral torsion is present not only in developmental hip dysplasia but also often accompanies impingement; it can be assessed reliably on axial MRI images covering the proximal and distal femur.
- MRI is the preferred imaging modality for characterizing the extent and severity of labral and cartilage lesions in developmental hip dysplasia and femoroacetabular impingement, providing essential information for treatment planning and outcome prediction.

Conflict of Interest I/We declare no competing interests as defined by Springer Nature or other interests that might be perceived to influence results and/or discussion reported in this manuscript.

References

1. Anderson MW, Greenspan A. Stress fractures. Radiology. 1996;199(1):1–12.
2. Bencardino JT, Palmer WE. Imaging of hip disorders in athletes. Radiol Clin North Am. 2002;40(2):267–87.
3. Blankenbaker DG, De Smet AA. Hip injuries in athletes. Radiol Clin North Am. 2010;48(6):1155–78.
4. Kim JW, et al. Subchondral fracture of the femoral head in healthy adults. Clin Orthop Relat Res. 2007;464:196–204.
5. Chen M, et al. Current research on subchondral insufficiency fracture of the femoral head. Clin Orthop Surg. 2022;14(4):477–85.
6. Vassalou EE, Spanakis M, et al. MR imaging of the hip: an update on bone marrow edema. Semin Musculoskelet Radiol. 2019;23(3):276–88.
7. Miyanishi K, Hara T, et al. Contrast-enhanced MR imaging of subchondral insufficiency fracture of the femoral head: a preliminary comparison with that of osteonecrosis of the femoral head. Arch Orthop Trauma Surg. 2009;129(5):583–9.
8. Sheehan SE, et al. Proximal femoral fractures: what the orthopedic surgeon wants to know. Radiographics. 2015;35(5):1563–84.
9. Yoon BH, Mont MA, Koo KH, et al. The 2019 revised version of association research circulation osseous staging system of osteonecrosis of the femoral head. J Arthroplast. 2020;35(4):933–40.
10. Hines JT, Jo WL, Cui Q, et al. Osteonecrosis of the femoral head: an updated review of ARCO on pathogenesis, staging and treatment. J Korean Med Sci. 2021;36(24):e177.
11. Mourad C, Vande Berg B. Osteoarthritis of the hip: is radiography still needed? Skeletal Radiol. 2023;52(11):2259–70.
12. Parker EA, Meyer AM, Nasir M, et al. Abnormal femoral anteversion is associated with the development of hip osteoarthritis: a systematic review and meta-analysis. Arthrosc Sports Med Rehabil. 2021;3(6):e2047–58.
13. Bensler S, Agten CA, Pfirrmann CWA, Sutter R. Osseous spurs at the fovea capitis femoris—a frequent finding in asymptomatic volunteers. Skeletal Radiol. 2018;47(1):69–77.
14. Sutter R, Dietrich TJ, Zingg PO, et al. How useful is the alpha angle for discriminating between symptomatic patients with cam-type femoroacetabular impingement and asymptomatic volunteers? Radiology. 2012;264(2):514–21.
15. Sutter R, Dietrich TJ, Zingg PO, Pfirrmann CWA. Femoral antetorsion: comparing asymptomatic volunteers and patients with femoroacetabular impingement. Radiology. 2012;263(2):475–83.
16. Schmaranzer F, Meier MK, Sutter R. Femoroacetabular impingement: preoperative planning and postoperative MR imaging evaluation. Magn Reson Imaging Clin N Am. 2025;33(1):29–41.
17. Schmaranzer F, Kheterpal AB, Bredella MA. Best practices: hip femoroacetabular impingement. AJR Am J Roentgenol. 2021;216(3):585–98.
18. Burke CJ, Walter WR, Gyftopoulos S, et al. Real-time assessment of femoroacetabular motion using radial gradient echo magnetic resonance arthrography at 3 tesla in routine clinical practice: a pilot study. Arthroscopy. 2019;35(8):2366–74.
19. Koles SL, Salat P, et al. Current concepts in extra-articular impingement of the hip: clinical diagnosis, imaging, and treatment. Semin Musculoskelet Radiol. 2017;21(5):547–60.
20. Hetsroni I, Larson CM, et al. Anterior inferior iliac spine deformity as an extra-articular source for hip impingement: a series of 10 patients treated with arthroscopic decompression. Arthroscopy. 2012;28(11):1644–53.
21. Samim M, Walter WR, et al. MRI assessment of subspine impingement: features beyond the anterior inferior iliac spine morphology. Radiology. 2019;293(2):412–21.
22. Agricola R, Heijboer MP, et al. A cam deformity is gradually acquired during skeletal maturation in adolescent and young male soccer players: a prospective study with minimum 2-year follow-up. Am J Sports Med. 2014;42(4):798–806.
23. Torriani M, Souto SC, et al. Ischiofemoral impingement syndrome: an entity with hip pain and abnormalities of the quadratus femoris muscle. AJR Am J Roentgenol. 2009;193(1):186–90.
24. Torriani M. Ischiofemoral impingement syndrome in 2024: updated concepts and imaging methods. Magn Reson Imaging Clin N Am. 2025;33(1):63–73.
25. Blankenbaker DG, Tuite MJ. Non-femoroacetabular impingement. Semin Musculoskelet Radiol. 2013;17(3):279–85.
26. Hernando MF, Cerezal L, et al. Deep gluteal syndrome: anatomy, imaging, and management of sciatic nerve entrapments in the subgluteal space. Skeletal Radiol. 2015;44(7):919–34.
27. Harris JD, Gerrie BJ, et al. Microinstability of the hip and the splits radiograph. Orthopedics. 2016;39(1):e169–75.
28. Harris JD, Lewis BD, et al. Hip Dysplasia. Clin Sports Med. 2021;40(2):271–88.
29. Barrera CA, Cohen SA, et al. Imaging of developmental dysplasia of the hip: ultrasound, radiography and magnetic resonance imaging. Pediatr Radiol. 2019;49(12):1652–68.
30. Paliobeis CP, Villar RN. The prevalence of dysplasia in femoroacetabular impingement. Hip Int. 2011;21(2):141–5.

Groin and Pelvic Pain in Athletes

6

Ara Kassarjian and Kenneth Lee

Learning Objectives
- Define the clinical entity of groin pain in athletes.
- Review the anatomy in the parasymphyseal region.
- Explore the clinical and imaging characteristics of groin pain in athletes.
- Briefly address management strategies and implications.

6.1 Introduction

Groin pain associated with athletic activity is a widely recognized clinical entity that continues to pose a significant challenge to medical teams in terms of both diagnosis and management. Over the years, terminology has evolved, and the term "groin pain in athletes" is now the most appropriate to describe this condition, reflecting its multifactorial etiology and the need for a multidisciplinary approach [1]. This condition is particularly prevalent in high-intensity sports involving rapid changes in direction, twisting, pivoting, and kicking, with soccer exhibiting the highest incidence among team sports [2, 3].

Epidemiological studies suggest that nearly one-third of soccer players will experience groin pain at some point in their careers, with a higher prevalence in men [4, 5]. Groin pain in athletes can lead to substantial disability, reduced performance, prolonged absence from training and competition, and in some cases career-threatening consequences if inadequately diagnosed or managed.

A. Kassarjian (✉)
Elite Sports Imaging, Madrid, Spain

Head of Radiology, Olympia Medical-Surgical Center, Madrid, Spain
e-mail: akassarjian@gmail.com

K. Lee
University of Wisconsin School of Medicine and Public Health, Musculoskeletal Imaging and Intervention, Madison, WI, USA
e-mail: klee2@uwhealth.org

Radiologists and clinicians encounter two typical presentations in athletes with groin pain:

1. Acute groin pain: Usually associated with a clear mechanism of injury, such as sudden directional changes, forceful muscle contractions, overstretching, or, less commonly, direct trauma. Imaging findings in acute cases are typically straightforward.
2. Chronic or insidious groin pain: Often resulting from repetitive microtrauma, overuse, or biomechanical imbalances. Clinical symptoms are less specific, and imaging findings can be subtle or multifactorial, complicating accurate diagnosis.

The challenges in diagnosis stem from the anatomical complexity of the groin region, the variable terminology historically used, and incomplete understanding of the pathophysiology underlying groin pain. These factors contribute to inconsistencies in clinical assessment, imaging interpretation, and treatment strategies [6].

To address these issues, an expert panel consisting of sports medicine physicians, physiotherapists, general and orthopedic surgeons, and radiologists convened in Doha in 2014, establishing a standardized framework for groin pain in athletes. They emphasized the use of "clinical entities" rather than ambiguous terms such as osteitis pubis, athletic pubalgia, pubic instability, or sports hernia [6–8].

The Doha Agreement categorized groin pain into three primary groups based on clinical presentation:

1. Defined clinical entities for groin pain: adductor-related, pubic-related, inguinal-related, and iliopsoas-related groin pain
2. Hip-related groin pain
3. Other causes of groin pain in athletes

Although imaging was not a central focus during the Doha meeting, the development of standardized imaging protocol was recommended to enhance diagnostic accuracy and guide patient management. MRI has since become the imaging modality of choice, due to its superior spatial resolution and tissue contrast.

6.2 Anatomical Considerations

The groin is an anatomically complex region where multiple muscular, tendinous, and ligamentous structures converge in a compact area. Detailed knowledge of this anatomy is crucial for accurate imaging interpretation [9, 10] (Fig. 6.1).

6.2.1 Symphysis Pubis and Capsuloligamentous Complex

The symphysis pubis is an amphiarthrodial joint formed by the convergence of the pubic rami and stabilized by four ligaments: superior, inferior (arcuate), anterior, and posterior pubic ligaments. Its fibrocartilaginous disc resembles an intervertebral disc, with a peripheral anulus fibrosus and a posterosuperior cleft [2].

The anterior abdominal muscles and adductors converge at the symphysis pubis. The rectus abdominis and adductor longus serve as primary stabilizers, with the anterior pubic ligament fusing with their aponeuroses to form the prepubic aponeurotic complex (P-PAC) [11]. Recent studies highlight the pyramidalis muscle, situated anterior to the rectus abdominis, as a key connector in the pyramidalis-anterior pubic ligament-adductor longus complex (PLAC), emphasizing the intricate fiber interconnections within this region [12, 13].

6.2.2 Inguinal Canal

The inguinal canal extends from the inferomedial abdominal wall to the peritoneum. It contains the spermatic cord in males or the round ligament in females, along with neurovascular structures. Key anatomical landmarks include the deep inguinal ring, an opening in the transversalis fascia above the midpoint of the inguinal ligament, and the superficial inguinal ring, an opening in the external oblique aponeurosis above the pubic tubercle [3, 14, 15]. These structures are critical in evaluating inguinal-related groin pain.

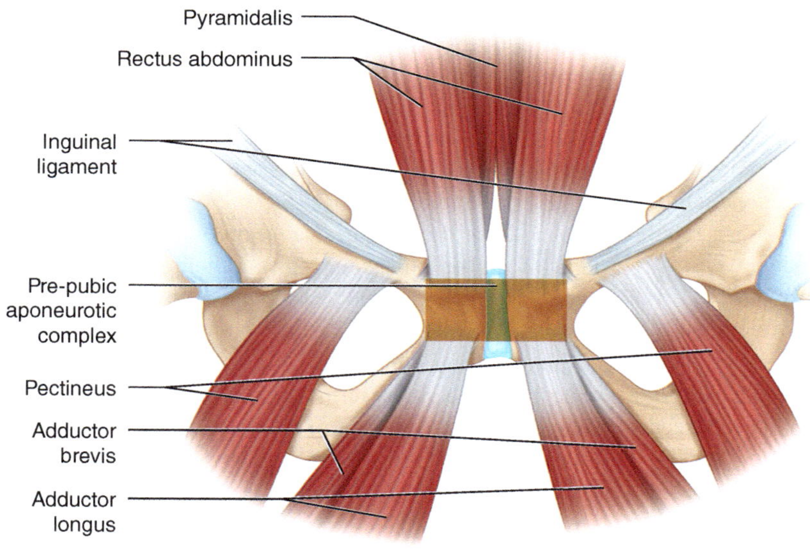

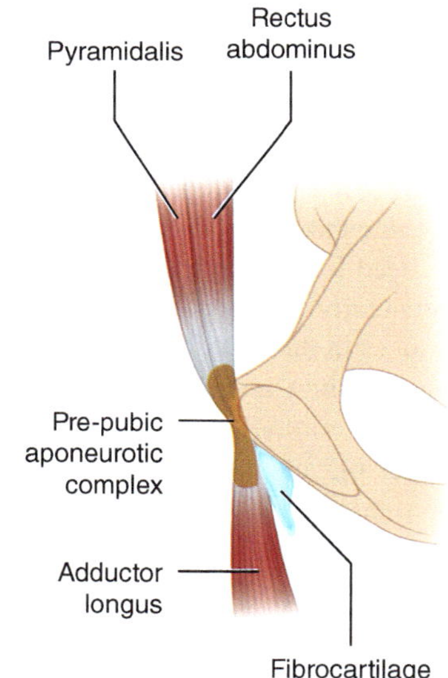

Fig. 6.1 Anatomy of the symphysis pubis

6.3 Biomechanical Considerations

The symphysis pubis functions as a pivot for forces generated by the adductor muscles and anterior abdominal wall. The rectus abdominis exerts a posterior and cranial pull during trunk rotation and extension, while the adductors exert an opposing downward and forward vector during hip adduction, sudden directional changes, and kicking [2, 3, 9, 16].

Imbalances between these opposing forces can compromise pubic stability, leading to chronic overload, microtrauma, and increased susceptibility to both acute and chronic injuries [1, 17, 18]. Understanding these biomechanics is essential for diagnosis, imaging interpretation, and rehabilitation planning.

6.4 Clinical Considerations

6.4.1 Presentation

Most athletes present with insidious, poorly localized pain that worsens with activity and improves at rest. Acute disabling pain is less frequent but more readily diagnosable due to a clear mechanism of injury [19, 20].

6.4.2 Examination

A multidisciplinary evaluation, combining history, physical examination, and imaging, is critical for accurate diagnosis. Assessment often involves palpation of the adductor origin, rectus abdominis, inguinal canal, and hip, with functional tests such as resisted adduction, trunk flexion, and hip flexion against resistance. Comparison with prior imaging and clinical signs and symptoms enhances diagnostic accuracy.

6.4.3 Clinical Entities

The Doha Agreement defines four primary clinical entities of groin pain:

1. Adductor-related: Pain near the adductor origin, tenderness on palpation, pain with resisted adduction, or stretching
2. Pubic-related: Local pain over the symphysis pubis, often with bone marrow edema or degenerative changes
3. Inguinal-related: Pain in the inguinal canal, exacerbated by Valsalva maneuver, often without a hernia
4. Iliopsoas-related: Less common; pain triggered by rising from squatting or resisted hip flexion

6.5 Diagnostic Algorithm

MRI is the first-line imaging modality, complemented by ultrasound and plain radiography where indicated (Fig. 6.2). MRI protocols typically involve the following:

- Large FOV coronal or axial sequences to localize injuries and detect unsuspected pathology (stress fractures, avulsions)
- High-resolution small FOV sequences in coronal, sagittal, axial, and oblique planes to evaluate the P-PAC/PLAC,

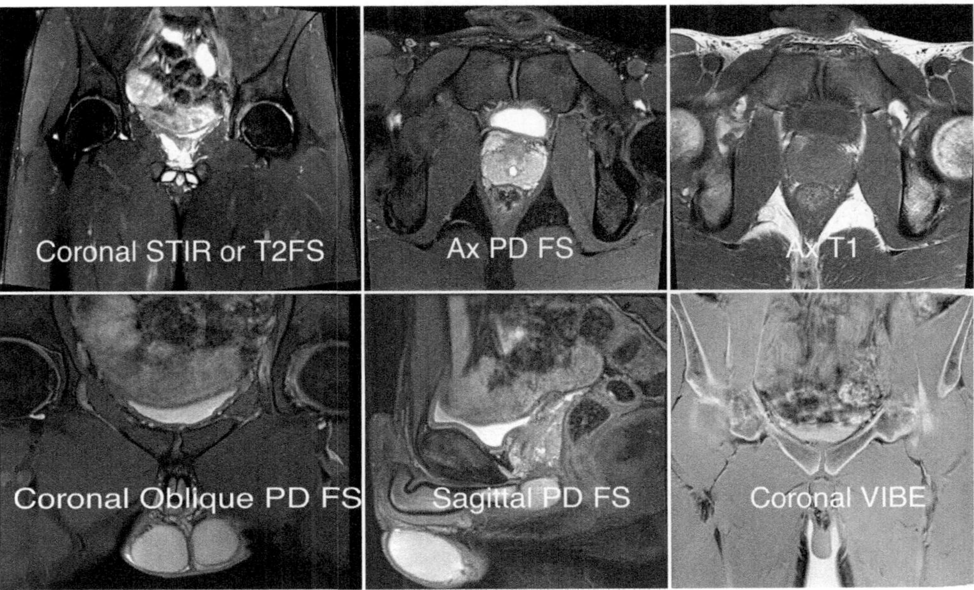

Fig. 6.2 MRI protocol for athletic groin pain. Coronal STIR or T2 FS of the pelvis, axial T1, axial PD FS, sagittal PD FS, and coronal oblique PD FS of the parasymphyseal region. Optional VIBE sequence with pseudo-CT

adductors, rectus abdominis, pubic symphysis, and inguinal region
- Optional three-dimensional gradient echo sequences (VIBE) for osseous lesions

Dynamic ultrasound is particularly useful for evaluating inguinal wall weakness, real-time tendon or muscle pathology, and patient-specific symptom reproduction [14, 21].

6.6 Pathology and Imaging

6.6.1 Aponeurotic Injuries

Lesions of the P-PAC/PLAC are frequent and may coexist with adductor or rectus abdominis injuries (Fig. 6.3). Fluid-sensitive sequences on MRI detect tears, enthesopathy, edema, and fatty infiltration. Classic signs include the following:

- Secondary cleft sign: Inferior extension of the interpubic cleft along the anteroinferior symphysis, indicating adductor tendon or gracilis injury [22–24]
- Superior cleft sign: Horizontal tear at the rectus-adductor junction, parallel to the superior pubic ramus [22, 25]

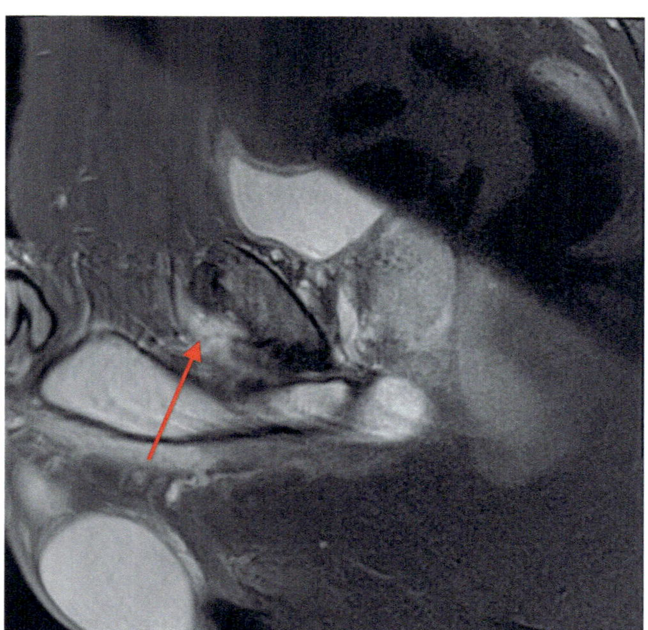

Fig. 6.3 Sagittal PD FS image demonstrates a tear of the P-PAC (arrow)

6.6.2 Bone and Symphyseal Changes

Bone marrow edema (BME) is common, often reflecting chronic overload or adaptive changes. Parasymphyseal fatigue fractures and apophyseal stress injuries occur from repetitive loading [17, 26]. In these cases, MRI reveals linear hypointensities and associated edema (Fig. 6.4). Chronic degeneration, disc protrusion, osteophytes, and subchondral cysts may also be present [2, 9, 27].

6.6.3 Tendon and Muscle Injuries

The proximal adductor longus is most commonly affected (Fig. 6.5). MRI findings include the following:

- Tendinopathy (thickening, increased signal)
- Partial or complete tears with tendon gap, loss of tension, or retraction
- Myotendinous injuries with "feather-like" edema patterns involving the myotendinous junction [28]

6.6.4 Iliopsoas and Inguinal Injuries

Iliopsoas injuries are less frequent and may be associated with bursitis and fluid distention of the bursa on MRI or US (Fig. 6.6). Inguinal-related pain often corresponds to abdominal wall weakness without true hernia, best assessed with dynamic ultrasound and Valsalva maneuvers [3, 29].

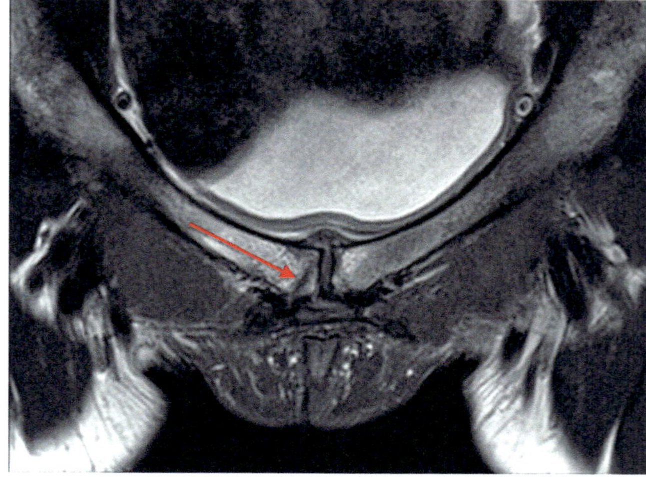

Fig. 6.4 Coronal oblique PD FS image demonstrates a right parasymphyseal fatigue fracture (arrow)

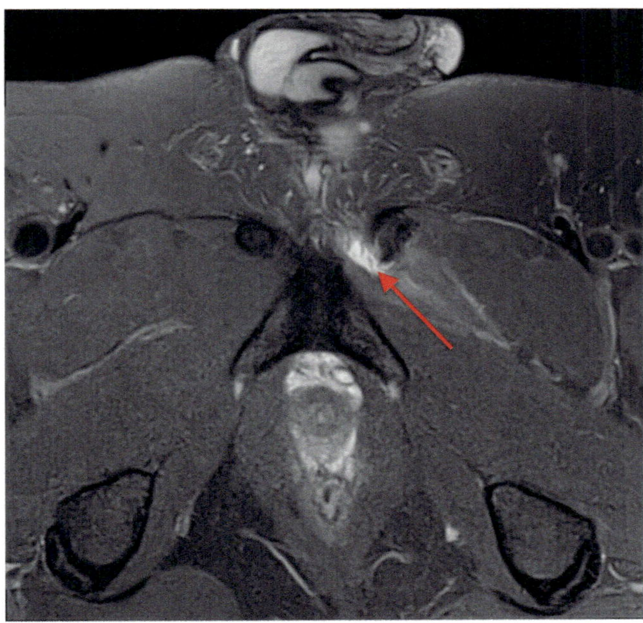

Fig. 6.5 Axial PD FS image demonstrates a tear and distal retraction of the left adductor longus tendon with underlying tendinopathy as evidenced by thickening of the tendon (arrow)

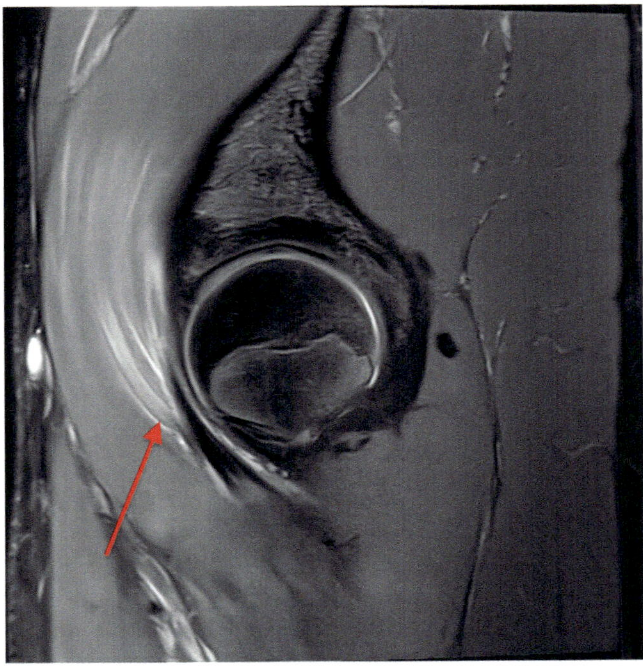

Fig. 6.6 Sagittal PD FS image demonstrates a mild myotendinous strain of the psoas (arrow)

6.7 Management Implications

Early and accurate diagnosis influences return-to-play timelines, which vary depending on lesion type, size, chronicity, and associated injuries. Multidisciplinary management integrates the following:

- Rest and activity modification
- Physiotherapy targeting core stabilization and hip and groin strengthening
- Interventional approaches (injections, PRP, surgery) in refractory cases
- Imaging follow-up to guide rehabilitation progression

6.8 Conclusion

Groin pain in athletes is a complex, multifactorial condition requiring precise clinical and imaging assessment. Adoption of Doha clinical entities, along with high-resolution MRI protocols, improves diagnostic accuracy, facilitates communication among healthcare professionals, and enhances patient outcomes. A structured, multidisciplinary approach is essential, given the frequent coexistence of symptomatic and asymptomatic lesions, biomechanical contributors, and sport-specific demands.

6.9 Posterior Pelvis

Learning Objectives

- Highlight relevant anatomy and imaging findings of hamstring injuries.
- Understand the most common cause of lateral pelvis pain and imaging features.

In the *posterior pelvis*, the hamstring tendons and muscles are the anatomic structures most affected by pathology and important for radiologists to understand. Hamstring injuries are one of the most common in sports and account for significant lost time off the field. The incidence in field-based team sports is 0.81 per 1000 exposure hours, and the prevalence is 13% for a nine-month period [30]. Field-based team sports that require sprinting and cutting maneuvers include soccer,

American football, rugby, Australian football, Gaelic football, and field hockey. The average time loss is approximately 18–24 days and a recurrence rate of up to 33%, with 17% of reinjuries within 12 months [31, 32]. Hamstring injuries pose a significant challenge to medical teams in management and return-to-play timeline. Imaging, both MRI and ultrasound (US), are playing increasingly important roles in diagnosis and treatment. MRI offers excellent resolution and detailed assessment of connective tissue and is essential for ruling out avulsion injuries [33]. US provides real-time, dynamic assessment and is valuable for follow-up and detecting fluid collections [34]. Therefore, it is important for radiologists to understand the imaging appearance of hamstring injuries especially in sports.

6.10 Mechanism of Injury

Hamstring tears typically occur by a noncontact mechanism. Two injury mechanisms were described that lead to tears at different sites: sprinting and hyperstretching [35, 36]. The sprint gait is divided into two phases: the support phase when one foot is on the ground and the swing phase in which both feet are on the ground [37]. Sprint-related hamstring muscle injury (biceps femoris) usually occurs in this swing phase, during active lengthening, right before the foot hits the ground [35]. Hyperstretching injuries occur when the hamstring is maximally stretched with a combination of hip flexion and knee extension, movements often seen in gymnastics or waterskiing [36]. Typically, the semimembranosus muscle is involved along the proximal tendon [38]. Risk factors for hamstring injuries include overload, fatigue, strength imbalance, low flexibility, dehydration, and poor core muscle stability [39]. And the most important risk factor is a previous hamstring injury [39].

6.11 Anatomy and Biomechanics

The hamstring muscle complex is made up of the biceps femoris (BF) long and short heads, semitendinosus and semimembranosus, which act to extend the hip and flex the knee [34] (Fig. 6.7). All muscles except the short head originate from the ischial tuberosity. The biceps femoris long head and semitendinosus are attached proximally by a conjoint tendon [40]. The biceps femoris short head originates distally from the linea aspera [40]. The biceps femoris attaches distally along the lateral aspect of the fibular head and the semimembranosus and semitendinosus at the tibia [40]. The sciatic nerve courses close to the hamstring origin. A primary function of the hamstring muscles is deceleration by eccentric contraction during running/kicking, placing the muscle under high strain during high stretch [41].

Injuries to the hamstring tendon and/or muscle can be well depicted on MRI. Tears may manifest as stretch injuries to complete avulsions from the ischial tuberosity attachment [42]. But most tears are characterized as partial or complete tears with tendon gap [42]. Awareness of myoconnective tissue anatomy is important for radiologists to be aware of since tears also occur at these locations. Myoconnective tissue anatomy includes the *myotendinous* junction (Fig 6.8a) and the *myofascial/aponeurotic* junction (Fig. 6.8b) [43].

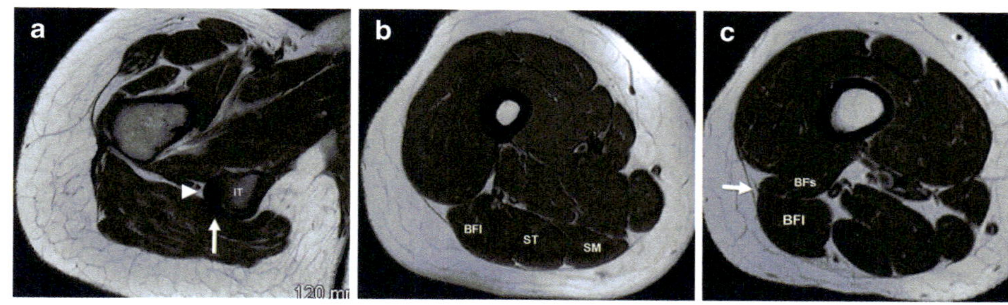

Fig. 6.7 Normal hamstring MRI anatomy of the right thigh. (**a**) Proximal thigh showing the ischial tuberosity (IT), conjoint tendon (arrow), semimembranosus (arrowhead), and sciatic nerve. (**b**) Mid-thigh showing the bicep femoris long head (BFl), semitendinosus (ST), and semimembranosus (SM) muscles. (**c**) Distal thigh showing the biceps femoris shorth head (BFs), biceps femoris long head (BFl), and the T-junction (arrow)

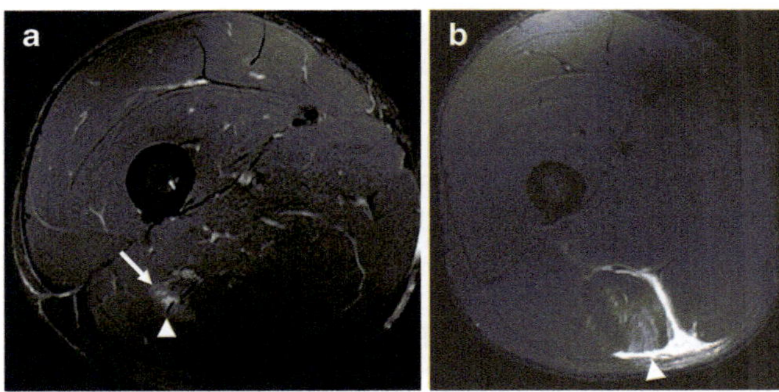

Fig. 6.8 Myoconnective tissue injury on MRI. (**a**) Axial T2-weighted fat-saturated MRI image of the thigh showing high T2 signal of the muscle (arrow) adjacent to the biceps femoris tendon (arrowhead) indicating a myotendinous junction tear. (**b**) Axial T2-weighted fat-saturated MRI image shows a fascial/aponeurotic tear (arrowhead) of the semitendinosus

6.12 Hamstring Injury Classification

Hamstring injuries were typically graded as 1, mild; 2, moderate; and 3, severe. Grade 1 involves minor muscle fiber damage with minimal pain and functional loss. Grade 2 involves partial tear with moderate pain and functional loss. Finally, grade 3 indicates complete muscle rupture with severe pain and functional loss [41]. However, traditional classification systems have gotten more sophisticated over the years after routine application of advanced imaging [43]. Peetrons was one of the first to add MRI to the traditional 1–3 grading of muscle injury [44]. Although accurate and reliable, the modified Peetrons classification's ordinal scale provided limited information regarding tear length, distance from origin, edema cross-sectional area, and tendon involvement [43]. This classification system is easy to use for daily clinical practice. However, as elite professional sports teams sought prognostic information for return-to-play, the British Athletics Muscle Injury Classification (BAMIC) system was adopted [43]. BAMIC uses MRI to further categorize injuries based on extent and anatomic location [43]. BAMIC grading has also been shown to significantly correlate to return-to-play (RTP) and has shown high intra and interrater reliability [32, 45]. Specifically, intratendinous ("c") injuries are associated with longer time to RTP and significantly higher reinjury rates, while grade 0 injuries predict a shorter time to RTP [46]. Thus, there has been a significant shift by sports medicine teams toward using the BAMIC grading system utilizing MRI [32]. Important to note, however, that RTP decisions are multifactorial, integrating MRI findings with clinical presentation, rehabilitation progress, and athlete performance metrics [32].

Table 6.1 British Athletics Muscle Injury Classification (BAMIC)

Injury severity	
Grade 0	MRI negative
Grade 1	Small tear, <10% CA, <5 cm CC
Grade 2	Moderate tear, 10–50% CA, 5–15 cm CC
Grade 3	Extensive, > 50% CA, > 15 cm CC
Grade 4	Complete tear with retraction
Anatomic grading	
Grade a	Myofascial
Grade b	Musculotendinous
Grade c	Intratendinous

CA cross-sectional area, *CC* cranial caudal distance

The BAMIC grading system uses numbers for injury severity and letters for anatomic site (Table 6.1). Given the anatomical proximity of the hamstring tendons to the sciatic nerve, acute hamstring injuries often result in irritation of the adjacent sciatic nerve from surrounding edema or hematoma. A prior study described sciatic nerve involvement in 30.6% of all HSIs and 81.3% of complete hamstring tendon injuries in American football players [47]. Current grading systems for hamstring injuries, including BAMIC, do not take sciatic nerve involvement into account [41, 43]. Previous studies have predominantly focused on sciatic nerve involvement in the case of complete hamstring tears and those requiring surgical management [48, 49]. Radiologists should carefully evaluate the sciatic nerve in the setting of hamstring injury.

6.13 Imaging Findings

MRI and US are the imaging tools often used to evaluate hamstring injuries. The two modalities should complement each other to ensure rapid diagnosis and treatment. MRI is the most effective diagnostic tool within the first 24 h of the injury [34]. An acute hamstring injury is best detected using fluid-sensitive sequences [34]. Hamstring injuries present with high T2 or STIR signal edema and hemorrhage involving the muscle and/or tendon. The extent and location of the abnormal signal involving the muscle belly, tendon, or myoconnective tissue is how MRI helps to classify and grade hamstring injuries and help predict recovery [43].

US, ideally performed between 2 and 48 h after injury, is well suited for detecting edema/hemorrhage and fluid collections associated with the injured muscle [44]. Additional advantages of US in hamstring evaluation include accessibility by portable ultrasound devices and quick diagnosis on the playing field. US can determine the location and extent of the injury (Fig 6.9a) but is limited by evaluation of deep structures [34]. US also plays a role in minimally invasive hamstring treatments (Fig 6.9b).

Proximal hamstring injuries include chronic tendinosis and acute hamstring avulsion from the ischial tuberosity. MRI is the ideal diagnostic tool for proximal hamstring injury evaluation [48]. It can diagnose tendinosis, tears, the amount of retraction, and sciatic nerve involvement (Fig. 6.10) [48]. Fast and accurate diagnosis is critical in the setting of acute avulsion injury, especially in elite athletes, for surgical management.

In the mid-hamstring complex, the biceps femoris is the most commonly injured muscle, followed by the semimembranosus and semitendinosus [34]. Tendon injury is important to recognize since it carries a worse prognosis compared to muscle or musculotendinous injuries. For example, a BAMIC 3c injury is the most extensive involvement of muscle and with tendon involvement (Fig. 6.11). The return-to-play is delayed with this injury grade as well as risk of reinjury [34].

In the distal hamstring complex, the distal musculotendinous T-junction injuries occur between the biceps femoris long head and short head muscles [34]. The "T-junction" is a confluence of the epimysium of the anterolateral long head and posteromedial short head and have been reported to have a high reinjury rate (Fig. 6.12) [50].

The role of MRI and US continue to expand, especially in elite athletes who require efficient and accurate diagnosis for a quicker return to play. MRI-grading system helps prognosis and estimate return to play.

Key Point

- Hamstring injuries are well evaluated by MRI. BAMIC is an emerging MRI-based classification system and has been shown to predict return-to-play.

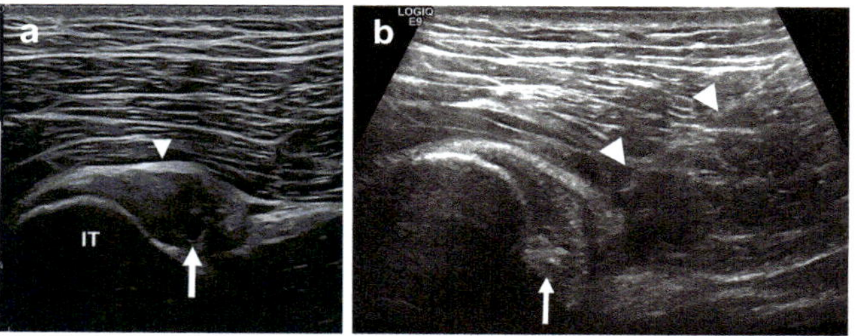

Fig. 6.9 Ultrasound as complementary tool. A 35-year-old woman runner with hamstring origin pain. (**a**) Short-axis sonogram shows thickening of the hamstring origin (arrowhead) and hypoechoic partial tear (arrow) of the semimembranosus tendon. Ischial tuberosity (IT). (**b**) Short-axis sonogram during US-guided platelet-rich plasma injection for treatment of the partial tear. 22G needle (arrowheads) in plane with the transducer from a lateral to medial approach, injecting into the tear defect (arrow)

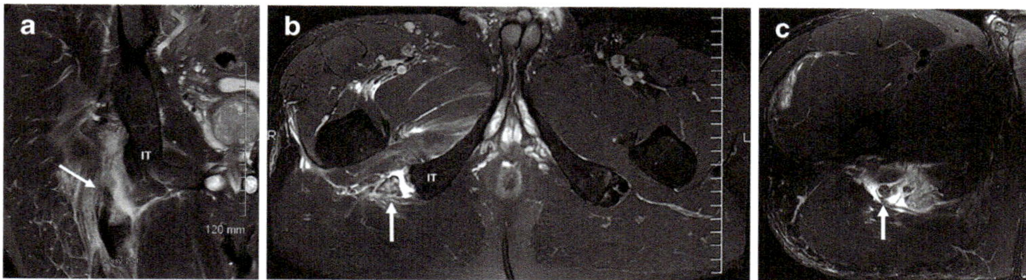

Fig. 6.10 Proximal hamstring avulsion and sciatic nerve involvement. (**a**) Coronal T2-weighted fat-saturated MRI image of the right hip shows a complete avulsion and retraction of the proximal hamstring origin (arrow). Ischial tuberosity (IT). (**b**) Axial T2-weighted fat-saturated MRI image of the bony pelvis shows absence of the right hamstring origin and retracted torn tendon end (arrow). (**c**) Axial T2-weighted fat-saturated MRI image of the right proximal thigh showing edema completing surrounding a thickened sciatic nerve (arrow)

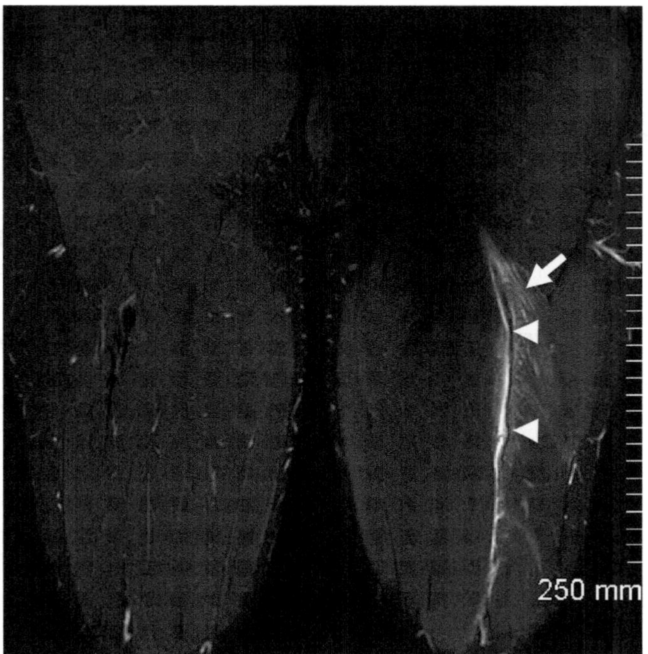

Fig. 6.11 BAMIC 3c injury. Coronal T2-weighted fat-saturated MRI image of the left mid-thigh showing a wavy biceps femoris tendon (arrowheads) and extensive feathery muscle edema of the biceps femoris muscle (arrow)

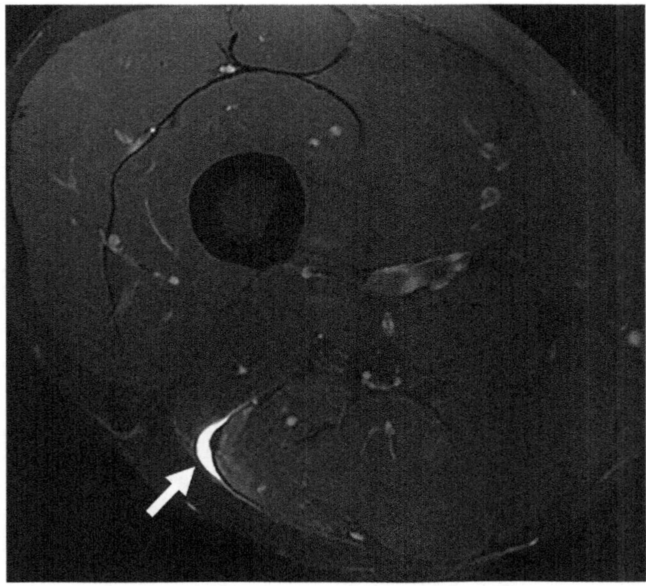

Fig. 6.12 T-junction injury. Axial T2-weighted fat-saturated MRI image of the right distal thigh showing a fascial tear (arrow) and associated edema at the junction between the biceps femoris long and short heads

6.14 Lateral Pelvis

The most common cause of lateral pelvis pain is a clinical entity referred to as greater trochanteric pain syndrome (GTPS) [51]. The underlying pathology is typically hip abductor tendon or gluteus medius and/or gluteus minimus tendinosis or tear from chronic repetitive injury, overload, or degenerative change [51]. The largest bursa is called the greater trochanteric bursa proper and overlies the posterior facet [52]. Bursal inflammation is often associated with tendon disease or mechanical friction. A less common cause of lateral hip pain is iliotibial band friction from compression or snapping over the greater trochanter and hip abductors.

6.15 Anatomy

The gluteus medius and minimus muscles arise from the external iliac fossa with a wide muscular attachment. The gluteus medius tendon inserts on the lateral facet while the gluteus minimus tendon inserts on the anterior facet (Fig. 6.13) [52]. The gluteus medius tendon has two parts—a thinner anterior attachment onto the lateral facet and a thicker posterior attachment onto the superoposterior facet [52].

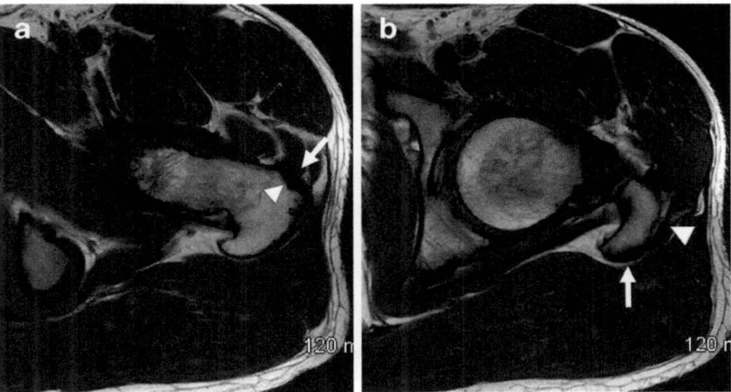

Fig. 6.13 Lateral pelvis MRI anatomy. (**a**) Axial T1-weigthed MRI images of the left hip shows the gluteus minimus tendon (arrow) attachment onto the anterior facet of the greater trochanter (arrowhead). (**b**) Axial T1-weighted MRI image, more cranially, showing the two parts to the gluteus medius tendon—thinner more lateral tendon (arrowhead) inserting on the lateral facet and the thicker posterior band (arrow) inserting on the superoposterior facet

6.16 Injury Biomechanics

Gluteal tendon injuries are associated with age and four times more frequent in women [53]. Injuries progress from tendinosis to tears [53]. Gluteus medius tendon tears most commonly start as partial thickness tears at the lateral facet and located anteriorly [53]. This can progress to full-thickness tears by continuing posteriorly [53]. Gluteus minimus tendon injury most commonly presents as degenerative tendinosis with associated edema. Partial tearing can occur with repetitive tensile loading and compressive stress on the deep tendon fibers, which can progress to complete tears.

6.17 Imaging Findings

MRI and US are well suited for evaluating the lateral pelvis. On MRI, symptomatic gluteal tendinosis will show increased signal intensity on T2-weighted images and tendon thickening (Fig. 6.14) [54]. There may also be associated peritendon soft tissue edema. However, not all peritrochanteric edema and tendon thickening is symptomatic [54]. Therefore, it is important to look for other causes of lateral hip pain such as spinal, arthritis, or nerve-related pain. A focal defect of the tendon fibers is seen with partial tears and an absent tendon, or "bald" facet sign, with complete tears (Fig. 6.15) [51]. Fatty atrophy of the gluteal muscles is a secondary sign of chronic tendon tears. In particular, gluteus muscle fatty atrophy, termed the "intergluteal fat strip" sign, is associated with symptomatic GTPS (Fig. 6.16) [55]. On US, gluteus tendinosis appears as tendon thickening and hypoechogenicity [51]. Hyperemia on power Doppler and bursitis may also be associated with tendinosis but not typically present [51]. Anechoic defects within the tendon are seen with tears [51]. Conservative treatment measures include rest, ice, and nonsteroidal anti-inflammatory drugs but also US-guided corticosteroid injection into the bursa (Fig. 6.17) [56].

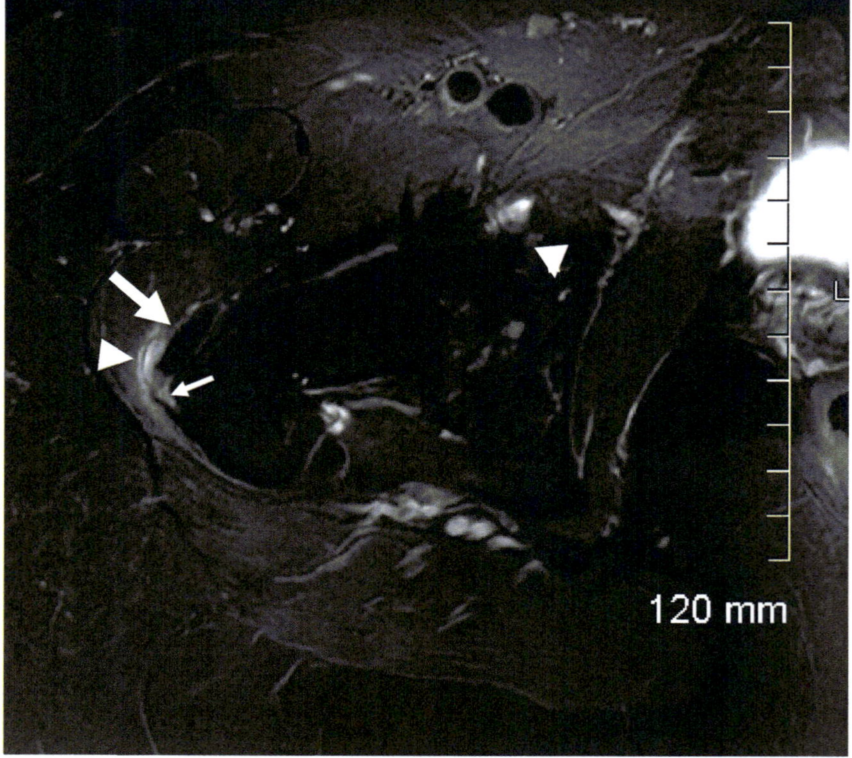

Fig. 6.14 Gluteal tendinosis. Axial T2-weighted fat-saturated MRI image of the right hip showing thickening of the gluteus minimus tendon (arrow) and peritendinous edema (arrowhead). Also a partial tear of the anterior gluteus medius tendon (small arrow)

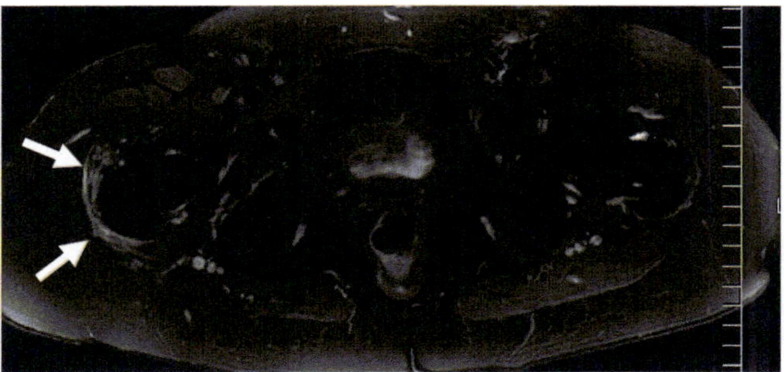

Fig. 6.15 Gluteal tendon tears. Axial T2-weighted fat-saturated MRI image of the bony pelvis showing complete tears ("bald" facet sign) of both the right gluteus medius and minimus tendons (arrows)

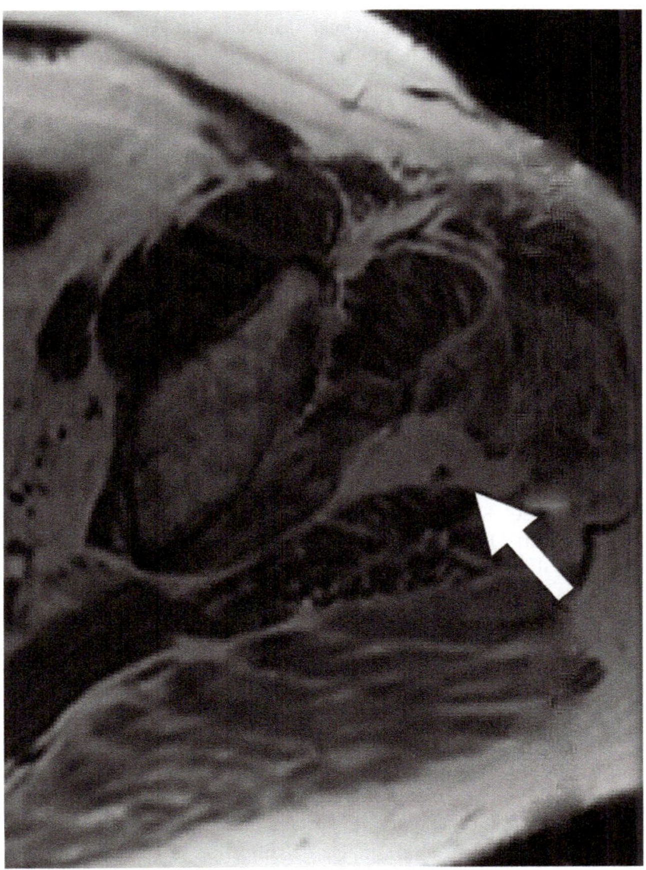

Fig. 6.16 Intergluteal fat strip sign. Axial T1-weighted MRI image of the left hip showing fatty atrophy of the gluteus medius muscle (arrow), a pattern seen in painful GTPS

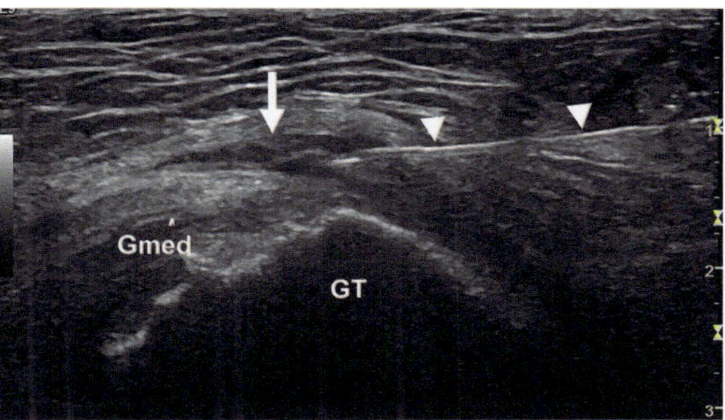

Fig. 6.17 US-guided greater trochanteric bursal corticosteroid injection. Short-axis sonogram of the left hip showing a 25-gauge, 3.5-inch needle (arrowhead) inplane with the transducer with tip placed into the greater trochanteric bursa proper (arrow). Gluteus medius tendon (Gmed) and greater trochanter (GT)

Key Point

- Most common causes of lateral pelvis pain involves disorders of the hip abductor tendons. MRI and US are well suited for evaluating and treating disorders of the hip abductor tendons.

Take-Home Message

- Hamstring injuries are one of the most common in sports and account for significant lost time off the field.
- British Athletics Muscle Injury Classification (BAMIC) system uses MRI to categorize hamstring injuries and correlates to return-to-play.
- MRI and US are complementary tools well suited for diagnosing and treating disorders of the lateral pelvis abductor tendons.

Conflict of Interest I/We declare no competing interests as defined by Springer Nature or other interests that might be perceived to influence results and/or discussion reported in this manuscript.

References

1. Hodler J, Kubik-Huch RA, Von GK, Musculoskeletal S, Von Schulthess GK. IDKD Springer Series Series Editors. Available from: http://www.springer.com/series/15856
2. Nelson EN, Kassarjian A, Palmer WE. MR imaging of sports-related groin pain. Magn Reson Imaging Clin N Am. 2005;13:727–42.
3. Chopra A, Robinson P. Imaging athletic groin pain. Radiol Clin North Am. 2016;54:865–73.
4. Koulouris G. Imaging review of groin pain in elite athletes: an anatomic approach to imaging findings. Am J Roentgenol. 2008;191:962–72.
5. Thorborg K, Reiman MP, Weir A, Kemp JL, Serner A, Mosler AB, et al. Clinical examination, diagnostic imaging, and testing of athletes with groin pain: an evidence-based approach to effective management. J Orthop Sports Phys Ther. 2018;48:239–49.
6. Candela V, De Carli A, Longo UG, Sturm S, Bruni G, Salvatore G, Denaro V. Hip and groin pain in soccer players. Joints. 2019;7(04):182–7.
7. Weir A, Brukner P, Delahunt E, Ekstrand J, Griffin D, Khan KM, et al. Doha agreement meeting on terminology and definitions in groin pain in athletes. Br J Sports Med. 2015;49(12):768–74.
8. Hölmich P. Long-standing groin pain in sportspeople falls into three primary patterns, a "clinical entity" approach: a prospective study of 207 patients. Br J Sports Med. 2007;41(4):247–52.
9. Coker DJ, Zoga AC. The role of magnetic resonance imaging in athletic pubalgia and core muscle injury. Top Magn Reson Imaging. 2015;24(4):183–91.
10. Zoga AC, Mullens FE, Meyers WC. The spectrum of MR imaging in athletic Pubalgia. Radiol Clin North Am. 2010;48:1179–97.
11. Mercouris P. Sports hernia: a pictorial review. South Afr J Radiol. 2014;18
12. Schilders E, Mitchell AWM, Johnson R, Dimitrakopoulou A, Kartsonaki C, Lee JC. Proximal adductor avulsions are rarely isolated but usually involve injury to the PLAC and pectineus: descriptive MRI findings in 145 athletes. Knee Surg Sports Traumatol Arthrosc. 2021;29(8):2424–36.
13. Schilders E, Bharam S, Golan E, Dimitrakopoulou A, Mitchell A, Spaepen M, et al. The pyramidalis–anterior pubic ligament–adductor longus complex (PLAC) and its role with adductor injuries: a new anatomical concept. Knee Surg Sports Traumatol Arthrosc. 2017;25(12):3969–77.
14. Slavotinek JP, Verrall GM, Fon GT, Sage MR. Groin pain in footballers: the association between preseason clinical and pubic bone magnetic resonance imaging findings and athlete outcome. Am J Sports Med. 2005;33(6):894–9.
15. Madani H, Robinson P. Top-ten tips for imaging groin injury in athletes. Semin Musculoskelet Radiol. 2019;23(4):361–75.
16. Cunningham PM, Brennan D, O'Connell M, MacMahon P, O'Neill P, Eustace S. Patterns of bone and soft-tissue injury at the symphysis pubis in soccer players: observations at MRI. AJR Am J Roentgenol. 2007;188(3)
17. Paajanen H, Hermunen H, Karonen J. Effect of heavy training in contact sports on MRI findings in the pubic region of asymptomatic competitive athletes compared with non-athlete controls. Skeletal Radiol. 2011;40(1):89–94.
18. Davies AG, Clarke AW, Gilmore J, Wotherspoon M, Connell DA. Review: imaging of groin pain in the athlete. Skeletal Radiol. 2010;39:629–44.
19. Omar IM, Zoga AC, Kavanagh EC, Franzcr GK, Bergin D, Gopez AG, et al. Athletic pubalgia and "sports hernia": optimal MR imaging technique and findings. Radiographics. 2008;28(5):1415–38.
20. Koh E, Boyle J. Pubic apophysitis in elite Australian rules football players: MRI findings and the utility of VIBE sequences in evaluating athletes with groin pain. Clin Radiol. 2020;75(4):293–301.
21. Schilders E, Talbot JC, Robinson P, Dimitrakopoulou A, Gibbon WW, Bismil Q. Adductor-related groin pain in recreational athletes. Role of the adductor enthesis, magnetic resonance imaging, and entheseal pubic cleft injections. J Bone Joint Surg. 2009;91(10):2455–60.
22. Saito M, Niga S, Nihei T, Uomizu M, Ikezawa Y, Tsukada S. The cleft sign may be an independent factor of magnetic resonance imaging findings associated with a delayed return-to-play time in athletes with groin pain. Knee Surg Sports Traumatol Arthrosc. 2021;29(5):1474–82.
23. Byrne CA, Bowden DJ, Alkhayat A, Kavanagh EC, Eustace SJ. Sports-related groin pain secondary to symphysis pubis disorders: correlation between MRI findings and outcome after fluoroscopy-guided injection of steroid and local anesthetic. Am J Roentgenol. 2017;209(2):380–8.
24. Zoga AC, Kavanagh EC, Omar IM, Morrison WB, Koulouris G, Lopez H, et al. Athletic pubalgia and the "sports hernia": MR imaging findings. Radiology. 2008;247(3):797–807.
25. Ooi MWX, Marzetti M, Rowbotham E, Bertham D, Robinson P. MRI findings in athletic groin pain: correlation of imaging with history and examination in symptomatic and asymptomatic athletes. Skeletal Radiol. 2024;54:841.
26. Branci S, Thorborg K, Nielsen MB, Hölmich P. Radiological findings in symphyseal and adductor-related groin pain in athletes: a critical review of the literature. Br J Sports Med. 2013;47:611–9.
27. Balius R, Blasi M, Pedret C, Alomar X, Peña-Amaro J, Vega JA, et al. A histoarchitectural approach to skeletal muscle injury: searching for a common nomenclature. Orthop J Sports Med. 2020;8(3)
28. Balius R, Alomar X, Pedret C, Blasi M, Rodas G, Pruna R, et al. Role of the extracellular matrix in muscle injuries: histoarchitectural considerations for muscle injuries. Orthop J Sports Med. 2018;6(9)
29. Falvey ÉC, King E, Kinsella S, Franklyn-Miller A. Athletic groin pain (part 1): a prospective anatomical diagnosis of 382 patients – clinical findings, MRI findings and patient-reported outcome measures at baseline. Br J Sports Med. 2016;50(7):423–30.
30. Maniar N, Carmichael DS, Hickey JT, Timmins RG, San Jose AJ, Dickson J, et al. Incidence and prevalence of hamstring injuries in field-based team sports: a systematic review and meta-analysis of 5952 injuries from over 7 million exposure hours. Br J Sports Med. 2023;57(2):109–16.
31. Danielsson A, Horvath A, Senorski C, Alentorn-Geli E, Garrett WE, Cugat R, et al. The mechanism of hamstring injuries – a systematic review. BMC Musculoskelet Disord. 2020;21(1):641.
32. Tears C, Rae G, Hide G, Sinha R, Franklin J, Brand P, et al. The British athletics muscle injury classification grading system as a predictor of return to play following hamstrings injury in professional football players. Phys Ther Sport. 2022;58:46–51.
33. Isern-Kebschull J, Mechó S, Pruna R, Kassarjian A, Valle X, Yanguas X, et al. Sports-related lower limb muscle injuries: pattern recognition approach and MRI review. Insights Imaging. 2020;11(1):108.
34. Marrero AM, Mazza LA, Cedola N, Neville MF, Trueba RH, Napoli A, et al. MRI and US in hamstring sports injury assessment: anatomy, imaging findings, and mechanisms of injury. Radiogr Rev Publ Radiol Soc N Am Inc. 2025;45(5):e240061.
35. Askling CM, Tengvar M, Saartok T, Thorstensson A. Acute first-time hamstring strains during high-speed running: a longitudinal

study including clinical and magnetic resonance imaging findings. Am J Sports Med. 2007;35(2):197–206.
36. Askling CM, Tengvar M, Saartok T, Thorstensson A. Acute first-time hamstring strains during slow-speed stretching: clinical, magnetic resonance imaging, and recovery characteristics. Am J Sports Med. 2007;35(10):1716–24.
37. Kapri E, Mehta M, S K. Biomechanics of running: an overview on gait cycle. Int J Phys Educ Fit Sports. 2021:1–9.
38. Heiderscheit BC, Sherry MA, Silder A, Chumanov ES, Thelen DG. Hamstring strain injuries: recommendations for diagnosis, rehabilitation, and injury prevention. J Orthop Sports Phys Ther. 2010;40(2):67–81.
39. Ahmad CS, Redler LH, Ciccotti MG, Maffulli N, Longo UG, Bradley J. Evaluation and management of hamstring injuries. Am J Sports Med. 2013;41(12):2933–47.
40. Koulouris G, Connell D. Hamstring muscle complex: an imaging review. Radiogr Rev Publ Radiol Soc N Am Inc. 2005;25(3):571–86.
41. Larson JH, Fenn TW, Allahabadi S, Nho SJ. Hamstring strains: classification and management. Sports Health. 2024;16(4):661–3.
42. Lee JC, Mitchell AWM, Healy JC. Imaging of muscle injury in the elite athlete. Br J Radiol. 2012;85(1016):1173–85.
43. Pollock N, James SLJ, Lee JC, Chakraverty R. British athletics muscle injury classification: a new grading system. Br J Sports Med. 2014;48(18):1347–51.
44. Peetrons P. Ultrasound of muscles. Eur Radiol. 2002;12(1):35–43.
45. Wangensteen A, Tol JL, Roemer FW, Bahr R, Dijkstra HP, Crema MD, et al. Intra- and interrater reliability of three different MRI grading and classification systems after acute hamstring injuries. Eur J Radiol. 2017;89:182–90.
46. Pollock N, Patel A, Chakraverty J, Suokas A, James SLJ, Chakraverty R. Time to return to full training is delayed and recurrence rate is higher in intratendinous ('c') acute hamstring injury in elite track and field athletes: clinical application of the British athletics muscle injury classification. Br J Sports Med. 2016;50(5):305–10.
47. Day MA, Karlsson LH, Herzog MM, Weiss LJ, McGonegle SJ, Greditzer HG, et al. Correlation of player and imaging characteristics with severity and missed time in National Football League Professional Athletes with hamstring strain injury: a retrospective review. Am J Sports Med. 2024;52(11):2709–17.
48. Lin Y, Sahr M, Lan R, Nguyen J, Tan ET, Sneag DB. MRI findings correlate with difficult dissection during proximal hamstring repair and with postoperative sciatica. Skeletal Radiol. 2024;53(11):2449–57.
49. Wilson TJ, Spinner RJ, Mohan R, Gibbs CM, Krych AJ. Sciatic nerve injury after proximal hamstring avulsion and repair. Orthop J Sports Med. 2017;5(7):2325967117713685.
50. Pedret C. Hamstring muscle injuries: MRI and ultrasound for diagnosis and prognosis. J Belg Soc Radiol. 2021;105(1):91.
51. Hegazi TM, Belair JA, McCarthy EJ, Roedl JB, Morrison WB. Sports injuries about the hip: what the radiologist should know. Radiographics. 2016;36(6):1717–45.
52. Pfirrmann CW, Chung CB, Theumann NH, Trudell DJ, Resnick D. Greater trochanter of the hip: attachment of the abductor mechanism and a complex of three bursae – MR imaging and MR bursography in cadavers and MR imaging in asymptomatic volunteers. Radiology. 2001;221(2):469–77.
53. Dishkin-Paset JG, Salata MJ, Gross CE, Manno K, Shewman EF, Wang VM, et al. A biomechanical comparison of repair techniques for complete gluteus medius tears. Arthrosc J Arthrosc Relat Surg. 2012;28(10):1410–6.
54. Blankenbaker DG, Ullrick SR, Davis KW, De Smet AA, Haaland B, Fine JP. Correlation of MRI findings with clinical findings of trochanteric pain syndrome. Skeletal Radiol. 2008;37(10):903–9.
55. Pfirrmann CWA, Notzli HP, Dora C, Hodler J, Zanetti M. Abductor tendons and muscles assessed at MR imaging after total hip arthroplasty in asymptomatic and symptomatic patients. Radiology. 2005;235(3):969–76.
56. McEvoy JR, Lee KS, Blankenbaker DG, del Rio AM, Keene JS. Ultrasound-guided corticosteroid injections for treatment of greater trochanteric pain syndrome: greater trochanter bursa versus subgluteus medius bursa. AJR Am J Roentgenol. 2013;201(2):W313–7.

Suggested Reading

Vasileff WK, Nekhline M, Kolowich PA, Talpos GB, Eyler WR, Van Holsbeeck M. Inguinal hernia in athletes: role of dynamic ultrasound. Sports Health. 2017;9(5):414–21.

Santilli OL, Nardelli N, Santilli HA, Tripoloni DE. Sports hernias: experience in a sports medicine center. Hernia. 2016;20(1):77–84.

Schilders E, Bismil Q, Robinson P, O'Connor PJ, Gibbon WW, Talbot JC. Adductor-related groin pain in competitive athletes: role of adductor enthesis, magnetic resonance imaging, and entheseal pubic cleft injections. J Bone Joint Surg. 2007;89:2173–8.

Murphy G, Foran P, Murphy D, Tobin O, Moynagh M, Eustace S. "Superior cleft sign" as a marker of rectus abdominus/adductor longus tear in patients with suspected sportsman's hernia. Skeletal Radiol. 2013;42(6):819–25.

Kunduracioglu B, Yilmaz C, Yorubulut M, Kudas S. Magnetic resonance findings of osteitis pubis. J Magn Reson Imaging. 2007;25(3):535–9.

Brandon CJ, Jacobson JA, Fessell D, Dong Q, Morag Y, Girish G, et al. Groin pain beyond the hip: how anatomy predisposes to injury as visualized by musculoskeletal ultrasound and MRI. Am J Roentgenol. 2011;197(5):1190–7.

Isern-Kebschull J, Mechó S, Pruna R, Kassarjian A, Valle X, Yanguas X, et al. Sports-related lower limb muscle injuries: pattern recognition approach and MRI review. Insights. Imaging. 2020;11(1)

Lovell G. The diagnosis of chronic groin pain in athletes: a review of 189 cases. Aust J Sci Med Sport. 1995;27(3):76–9.

Caudill P, Nyland J, Smith C, Yerasimides J, Lach J. Sports hernias: a systematic literature review. Br J Sports Med. 2007;42(12):954–64.

Muschaweck U, Berger LM. Sportsmen's groin-diagnostic approach and treatment with the minimal repair technique: a single-center uncontrolled clinical review. Sports Health. 2010;2(3):216–21.

Bou Antoun M, Reboul G, Ronot M, Crombe A, Poussange N, Pesquer L. Imaging of inguinal-related groin pain in athletes. Br J Radiol. 2018;91(1092):20170856.

7 MRI of the Knee

J. Fritz and L. White

> **Learning Objectives**
> - Understand optimal MRI protocols and sequences for comprehensive evaluation of the knee.
> - Recognize characteristic MRI findings of meniscal, ligamentous, and chondral pathologies.
> - Apply pattern recognition to identify combined and multiligamentous injuries.
> - Identify common pitfalls and technical limitations in knee MRI interpretation.

7.1 Introduction

The knee joint represents one of the most frequently imaged anatomic regions in musculoskeletal radiology, with MRI serving as the definitive noninvasive modality for comprehensive evaluation of internal derangement [1]. The superior soft tissue contrast resolution and multiplanar capabilities of MRI enable detailed visualization of menisci, ligaments, cartilage, and osseous structures that cannot be adequately assessed through conventional radiography or clinical examination alone [2].

Traditional knee MRI protocols have historically required 20–25 min of acquisition time, presenting challenges for patient throughput, motion artifacts, and healthcare economics [1]. Recent technological advances have revolutionized knee imaging through accelerated acquisition techniques. Parallel imaging (PI) exploits k-space symmetry by undersampling phase-encoding steps, achieving two- to threefold acceleration [3]. Simultaneous multislice (SMS) acquisition excites multiple slices concurrently using multifrequency pulses, providing multiplicative acceleration when combined with PI [4].

The integration of deep learning (DL) reconstruction algorithms represents a paradigm shift in accelerated imaging. These convolutional neural networks enhance image quality by reducing noise and artifacts inherent to highly accelerated acquisitions [5]. Validation studies using arthroscopic correlation have demonstrated that sixfold accelerated protocols with DL reconstruction maintain diagnostic performance comparable to standard protocols while reducing acquisition time to under 5 min [6, 7] (Table 7.1).

This technological evolution has profound implications for clinical practice. Rapid protocols improve patient comfort, reduce motion-related artifacts, and enhance departmental workflow efficiency. The ability to obtain high-quality diagnostic images in less than 5 min makes MRI more accessible for claustrophobic patients and pediatric populations while maintaining the diagnostic confidence required for treatment planning [8].

J. Fritz (✉)
Department of Radiology, Grossman School of Medicine, New York University, New York, NY, USA
e-mail: Jan.fritz@nyulangone.org

L. White
Department of Medical Imaging, Division of Musculoskeletal Imaging, University of Toronto, Toronto, ON, Canada

Joint Department of Medical Imaging, University Health Network, Toronto, ON, Canada

Department of Surgery, University of Toronto, Toronto, ON, Canada
e-mail: lawrence.white@uhn.ca

Table 7.1 Sub-5-min 3-Tesla sixfold SMSx2-PATx3-accelerated knee MRI protocol with deep learning superresolution image reconstruction

Parameter	Ax T2 FS	Cor PD	Cor PD FS	Sag T2 FS	Sag PD
Gradient performance	High	High	High	High	High
Radiofrequency speed	Fast	Fast	Fast	Fast	Fast
Repetition/echo time [ms]	3600/57	3700/24	3700/35	3700/56	3700/24
PI	3	3	3	3	3
SMS/FOV shift	2/2	2/2	2/2	2/2	2/2
Echo-train length	13	13	13	13	13
Bandwidth [Hz/pixel]	296	354	301	299	354
Echo spacing [ms]	7.1	8.0	7.1	8.0	8.0
FOV [mm]	140 × 140	140 × 140	140 × 140	140 × 140	140 × 140
Matrix	272 × 204	336 × 252	272 × 204	304 × 228	336 × 252
Slice thickness [mm]	3	3	3	3	3
Slices	38	36	36	38	38
Phase direction	Right-to-left	Head-to-foot	Head-to-foot	Head-to-foot	Head-to-foot
Flip angle [°]	125	125	125	125	125
Acquisition time [mm:ss]	00:43	01:00	00:53	00:57	01:01

Ax axial, *Cor* coronal, *Sag* sagittal, *PD* proton density weighted, *FS* fat suppression, *PI* parallel imaging acceleration factor, *SMS* simultaneous multislice acquisition acceleration factor, *FOV* field of view

7.2 MRI Technique and Protocols

Comprehensive knee MRI evaluation requires strategic sequence selection balancing diagnostic yield with acquisition efficiency. The standard protocol incorporates multiple tissue contrasts across three orthogonal planes to optimize visualization of specific anatomic structures.

Essential sequences include sagittal proton density (PD) for meniscal evaluation, sagittal and coronal PD fat-saturated (FS) for ligamentous and cartilaginous assessment, and axial T2-weighted imaging for patellofemoral evaluation and joint effusions [9]. The combination of intermediate-TE sequences (PD, PD FS) with long-TE fluid-sensitive sequences (T2) maximizes both sensitivity and specificity for detecting internal derangement.

Three-dimensional isotropic acquisitions can supplement or replace two-dimensional sequences, offering multiplanar reformation capabilities with reduced partial volume effects. These sequences particularly benefit cartilage assessment and enable the creation of thin contiguous slices for improved visualization of small structures [4].

Accelerated protocols leverage multiple technologies synergistically. Parallel imaging reduces acquisition time through k-space undersampling, with acceleration factors of 2–3x routinely achievable using dedicated multichannel knee coils. Simultaneous multislice techniques provide additional acceleration by exciting multiple slices concurrently, achieving combined acceleration factors of 4–6x when integrated with parallel imaging [7].

Deep learning reconstruction addresses the signal-to-noise penalty inherent to acceleration. These algorithms, trained on large datasets of paired low- and high-resolution images, restore image quality through intelligent denoising and artifact reduction. Recent validation studies demonstrate that sixfold accelerated protocols with DL reconstruction achieve diagnostic performance equivalent to standard protocols for meniscal, ligamentous, and cartilaginous pathology detection [6, 7].

Patient positioning and coil selection significantly impact image quality. The knee should be positioned in 10–15 degrees of flexion using appropriate padding, with the patella centered within the coil. This positioning optimizes visualization of the anterior cruciate ligament and reduces motion artifacts.

Postoperative MRI presents unique challenges requiring protocol modifications. Often, modifying the two-dimensional turbo spin echo pulse sequence protocol by increasing the receiver bandwidth and using STIR instead of spectral fat suppression is sufficient. Metal artifact reduction sequences, such as slice encoding for metal artifact correction (SEMAC) and multiacquisition variable-resonance image combination (MAVRIC), can be applied to challenging cases to minimize susceptibility artifacts from large or highly susceptible orthopedic hardware but at the expense of spatial detail [1].

Key Point

Essential sequences for comprehensive knee MRI evaluation include sagittal, coronal, and axial nonfat-suppressed and fat-suppressed PD and T2-weighted fast and turbo spin echo pulse sequences and optionally three-dimensional isotropic sequences. Modern accelerated protocols achieve diagnostic quality in under 5 min through combined parallel imaging, simultaneous multislice, and deep learning reconstruction.

7.3 Meniscal Abnormalities

The menisci serve critical biomechanical functions in load distribution, shock absorption, and joint stability. Their fibrocartilaginous composition produces characteristic low-signal intensity on all pulse sequences in the normal state, appearing as triangular structures on sagittal images and bow-tie configurations on coronal acquisitions [10].

7.3.1 Diagnostic Criteria

Meniscal tear diagnosis relies on strict imaging criteria to distinguish pathologic signal from normal variations. The fundamental criterion requires abnormal signal intensity extending to the articular surface on at least two consecutive images or in two different imaging planes [11]. This "two-slice rule" differentiates true tears from volume averaging artifacts and normal intrameniscal signal variations. However, with improving image quality and deep learning-based superresolution, meniscus tears may also be diagnosed on single images if convincingly displayed.

Normal menisci may demonstrate an intrameniscal signal that does not reach the surface, representing mucoid degeneration without macroscopic tearing. This finding, particularly common in individuals over 40 years, correlates poorly with clinical symptoms and typically requires no intervention.

7.3.2 Tear Morphology and Patterns

Meniscal tears exhibit characteristic morphologic patterns that influence treatment decisions. Horizontal tears course parallel to the tibial plateau, dividing the meniscus into superior and inferior leaflets. These tears predominantly affect older patients and frequently result from degenerative changes rather than acute trauma.

Radial tears extend perpendicular to the circumferential fibers from the free edge toward the periphery. These tears disrupt the critical hoop stress mechanism, leading to altered load transmission and accelerated cartilage degeneration. Complete radial tears are functionally equivalent to total meniscectomy regarding biomechanical consequences [12].

Vertical longitudinal tears parallel the circumferential fibers and typically result from acute trauma in younger patients. When these tears extend through the peripheral vascular zone, they demonstrate favorable healing potential with appropriate surgical repair. Complex tears combine multiple tear patterns and generally indicate chronic degenerative processes.

7.3.3 Special Tear Patterns

Bucket-handle tears represent displaced vertical longitudinal tears with the inner fragment displacing into the intercondylar notch. The "double PCL sign" on sagittal images and the absent bow-tie sign on consecutive coronal images suggest this diagnosis (Fig. 7.1). These tears frequently cause mechanical symptoms requiring urgent surgical intervention [13].

Root tears involve the meniscal attachments and functionally destabilize the entire meniscus. Posterior root tears manifest as radial tears at the root insertion or "ghost meniscus" sign with meniscal extrusion exceeding 3 mm. These injuries significantly alter joint biomechanics and accelerate osteoarthritis progression [14].

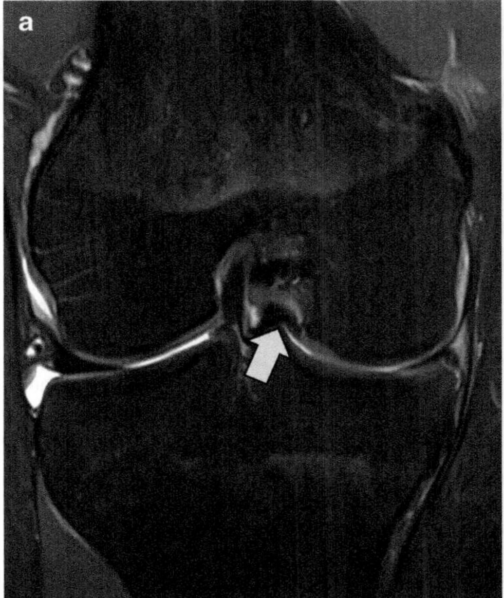

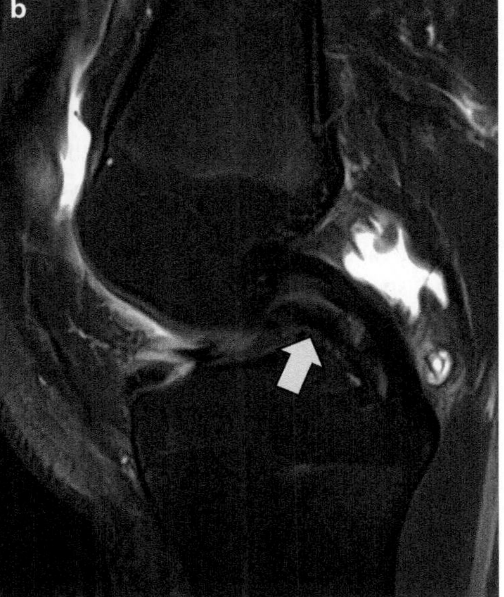

Fig. 7.1 Bucket-handle tear of the medial meniscus in a 24-year-old soccer player with knee locking. (**a**) Sagittal fat-suppressed T2-weighted image demonstrates the characteristic "double PCL sign" (arrow) with the displaced meniscal fragment lying parallel to the posterior cruciate ligament within the intercondylar notch. (**b**) Coronal proton density-weighted fat-suppressed image confirms the displaced meniscal fragment (arrow) and shows the donor site with an absent body segment of the medial meniscus. This injury pattern typically requires urgent arthroscopic reduction and repair

Ramp lesions represent peripheral tears of the posteromedial meniscocapsular junction associated with ACL injuries. These lesions appear as a vertical fluid signal at the posterior medial meniscus-capsule interface on sagittal images. Detection sensitivity improves with recognition of associated findings, including posterior medial tibial plateau bone contusions [15].

7.3.4 Pitfalls and Limitations

Several normal structures and artifacts mimic meniscal pathology. The transverse meniscal ligament, meniscofemoral ligaments, and popliteus tendon create linear signals potentially misinterpreted as tears. The magic angle phenomenon produces an increased signal in structures oriented 55 degrees to the main magnetic field, particularly affecting the posterior horn lateral meniscus.

Truncation artifacts generate a linear signal that parallels the meniscal surfaces in images with a low matrix size. Vascular structures within the peripheral third create punctate signal foci distinguished from tears by their characteristic location and morphology.

7.3.5 Clinical Correlation

Not all meniscal tears produce symptoms or require treatment. Asymptomatic tears occur in up to 63% of individuals over 50 years, particularly horizontal tears and signal abnormalities that do not meet strict tear criteria. Correlation with clinical findings, including mechanical symptoms and examination findings, guides management decisions.

Key Point

The "two-slice rule," requiring an abnormal signal extending to the articular surface on two consecutive images, remains important for meniscal tear diagnosis. However, with improving image quality and deep learning-based superresolution, there will be cases where small meniscal tears will only be visible on a single image. Recognition of tear morphology patterns, including horizontal, radial, vertical, complex, and special tears—such as bucket-handle, root, and ramp lesions—guides surgical planning.

7.4 Anterior Cruciate Ligament Injuries

The anterior cruciate ligament represents the most frequently disrupted major knee ligament, with an annual incidence of approximately 1 in 3500 individuals. Noncontact mechanisms account for 72% of injuries, typically occurring during deceleration with direction changes in sports requiring cutting and pivoting movements [16].

7.4.1 Primary MRI Signs

Complete ACL tears demonstrate characteristic primary signs, including fiber discontinuity, abnormal ligament orientation, and diffuse signal hyperintensity on fluid-sensitive sequences (Fig. 7.2). The normal ACL appears as a band of

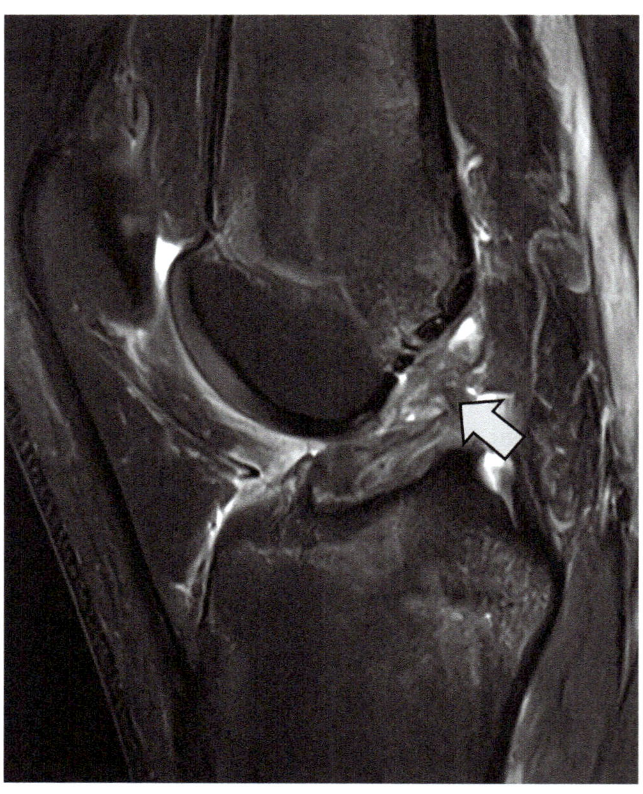

Fig. 7.2 Complete anterior cruciate ligament tear at the femoral attachment in a 19-year-old basketball player following a noncontact pivoting injury. Sagittal proton density fat-suppressed image shows complete disruption of ACL fibers at the femoral origin (arrow) with wavy, horizontally oriented ligament remnant and surrounding edema. The associated bone marrow edema at the lateral femoral condyle sulcus terminalis and posterior lateral tibial plateau (not shown) indicated a classic pivot-shift injury mechanism. The proximal tear location with good tissue quality makes this injury potentially amenable to primary repair

low-signal intensity fibers coursing parallel to Blumensaat's line on sagittal images. Acute tears disrupt this architecture, producing a horizontally oriented or absent ligament with amorphous high signal replacing normal fiber structure.

Tear location influences surgical management options. Proximal tears near the femoral attachment occur most frequently (90%), followed by midsubstance (7%) and distal tibial attachment tears (3%). Proximal tears with good tissue quality may be amenable to primary repair rather than reconstruction in selected patients.

7.4.2 Secondary Signs and Associated Injuries

The pivot-shift mechanism produces pathognomonic bone contusion patterns. Impaction between the lateral femoral condyle and posterior lateral tibial plateau creates characteristic edema at the sulcus terminalis and posterior tibial margin. The deep lateral femoral notch sign represents chronic osseous remodeling at this impaction site.

Secondary signs include anterior tibial translation exceeding 7 mm, posterior cruciate ligament buckling, and uncovering of the posterior horn lateral meniscus. These findings improve diagnostic confidence when primary signs remain equivocal.

Associated injuries occur in 70% of acute ACL tears. Meniscal injuries predominate, with lateral meniscus tears more common acutely and medial meniscus tears increasing with chronicity. Ramp lesions affect 15–40% of ACL injuries but may be subtle on preoperative imaging [17].

7.4.3 Partial Tears

Partial ACL tears, representing 10–27% of ACL injuries, present diagnostic challenges. Imaging features include focal signal abnormality with some intact fibers, ligament attenuation, and abnormal orientation without complete disruption. High-grade partial tears involving over 50% of fibers demonstrate increased risk of progression to complete tears and may warrant surgical intervention. Clinical correlation remains essential, as partial tears can appear morphologically intact on MRI.

7.5 Posterior Cruciate Ligament Injuries

The PCL, though stronger than the ACL, tears less frequently, with an incidence of 2 per 100,000 annually. Dashboard injuries producing posterior tibial translation on a flexed knee represent the classic mechanism, though hyperextension injuries also occur [18].

7.5.1 MRI Features

The normal PCL appears uniformly hypointense on all sequences with a smooth, curved contour. Acute tears manifest as focal or diffuse signal hyperintensity, fiber disruption, and ligament thickening (Fig. 7.3). Unlike ACL tears, partial PCL tears commonly maintain peripheral fiber continuity despite central disruption, appearing in 47–62% of cases. Scarred ligaments may appear morphologically intact despite persistent laxity, necessitating correlation with clinical stability testing.

7.5.2 Associated Injuries

Isolated PCL tears are uncommon, with multiligamentous injuries predominating. Combined injuries involving the posterolateral corner occur frequently and significantly impact surgical planning. Bone contusion patterns vary with mechanism—anterior tibial contusions in dashboard injuries

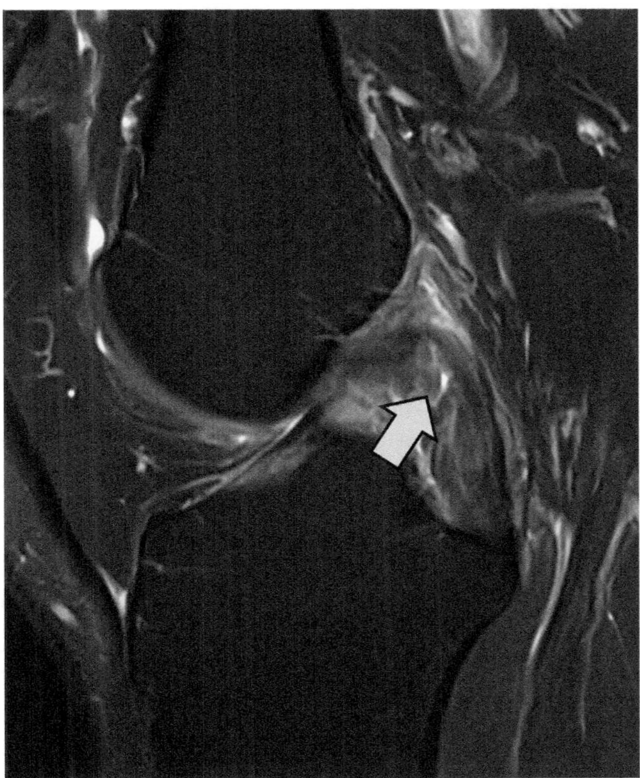

Fig. 7.3 Posterior cruciate ligament midsubstance tear in a 32-year-old patient following dashboard injury in a motor vehicle accident. Sagittal T2-weighted fat-suppressed image demonstrates focal disruption of PCL fibers at the midsubstance (arrow) with increased intraligamentous signal and thickening. Note the preserved peripheral fiber continuity, which is characteristic of partial PCL tears. Associated anterior tibial bone marrow edema (not shown) supported the dashboard injury mechanism

versus “kissing contusions” of the anterior femoral condyles and tibial plateaus in hyperextension. PCL avulsion fractures occur in 10% of injuries, more commonly at the tibial insertion. These injuries may be amenable to primary fixation when recognized acutely.

Key Point
Combined ligament injuries should be suspected when characteristic bone bruise patterns accompany primary ligamentous disruption. Recognition of multiligamentous involvement critically influences surgical timing and technique selection.

7.6 Collateral Ligaments and Corners

7.6.1 Medial Collateral Ligament

The MCL represents the most frequently injured knee ligament, typically resulting from valgus stress during contact sports or cutting maneuvers. The superficial MCL provides primary valgus stability while the deep fibers stabilize against rotation.

MRI evaluation optimally employs coronal and axial sequences to assess the superficial and deep MCL components. Grade 1 injuries demonstrate ligamentous edema without discretely depicted fiber disruption. Grade 2 injuries show partially disrupted and partially continuous fibers. Grade 3 tears exhibit complete discontinuity with ligament retraction (Fig. 7.4) [19].

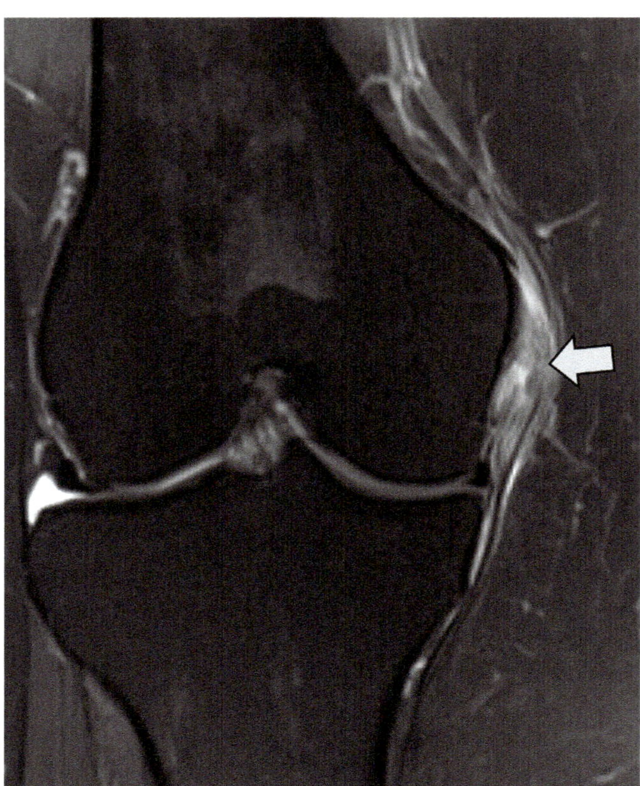

Fig. 7.4 Grade 3 medial collateral ligament tear in a 27-year-old football player who sustained valgus stress injury. Coronal proton density fat-suppressed image shows complete discontinuity of the superficial MCL fibers near the femoral attachment (arrow) with surrounding soft tissue edema and hemorrhage. The proximal tear location typically demonstrates favorable healing with conservative management, though the extent of retraction and associated injuries influence treatment decisions

Location significantly influences healing potential. Proximal femoral avulsions in isolation, representing the most common site, typically heal with conservative management. Distal tibial avulsions demonstrate poorer healing capacity, particularly when complicated by Stener-like lesions where torn fibers displace superficial to the pes anserinus tendons, preventing ligament-to-bone healing [20].

Associated injuries define specific patterns. O'Donoghue's “unhappy triad” combines ACL tear, MCL injury, and medial meniscus tear. Anteromedial rotatory instability results from combined ACL, MCL, and posteromedial corner disruption, requiring comprehensive surgical reconstruction.

7.6.2 Posterolateral Corner

The posterolateral corner provides critical stability against varus stress, external rotation, and posterior translation. Primary stabilizers include the fibular collateral ligament, popliteus tendon, and popliteofibular ligament. These structures work synergistically, with injury to multiple components required for clinical instability [21].

PLC injuries rarely occur in isolation, accompanying cruciate tears in nearly 90% of cases. Initial clinical diagnosis proves challenging, with up to 72% of injuries missed acutely. Unrecognized PLC injuries contribute to cruciate reconstruction failure, emphasizing the importance of comprehensive imaging evaluation.

MRI assessment requires a systematic evaluation of each component. FCL tears appear as fiber discontinuity with surrounding edema, most commonly at the fibular insertion (Fig. 7.5). Popliteus injuries typically involve the myotendinous junction with strain or partial tearing. The popliteofibular ligament, visible in only 50% of routine examinations, requires indirect signs, including edema between the popliteus and fibular styloid.

Arcuate fractures at the fibular styloid indicate PLC avulsion and suggest significant instability. Grade 3 injuries involving complete disruption of two or more primary stabi-

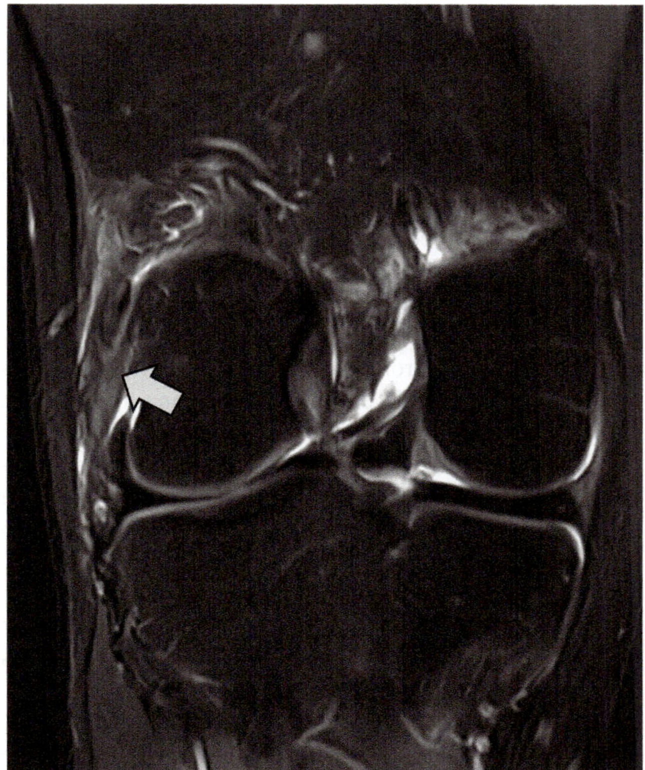

Fig. 7.5 Complete fibular collateral ligament tear as part of multiligamentous knee injury in a 35-year-old skier. Coronal proton density fat-suppressed image demonstrates complete disruption of the FCL at its fibular insertion (arrow) with ligament retraction and surrounding edema. This posterolateral corner injury was associated with complete ACL tear (not shown), requiring staged surgical reconstruction. Isolated FCL tears are rare; systematic evaluation for associated posterolateral corner and cruciate injuries is essential

lizers require surgical reconstruction within six weeks for optimal outcomes.

> **Key Point**
> Posterolateral corner injuries rarely occur in isolation, accompanying cruciate ligament tears in nearly 90% of cases. Unrecognized PLC injury represents a major cause of cruciate reconstruction failure.

7.7 Extensor Mechanism and Overuse

7.7.1 Extensor Mechanism Injuries

Quadriceps and patellar tendon ruptures represent distinct entities affecting different populations. Quadriceps tears typically occur in middle-aged males due to eccentric contraction during knee flexion. MRI demonstrates discontinuous low-signal fibers with retraction and wavy tendon morphology. Laminar anatomy evaluation guides surgical planning, with tears of two or more layers often requiring repair.

Patellar tendon ruptures affect younger athletes during explosive jumping activities. Proximal avulsions predominate (82%), appearing as tendon discontinuity with inferior patellar displacement. Complete ruptures mandate surgical repair, with MRI primarily confirming clinical diagnosis rather than influencing management.

The medial patellofemoral ligament provides primary restraint against lateral patellar instability. Lateral dislocation produces characteristic injury patterns, including MPFL disruption (95% of cases), impaction contusions at the medial patella and lateral femoral condyle, and potential osteochondral fractures. MPFL tears occur equally at patellar (37%) and femoral (37%) attachments, with midsubstance tears less common (16%) [22].

7.7.2 Overuse Syndromes

Patellar tendinopathy (“jumper’s knee”) affects up to 40–50% of elite jumping athletes. MRI reveals proximal patellar tendon thickening with intrasubstance signal, typically involving the medial fibers (Fig. 7.6). These changes may persist despite clinical improvement, limiting MRI utility in monitoring treatment response.

Iliotibial band syndrome produces lateral knee pain in runners and cyclists. A fluid signal deep to the ITB at the lateral epicondyle, sometimes with discrete bursitis, confirms the diagnosis. Associated findings include ITB thickening and epicondylar edema.

Quadriceps tendinopathy demonstrates similar imaging features to patellar tendinopathy but affects the quadriceps

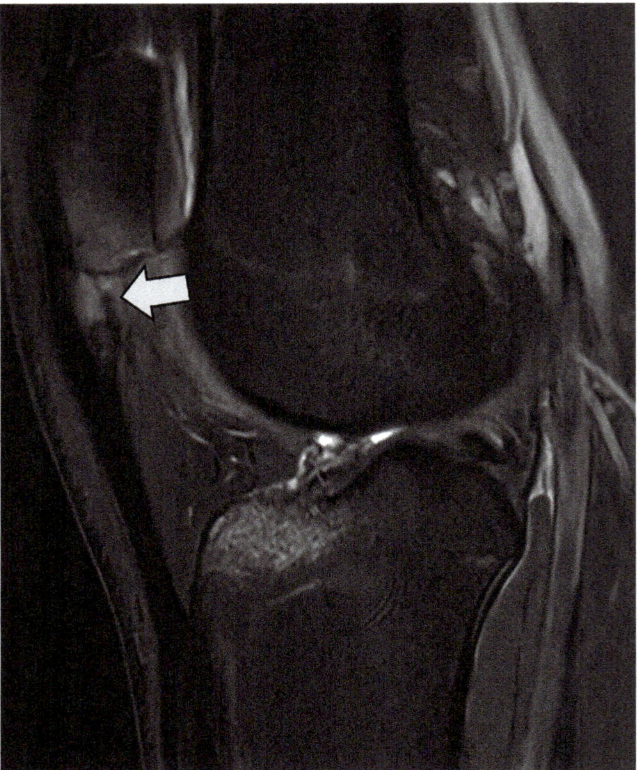

Fig. 7.6 Patellar tendinopathy (jumper's knee) in a 22-year-old volleyball player with chronic anterior knee pain. Sagittal T2 fat-suppressed image shows characteristic focal thickening and increased intrasubstance signal of the proximal patellar tendon at its patellar attachment (arrow), predominantly involving the deep articular-surface fibers. These findings may persist despite clinical improvement, limiting the utility of follow-up MRI in assessing treatment response. The absence of complete fiber disruption distinguishes tendinopathy from partial tear

insertion. Both entities may coexist in jumping athletes, necessitating a comprehensive evaluation of the extensor mechanism.

> **Key Point**
> MRI detects subtle overuse changes before structural failure occurs, enabling early intervention. However, MRI findings may persist after clinical resolution, necessitating correlation with symptoms.

7.8 Cartilage and Bone

Articular cartilage evaluation requires appropriate sequence selection and systematic assessment. Intermediate-weighted sequences provide optimal contrast between cartilage and joint fluid, while three-dimensional gradient-echo sequences enable thin-section evaluation with high spatial resolution [19].

Acute osteochondral injuries accompany ACL tears and patellar dislocations with high frequency. These injuries range from isolated cartilage delamination to displaced osteochondral fragments. Fragment size exceeding 10–15 mm and involvement of weight-bearing surfaces influence surgical decision-making. MRI precisely localizes donor sites and displaced fragments, guiding operative planning.

Bone marrow edema patterns provide insights into injury mechanisms and chronicity. Acute traumatic contusions demonstrate geographic edema corresponding to impaction sites. Stress-related edema appears more ill-defined, often linear, paralleling trabecular architecture. Subchondral insufficiency fractures manifest as linear low signal on all sequences with surrounding edema, requiring differentiation from osteonecrosis.

Cartilage assessment often employs modified Outerbridge grading, grading from signal alteration (Grade 1) through partial-thickness defects (Grades 2–3) to full-thickness loss with exposed bone (Grade 4). Quantitative techniques, including T2 mapping, detect early compositional changes before morphologic alterations, though clinical application remains limited [13].

7.9 Conclusions

MRI has evolved into an indispensable tool for comprehensive knee evaluation, providing unparalleled visualization of soft tissue and osseous pathology. Systematic assessment using appropriate sequences enables accurate diagnosis of meniscal, ligamentous, and cartilaginous injuries, guiding clinical management. The integration of accelerated imaging techniques, including parallel imaging, simultaneous multislice acquisition, and deep learning reconstruction, has overcome historical limitations of lengthy acquisition times without compromising diagnostic quality.

Recognition of injury patterns and associations enhances diagnostic accuracy. Understanding the relationships between mechanism, primary injury, and expected associated findings improves the detection of subtle pathology. The high prevalence of combined injuries, particularly in cruciate ligament disruptions, necessitates a comprehensive evaluation of all knee structures.

Future developments in quantitative imaging, artificial intelligence-assisted interpretation, and ultrafast protocols promise continued advancement in knee MRI capabilities. However, correlation with clinical findings remains paramount, as imaging abnormalities do not invariably correlate with symptoms or require intervention. The synergy between advanced imaging technology and clinical expertise will continue to drive improvements in the diagnosis and treatment of knee disorders.

Take-Home Messages

- Systematic evaluation of sagittal, coronal, and axial nonfat-suppressed and fat-suppressed PD and T2-weighted fast and turbo spin echo pulse sequences is essential for comprehensive knee assessment.
- Recognition of injury patterns and associations, particularly in ligamentous injuries, enhances diagnostic accuracy.
- Meniscal tear morphology and location directly influence surgical management decisions.
- Accelerated MRI protocols using combined parallel imaging, SMS, and deep learning enable diagnostic-quality imaging in under 5 min.
- Clinical correlation remains crucial, as many imaging abnormalities, particularly in older patients, may be asymptomatic.

Conflict of Interest I/We declare no competing interests as defined by Springer Nature or other interests that might be perceived to influence results and/or discussion reported in this manuscript.

References

1. Fritz J, Fritz B. MR imaging of acute knee injuries: systematic evaluation and reporting. Radiol Clin North Am. 2023;61:261–80.
2. Oei EHG, Nikken JJ, Verstijnen ACM, et al. MR imaging of the menisci and cruciate ligaments: a systematic review. Radiology. 2003;226:837–48.
3. Barth M, Breuer F, Koopmans PJ, et al. Simultaneous multislice (SMS) imaging techniques. Magn Reson Med. 2016;75:63–81.
4. Fritz J, Ahlawat S, Demehri S, et al. Simultaneous multislice accelerated turbo spin Echo magnetic resonance imaging: comparison and combination with in-plane parallel imaging acceleration for high-resolution magnetic resonance imaging of the knee. Investig Radiol. 2017;52:529–37.
5. Lin DJ, Walter SS, Fritz J. Artificial intelligence-driven ultra-fast superresolution MRI: 10-fold accelerated musculoskeletal turbo spin Echo MRI within reach. Investig Radiol. 2023;58:28–42.
6. Vosshenrich J, Carrino JA, Dyer GSM, et al. Arthroscopy-validated diagnostic performance of sub-5-min deep learning super-resolution 3T knee MRI in children and adolescents. Skeletal Radiol. 2025; (in press)
7. Walter SS, Fritz B, Kijowski R, et al. Deep learning super-resolution for simultaneous multislice parallel imaging-accelerated knee MRI using arthroscopy validation. Radiology. 2025;314:e241249.
8. Del Grande F, Rashidi A, Luna R, et al. Five-minute five-sequence knee MRI using combined simultaneous multislice and parallel imaging acceleration: comparison with 10-minute parallel imaging knee MRI. Radiology. 2021;299:635–46.
9. Fox MG. MR imaging of the meniscus: review, current trends, and clinical implications. Radiol Clin North Am. 2007;45:1033–53.
10. Mameri ES, Dashti Ardakani M, Kharazmi AB, et al. Review of meniscus anatomy and biomechanics. Curr Rev Musculoskelet Med. 2022;15:323–35.
11. Smet AAD, How I. Diagnose meniscal tears on knee MRI. Am J Roentgenol. 2012;199:481–99.
12. Wadhwa V, Omar H, Coyner K, et al. ISAKOS classification of meniscal tears-illustration on 2D and 3D isotropic spin echo MR imaging. Eur J Radiol. 2016;85:15–24.
13. Tomsan H, Cosgarea AJ, Joshi RP, et al. Knee MRI: meniscus roots, ramps, repairs, and repercussions. Radiographics. 2023;43:e220208.
14. Kopf S, Beaufils P, Hirschmann MT, et al. Management of traumatic meniscus tears: the 2019 ESSKA meniscus consensus. Knee Surg Sports Traumatol Arthrosc. 2020;28:1177–94.
15. Nguyen JC, De Smet AA, Graf BK, et al. MRI criteria for meniscal ramp lesions of the knee in children with anterior cruciate ligament tears. Am J Roentgenol. 2021;216:791–8.
16. Kobayashi H, Kanamura T, Koshida S, et al. Mechanisms of the anterior cruciate ligament injury in sports activities: a twenty-year clinical research of 1,700 athletes. J Sports Sci Med. 2010;9:669–75.
17. Thaunat M, Jan N, Fayard JM, et al. Ramp lesion subtypes: prevalence, imaging, and arthroscopic findings in 2156 anterior cruciate ligament reconstructions. Am J Sports Med. 2021;49:1813–21.
18. Schulz MS, Russe K, Weiler A, et al. Epidemiology of posterior cruciate ligament injuries. Arch Orthop Trauma Surg. 2003;123:186–91.
19. Fritz B, Fritz J. MR imaging of acute knee injuries: systematic evaluation and reporting. Radiol Clin North Am. 2023;61:261–80.
20. Alaia EF, Rosenberg ZS, Alaia MJ. Stener-like lesions of the superficial medial collateral ligament of the knee: MRI features. Am J Roentgenol. 2019;213:W272–6.
21. Rosas HG. Unraveling the posterolateral corner of the knee. Radiographics. 2016;36:1776–91.
22. Watts RE, Fritz B, Martel-Villagrán J, et al. Patellar tracking: an old problem with new insights. Radiographics. 2023;43:e220177.

The Ankle and Foot

8

Andrew J. Grainger and Marco Zanetti

Learning Objectives

By the end of this chapter, the reader should be able to:

1. Identify the appropriate imaging modalities for evaluating foot and ankle pathology.
2. Recognize and interpret imaging findings associated with common foot and ankle pathology.
3. Recognize imaging pitfalls including normal anatomical variants which can lead to confusion with pathology.

8.1 Introduction

The ankle joint or talocrural joint is formed by the articulation between the tibia and fibula, which form the mortice, which articulates with the talus. Anatomically the foot can be divided into the hindfoot, midfoot, and forefoot. The hindfoot, consisting of the calcaneus and talus, articulates with the midfoot through the midtarsal or Chopart joint, comprising the talonavicular and calcaneocuboid joints. The midfoot contains the navicular, cuboid, and the medial, intermediate, and lateral cuneiform bones, while the forefoot comprises the metatarsal bones and the phalanges. Tendons pass into the foot from the lower leg via the ankle. In addition, the foot has intrinsic muscles and tendons, which contribute to articular support and movement.

The foot and ankle are involved in a wide range of pathologies. The foot is frequently involved in systemic arthritides, given the numerous articulations and enthesis sites, and is also a common location for osteomyelitis, septic arthritis, and soft tissue infections. Additionally, the foot and ankle may be the site of primary or secondary bone and soft tissue tumors, as well as tumor-mimicking conditions. A detailed discussion of musculoskeletal infection, peripheral arthritis, and oncologic imaging is beyond the scope of this chapter but is covered in separate, dedicated modules.

Imaging of the foot and ankle must be tailored to the clinical question, with attention directed toward either the hindfoot and ankle, or the forefoot.

8.2 Imaging Techniques

Conventional radiographs remain the initial imaging modality, especially in acute trauma, as they allow rapid assessment of fractures, malalignment, gross osseous abnormalities, and static alignment of the foot and ankle. In the foot, fractures can be challenging to recognize due to the complex three-dimensional structure of the bone anatomy. Here computed tomography (CT) is frequently used to supplement radiographs for bone injury. Magnetic resonance imaging (MRI) and ultrasound (US) are indispensable for detailed evaluation of ligaments, tendons, fascia, and soft tissue lesions, while osteochondral lesions and marrow abnormalities are also well shown on MRI.

8.2.1 Conventional Radiographs

8.2.1.1 Standard Projections

Routine hindfoot radiographs include anteroposterior (AP) and lateral ankle views. The AP projection is typically obtained with 20° of internal rotation, creating the mortise view, which eliminates fibular overlap of the talus and optimizes visualization of the talar dome; without this adjustment, osteochondral lesions may be obscured by fibular superimposition. A 45° dorsoplantar (DP) oblique projection

A. J. Grainger (✉)
Department of Radiology, Cambridge University Hospitals, Cambridge, UK
e-mail: andrewgrainger@nhs.net

M. Zanetti
Department of Radiology, Cantonal Hospital Baden, Baden, Switzerland
e-mail: marco.zanetti@ksb.ch

J. Hodler et al. (eds.), *Musculoskeletal Diseases 2026-2029*, IDKD Springer Series,
https://doi.org/10.1007/978-3-032-17040-8_8

provides additional information about the midfoot, particularly the calcaneonavicular region, and is valuable in detecting occult fractures or tarsal coalitions.

8.2.1.2 Functional and Alignment Views

Weight-bearing radiographs are critical for evaluating the longitudinal arch and static alignment of the foot. For patients with chronic pain or suspected deformity, hindfoot alignment can be assessed with the Saltzman view, which provides reproducible depiction of varus or valgus angulation relative to the tibial axis [1].

8.2.2 CT

Computed tomography (CT) is indispensable for high-resolution assessment of the complex osseous anatomy and, thanks to its multiplanar reconstruction capabilities, is especially valuable for the evaluation of bone trauma. It also provides useful information for the surgical planning of corrective surgery for congenital coalitions and deformities.

8.2.3 US

The soft tissues of the foot and ankle tend to lie superficially which means US plays an important role in their assessment. Its real-time, dynamic capabilities make US highly effective for evaluating superficial tendons, ligaments, and peripheral nerves, as well as for guiding diagnostic and therapeutic interventions.

8.2.4 MRI

Magnetic resonance imaging (MRI) provides unparalleled soft tissue contrast and is the modality of choice for comprehensive evaluation of joint integrity, bone marrow abnormalities, soft tissue pathology, and occult fractures. MRI is particularly valuable in diagnosing ligamentous injuries, tendon pathology, osteomyelitis, and inflammatory arthropathies, as well as in assessing infection and neoplastic lesions.

8.2.4.1 MRI Protocols

Hindfoot Protocol

MRI sequences must be adapted to the suspected pathology. A comprehensive hindfoot protocol includes sagittal STIR, sagittal T1-weighted, coronal T2-weighted or proton-density (PD) fat-suppressed, axial T2-weighted, and an oblique 45° PD fat-suppressed sequence between coronal and axial planes to optimize visualization of the cross-sectional view of the flexor tendons and extensor tendons. For midfoot pathology, especially at the Lisfranc joint, add a PD fat-suppressed or STIR sequence oriented parallel to the metatarsals [2].

Forefoot Protocol

Forefoot imaging is best performed with the patient prone, allowing the toes to extend and widening intermetatarsal spaces. This positioning improves detection of Morton neuromas [3].

8.3 Imaging the Ankle and Hindfoot

8.3.1 Fractures

8.3.1.1 Radiography and Artificial Intelligence

Digital radiography enhances sensitivity for small or minimally displaced fractures. Computer-aided detection and artificial intelligence tools further improve fracture recognition, though radiologist oversight remains essential [4].

8.3.1.2 Classification Systems

The *Lauge-Hansen classification* (Table 8.1) is mechanism-based, describing four major injury patterns: supination–

Table 8.1 Lauge–Hansen classification of ankle fractures (mechanism-based)

Mechanism	Initial injury	Sequential lesions	Typical weber type
Supination–adduction (SA)	ATFL rupture or transverse fibular fracture	Vertical-oblique fracture of medial malleolus	Weber A
Supination–external rotation (SER) *(most common)*	AITFL rupture	Oblique spiral fibular fracture → posterior malleolus (Volkmann) fracture or PITFL injury → medial structures (transverse medial malleolus fracture or deltoid rupture)	Weber B
Pronation–abduction (PA)	Medial injury (deltoid ligament or medial malleolus)	Transverse fibular fracture above syndesmosis	Weber B/C (depending on height)
Pronation–external rotation (PER)	Medial injury (deltoid ligament or medial malleolus)	AITFL rupture → interosseous membrane tear → fibular fracture above syndesmosis → posterior malleolus (Volkmann) fracture or PITFL injury	Weber C

Table 8.2 Weber classification of fibular fractures (anatomic, syndesmosis-based)

Type	Fracture level	Stability features
A	Below syndesmosis	Usually stable
B	At level of syndesmosis	Variable stability (partial syndesmotic injury possible)
C	Above syndesmosis	Unstable (complete syndesmotic disruption with medial injury)

adduction, supination–external rotation, pronation–abduction, and pronation–external rotation, each correlating with predictable sequences of fracture and ligamentous injury [5]. The *Weber classification* (Table 8.2) is anatomic, categorizing fibular fractures by their relationship to the syndesmosis: type A (below), type B (at) (Fig. 8.1), and type C (above), with stability and ligamentous involvement varying accordingly [6].

8.3.2 MRI of Ankle Ligaments

Key Point

The anterior talofibular ligament (ATFL) is the ligament most commonly injured after an ankle sprain. Understanding the injury mechanism—for example, using the Lauge–Hansen classification—helps explain why the ATFL is often spared when the tibiofibular syndesmosis is disrupted.

8.3.2.1 Imaging Principles

On MRI, ligament tears are categorized as partial or complete, although functional competence may not be strictly correlated with imaging appearance. Criteria for injury include discontinuity, thickening with abnormal high signal, or nonvisualization (Table 8.3).

8.3.2.2 Lateral Ligament Complex

The anterior talofibular ligament (ATFL) is the most frequently injured ankle ligament and is best visualized on axial images as a thin low-signal band spanning the fibular tip to the talar neck (≈2 mm). Discontinuity or fluid-sensitive hyperintensity suggests injury. The calcaneofibular ligament (CFL) extends from the fibular tip to the lateral calcaneus, oblique in the coronal plane; sequential review of coronal and axial slices is required, and multiplanar reconstructions improve visualization [7]. The posterior talofibular ligament (PTFL) is the strongest lateral component, rarely injured except in severe dislocations, and is best depicted on axial sequences.

8.3.2.3 Tibiofibular Syndesmosis

The syndesmosis comprises the anterior inferior tibiofibular ligament (AITFL), posterior inferior tibiofibular ligament (PITFL), transverse tibiofibular ligament, and interosseous ligament. Given their obliquity, oblique axial and coronal planes are optimal [8]. Injury ("high ankle sprain") may be radiographically occult yet produce mortise widening and instability.

8.3.2.4 Medial (Deltoid) Ligament

The deltoid ligament complex consists of superficial (tibionavicular, tibiospring, tibiocalcaneal) and deep layers. The superficial layer is best seen on coronal imaging. The posterior tibiotalar ligament (Fig. 8.2) is the key deep stabilizer; loss of its normal striated appearance suggests acute injury or scarring, particularly relevant in younger patients. The anterior tibiotalar ligament is thin and variably present (~50%); nonvisualization should not be overcalled. Comprehensive MRI anatomy, injury patterns, and imaging pitfalls of the medial collateral complex—including criteria indicating medial mortise instability—are detailed by Mengiardi and colleagues [9].

8.3.2.5 Spring (Plantar Calcaneonavicular) Ligament Complex

The spring ligament includes superomedial, medioplantar oblique, and inferoplantar longitudinal components bridging the sustentaculum tali and navicular. It provides static support to the talar head and medial longitudinal arch; failure predisposes to progressive flatfoot. On MRI, it appears as a low-signal, bandlike structure best appreciated on coronal and axial planes, with tears most conspicuous distally in the tibiospring portion (Fig. 8.3). High-resolution MRI anatomy and pathology of the spring ligament subcomponents—and their interaction with posterior tibial tendon (PTT) dysfunction in adult-acquired flatfoot—are comprehensively reviewed by Mengiardi and colleagues [10].

8.3.3 MRI of Ankle Tendons (Table 8.4)

8.3.3.1 Extensor Tendons

Anterior to the ankle and stabilized by extensor retinacula, the tendons appear medial to lateral as tibialis anterior (TAT), extensor hallucis longus (EHL), and extensor digitorum longus (EDL). Tendinopathy manifests as thickening and increased fluid-sensitive signal; tenosynovitis presents with peritendinous fluid [11].

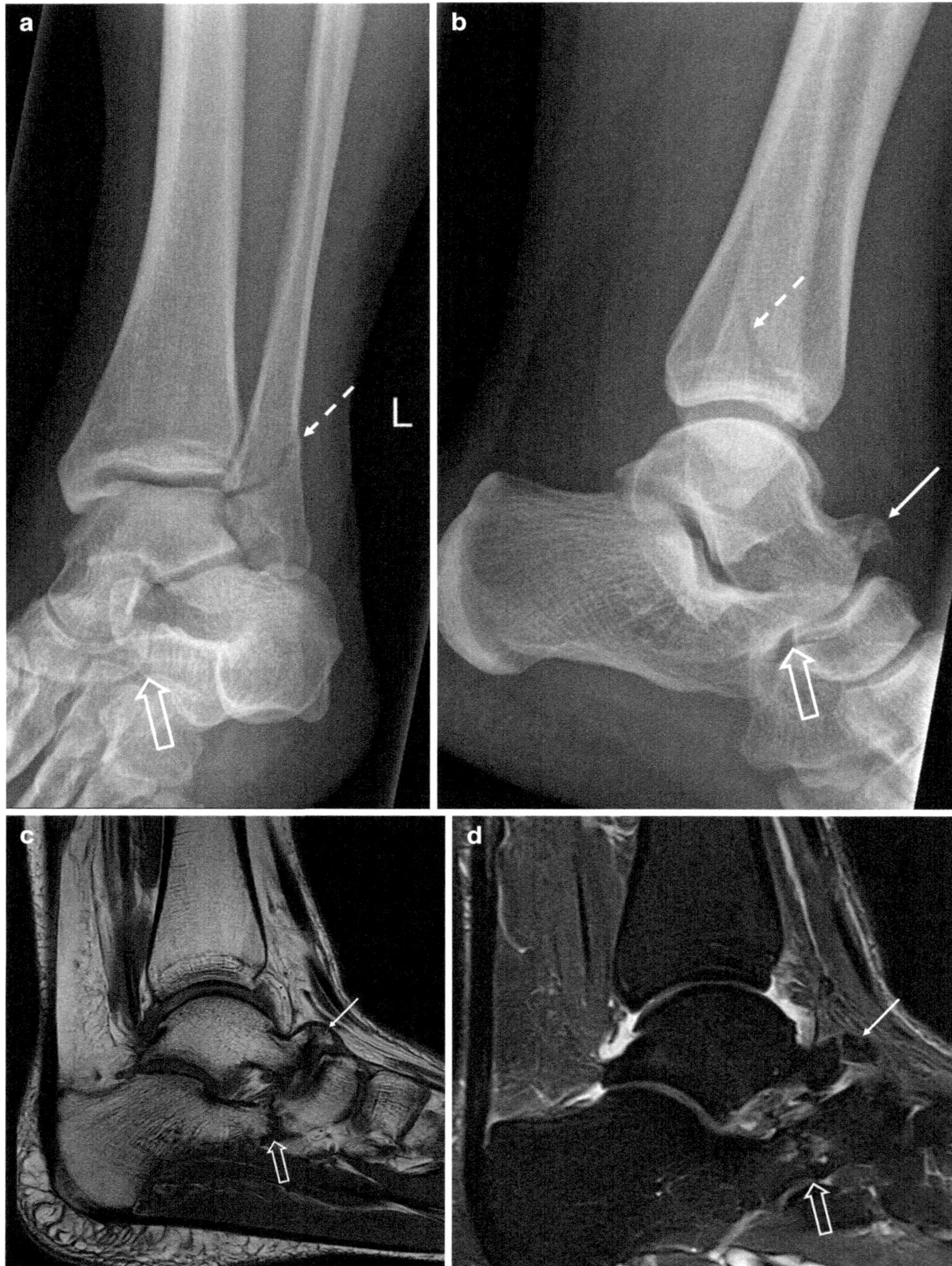

Fig. 8.1 Fracture of the lateral malleolus. (**a**) AP (Mortise) and (**b**) lateral radiographs along with (**c**) T1- and (**d**) STIR-weighted MRI demonstrate a Weber type B fracture (*broken arrow*). The patient also has a fibrous calcaneonavicular coalition (*open arrow*) with a characteristic talar beak (*solid arrow*)

Table 8.3 MRI evaluation of major ankle ligaments

Ligament	Orientation	Best MRI plane	Key imaging findings in injury
ATFL	Perpendicular to fibular axis	Axial	Thickening, discontinuity, high T2/STIR signal
CFL	Oblique (fibula → calcaneus)	Coronal ± oblique	Not fully in single slice, sequential/MPR imaging needed
PTFL	Perpendicular to fibula	Axial	Rarely torn except in dislocation
AITFL	Oblique, anterior tibia → fibula	Oblique axial	Fiber discontinuity, periligamentous edema
PITFL	Posterior tibia → fibula	Coronal/oblique	Thick, striated band; involvement = instability
Superficial deltoid	Medial malleolus → navicular/ spring/sustentaculum	Coronal	Thickening, edema, discontinuity
Deep deltoid (posterior tibiotalar)	Posterior colliculus → talus	Coronal	Absence of striations → instability
Spring ligament (superomedial, medioplantar oblique, inferoplantar longitudinal)	Sustentaculum tali → navicular	Coronal and axial	Tears most often distal tibiospring portion

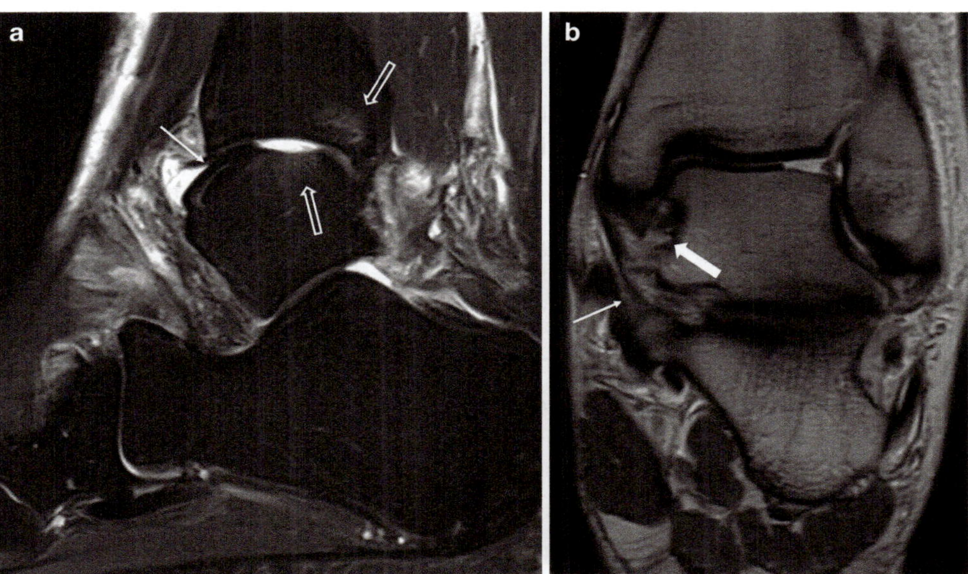

Fig. 8.2 (**a**) Sagittal STIR MRI shows an osteochondral defect at the lateral talar dome with an anteriorly displaced cartilage flap (*thin arrow*). There are bone bruises (*open arrows*) around the osteochondral defect and in the opposing dorsal aspect of the tibia (kissing lesion). (**b**) Coronal proton density-weighted MRI also shows there is a tear of the deep deltoid (posterior tibiotalar) ligament (*thick arrow*). The superficial tibiocalcaneal ligament is intact (*thin arrow*)

Table 8.4 Tendon compartments of the ankle (axial mnemonics)

Compartment	Order/ mnemonic	Tendons	Key MRI findings
Extensor (anterior)	Medial → lateral	Tibialis anterior, extensor hallucis longus, extensor digitorum longus	Small caliber; asymmetry or fluid → tendinopathy
Flexor (posteromedial)	**T**om, **D**ick, **A**nd **V**ery **N**ervous **H**arry	Tibialis posterior, flexor digitorum longus, tibial artery/vein, tibial nerve, flexor hallucis longus	Compare PTT:FDL (≈2:1); magic angle artifact common
Peroneal (lateral)	Anterior → posterior	Peroneus brevis, peroneus longus	PB split tear (“C-shape” encircling PL); PL attrition at cuboid tunnel
Posterior (Achilles/ plantar fascia)	–	Achilles tendon, plantar fascia	Midsubstance Achilles most often affected; central band thickening = plantar fasciitis

8.3.3.2 Flexor Tendons

Key Point
Compare PTT and FDL diameters at the same axial level (PTT ≈ 2× FDL); deviation suggests PTT disease. PB longitudinal splits can be deceptively subtle; tendon sheath effusion increases conspicuity. Small amounts of peritendinous fluid may be physiological in many compartments, but around the peroneal tendons, fluid more often indicates pathology [11].

Posteromedial tendons course behind the medial malleolus in the order: posterior tibial tendon (PTT), flexor digitorum longus (FDL), posterior tibial vessels, tibial nerve, and flexor hallucis longus (FHL). The *PTT* (Fig. 8.4) should be about twice the diameter of the *FDL*; reduced caliber suggests chronic disease. Magic-angle artifact is common and may simulate pathology [12, 13]. Chronic PTT dysfunction is the primary cause of adult-acquired flatfoot and is intimately linked with insufficiency of the spring ligament complex [10] (Fig. 8.3). The *FHL* is prone to stenosing tenosynovitis at the posterior talar tunnel, particularly in dancers.

8.3.3.3 Peroneal Tendons

Peroneus brevis (PB) lies anterior to peroneus longus (PL) in the retrofibular groove. Longitudinal splits of PB (Fig. 8.5) form a C-shaped tendon encircling PL; these may be subtle unless accompanied by sheath effusion [14]. PL commonly undergoes degenerative change at the cuboid tunnel; os peroneum fracture or cuboid marrow edema suggests mechanical overload [11].

8.3.3.4 Achilles Tendon and Plantar Fascia

Tendinosis of the Achilles tendon most often occurs 2–4 cm above its calcaneal insertion. MRI differentiates tendinopathy from partial tear [15]. In distal disease, evaluate for retrocalcaneal bursitis which can be associated with rheumatoid diseases or Haglund deformity. Plantar fasciitis presents with central band thickening and increased signal and is discussed further in Sect. 8.4.4.1 (Fig. 8.6) [16].

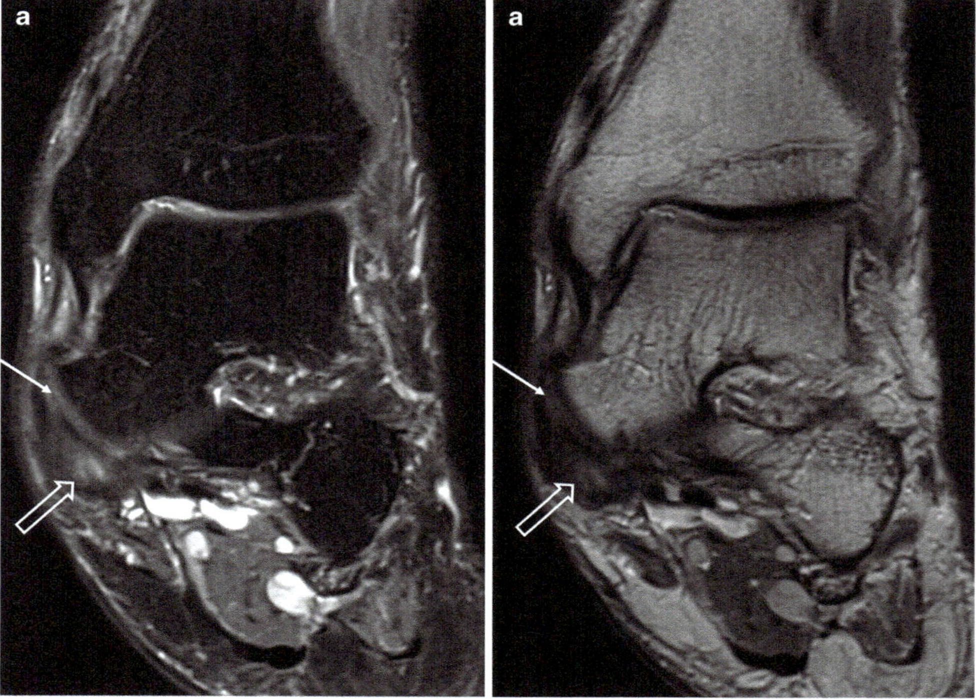

Fig. 8.3 Coronal proton density-weighted MRI (**a**) with and (**b**) without fat suppression demonstrates a tear of the spring ligament (*thin solid arrow*) and a partial tear of the posterior tibial tendon (*open arrow*)

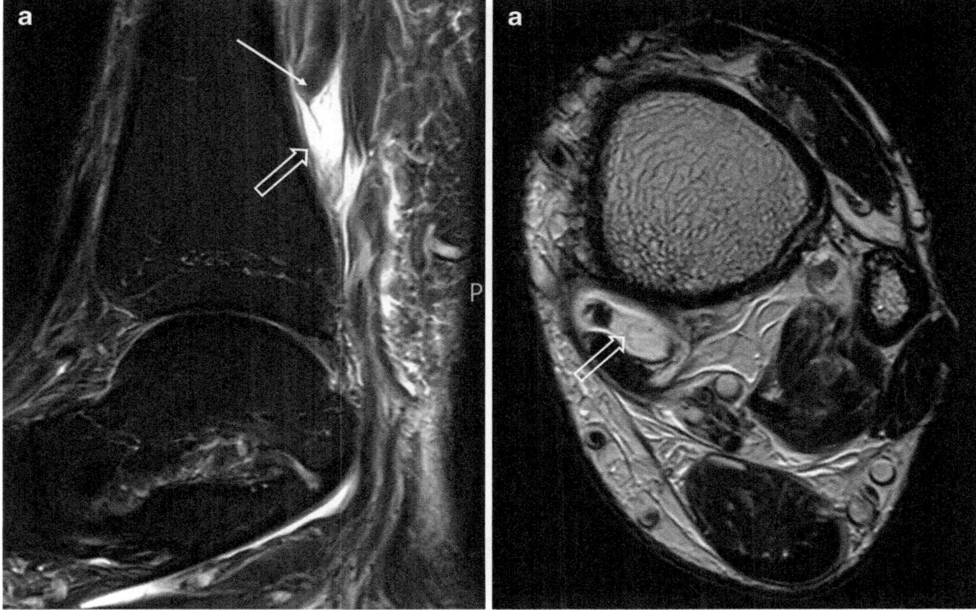

Fig. 8.4 (**a**) Sagittal STIR and (**b**) axial T2-weighted fat-suppressed MRI showing a complete tear of the posterior tibial tendon. The proximal tendon stump is seen 4 cm above the ankle joint (*solid arrow*). Distally the almost empty tendon sheath is seen (*open arrow*)

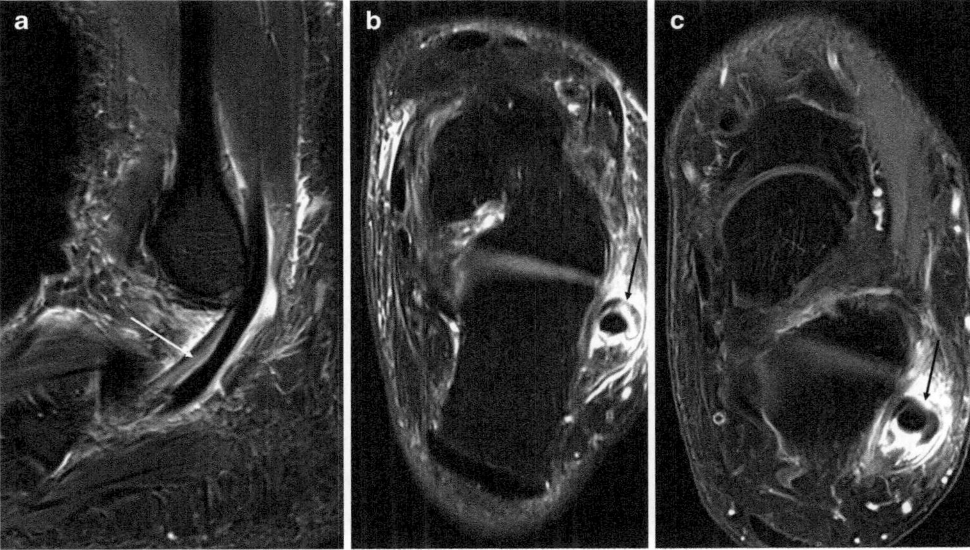

Fig. 8.5 (**a**) Sagittal STIR, (**b**) axial oblique proton density weighted with fat suppression and (**c**) post gadolinium axial T1-weighted fat-suppressed MRI images show a longitudinal split tear of the peroneus brevis tendon (*arrow*) with associated tenosynovitis

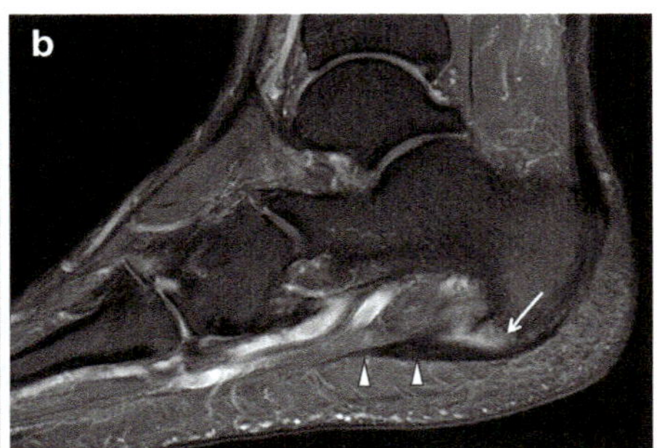

Fig. 8.6 Plantar fasciitis. (**a**) Ultrasound demonstrates a thickened and hyporeflective origin (*arrows*) to the central band of the plantar fascia as it arises from the calcaneus (*calc*). (**b**) In a different patient, T2-weighted MRI with fat suppression shows thickening of the central band of the plantar fascia with high-signal change in its substance (*arrow*) representing plantar fasciitis. *Arrowheads: plantar fascia*

8.4 Imaging the Foot

8.4.1 Congenital Foot Abnormalities

The foot is a common site for congenital deformities, and a full discussion of the variety and subtypes seen is beyond the scope of this text. The reader is referred to specialist texts on the subject. However, commonly seen conditions are discussed here, with the emphasis placed on radiological evaluation.

8.4.1.1 Congenital Talipes Equinovarus (TEV)

Also known as congenital clubfoot, this condition is a foot deformity where the forefoot is fixed in plantar flexion creating a high longitudinal arch. Four elements make up the deformity: an equinus position of the calcaneus, varus position of the hindfoot, adduction and varus deformity of the forefoot, and talonavicular subluxation. Several angles are described on the AP and lateral foot radiograph to assess the deformity, but a fundamental feature of TEV is the malalignment between the calcaneus and talus, which means the talocalcaneal angles provide a useful and relatively straightforward means to evaluate the condition. These are undertaken on the DP and lateral radiograph (Fig. 8.7). Both angles will be reduced in talipes equinovarus (<25 degrees). In addition, the longitudinal axis of the talus normally passes along the line of the first metatarsal or medial to it. In TEV the longitudinal axis of the talus will pass lateral to the axis of the first metatarsal.

Assessing the radiographic appearances after surgery is important to monitor progress and identify complications of the surgery, most commonly overcorrection giving a "rocker-bottom" flat foot deformity.

8.4.1.2 Congenital Vertical Talus (CVT) and Pes Planus

In congenital vertical talus (also known as rocker bottom foot), the talus assumes a downward directed and medial alignment, which on the lateral radiograph gives it the vertical alignment in the name. There is associated talonavicular dislocation, which distinguishes the condition from an acquired flatfoot deformity, but often the radiographic assessment for this condition is made before the navicular ossifies. The vertical alignment of the talus is apparent on the lateral radiograph (Fig. 8.8), and the DP radiograph typically shows an increased talocalcaneal angle. An important distinction between pes planovalgus and CVT is that a lateral radiograph in maximum plantar flexion will not show reduction of the talonavicular dislocation in CVT.

8.4.1.3 Tarsal Coalition

Key Point

Coalitions can lead to secondary osteoarthritis and most commonly are talocalcaneal or calcaneonavicular. Due to the complex three-dimensional anatomy, MRI and CT are often necessary for evaluating for the presence of coalition.

Tarsal coalition describes an abnormal congenital fusion between two or more tarsal bones which may be partial or complete. The fusion can be classified by the type of tissue involved as either osseous, fibrous, or cartilaginous coalitions. Such coalitions may be clinically silent in childhood, with symptoms emerging during adolescence or early adulthood, typically presenting as a painful flatfoot deformity. With time, the altered biomechanics can lead to the development of secondary osteoarthritis.

The most frequently encountered coalitions are between the calcaneus and navicular, where the majority of coalitions are nonosseous (Figs. 8.1 and 8.9) and between the talus and calcaneus, where all three subtypes are represented. Together, these two types account for approximately 90% of all tarsal coalitions.

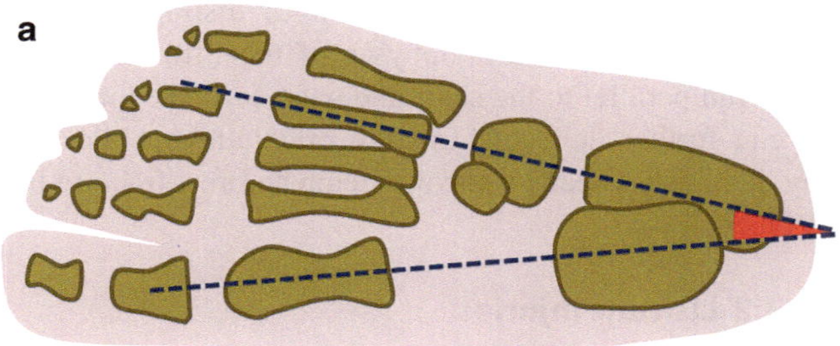

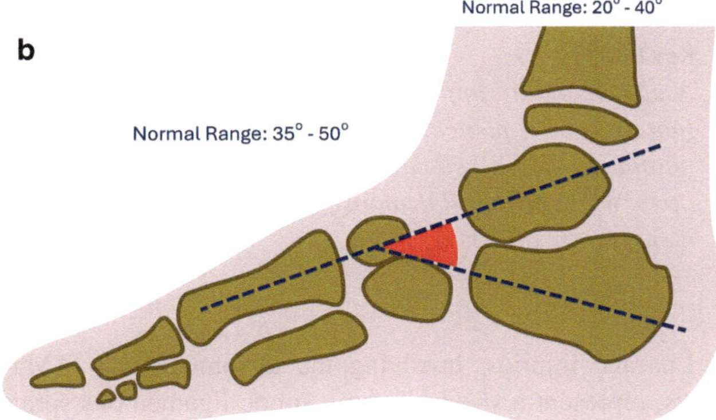

Fig. 8.7 Measurement of the talocalcaneal angles (*shown in red*) on (**a**) dorsoplantar and (**b**) lateral radiographs of the foot. In talipes equinovarus, both angles will be reduced (< 25 degrees)

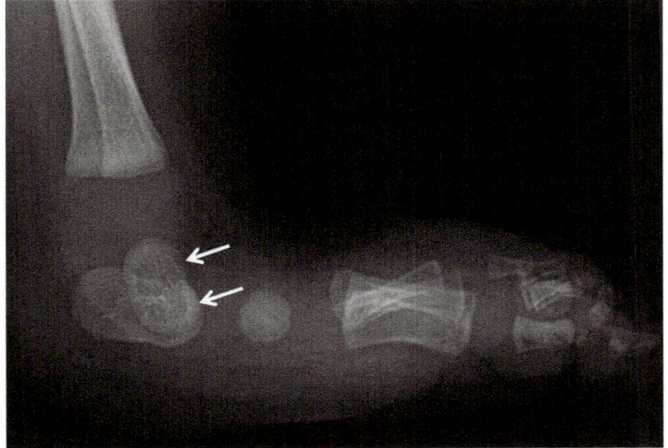

Fig. 8.8 Congenital vertical talus. The lateral radiograph demonstrates the vertical alignment of the talus (*arrows*)

Diagnosing tarsal coalitions using standard radiography can be challenging due to the complex three-dimensional arrangement of the tarsal bones. However, certain radiographic signs are considered characteristic:

Calcaneonavicular coalition: This often appears as an elongated anterior process of the calcaneus, producing the so-called anteater nose sign, most effectively visualized on the oblique (DP) foot view. Imaging may also demonstrate a hypoplastic talar head.

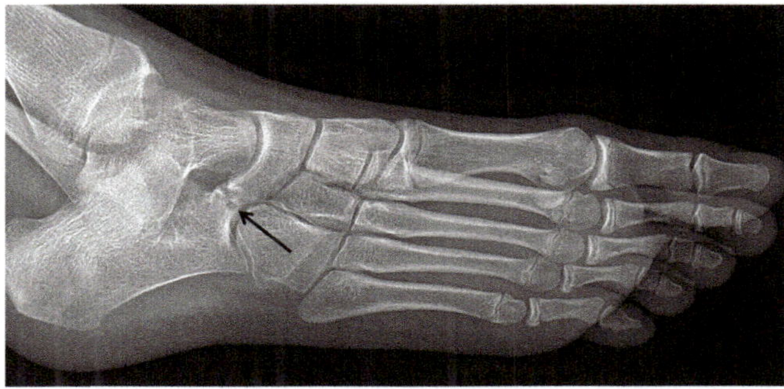

Fig. 8.9 Calcaneonavicular fibrous coalition. Dorsoplantar oblique radiograph demonstrates the prominent anterior calcaneal process leading to a decreased distance from the navicular (*arrow*). Note the bone irregularity either side of the fibrous union between the two bones

Talocalcaneal coalition: Typically involving the middle facet of the subtalar joint, this may manifest as localized sclerosis. *The C-sign*, representing a continuous C-shaped radiodense outline encircling the talus and sustentaculum tali, is another diagnostic clue. In talocalcaneal coalition, restricted subtalar mobility may lead to osteoarthritis at adjacent joints, particularly the talonavicular joint, where osteophyte may give rise to a so-called talar beak.

CT (computed tomography) is particularly useful for delineating osseous coalition, although fibrous and cartilaginous coalitions may be less conspicuous. Suggestive findings include joint space narrowing and reactive bone changes adjacent to the coalition.

MRI (magnetic resonance imaging) offers superior soft tissue contrast and is capable of detecting all types of coalitions—osseous, fibrous, and cartilaginous [17]. MRI can also demonstrate associated bone marrow edema and soft tissue inflammation, which can confirm the coalition as a symptomatic source. However, differentiating between synovial inflammation and fibrous coalition can sometimes be difficult on MRI [18, 19].

8.4.2 Bone Variants

Sesamoid bones represent bones within tendons, while accessory ossicles usually relate to unfused additional ossification centers.

Sesamoid bones are variable, but among the most important in the foot are the medial and lateral hallux sesamoids which are consistently seen at the first metatarsophalangeal joint (MTPJ) and the os peroneum. The hallux sesamoids lie within the flexor hallucis brevis tendons on the plantar aspect of the foot while the os peroneum lies on the lateral aspect of the foot in the peroneus longus, close to the calcaneocuboid joint. Common pathologies seen in the sesamoid bones include fracture and osteonecrosis. Where a fracture is seen

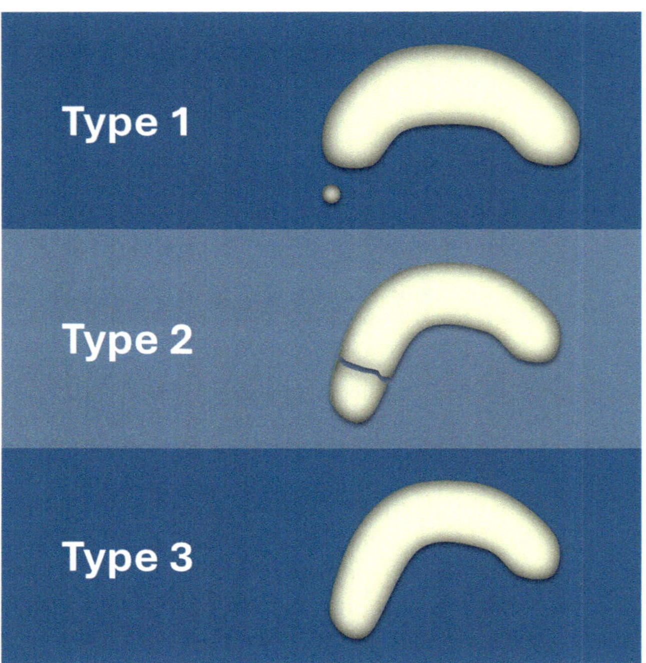

Fig. 8.10 Types of accessory navicular

it is possible that there may be disruption of the tendon the sesamoid lies in, and this possibility should be raised by the reporting radiologist. For instance, fractures of the os peroneum are likely to be associated with damage to the peroneus longus tendon.

Accessory ossicles are also variably located and it is important for the radiologist to be aware of their common locations. They can give rise to symptoms typically through impingement, for instance, the os trigonum on the dorsal aspect of the ankle may be a cause of posterior ankle impingement or through the development of a stress response across the synchondrosis attaching the accessory ossicle to the adjacent bones. Such stress response, due to instability at the synchondrosis, is best detected on MRI and can also be seen with the os trigonum. Other sites of symptomatic accessory ossicles include the accessory navicular, of which three types are recognized (Fig. 8.10).

8.4.3 Bone Trauma

Common fracture patterns include the following:

8.4.3.1 Fifth Metatarsal Base Fractures

Fractures of the base of the fifth metatarsal are among the most common foot injuries. Precise classification is essential, as prognosis and management differ considerably according to fracture location. These fractures are divided into three main types (Table 8.5) [20].

Radiographically, it is important to distinguish acute fractures from unfused apophyses of the fifth metatarsal, which run parallel to the shaft and have corticated margins. CT can further delineate fracture orientation, while MRI may demonstrate early marrow edema before a fracture line becomes visible.

8.4.3.2 Lisfranc Injuries

> **Key Point**
> *A multimodality approach is required to imaging the foot as a consequence of its complex three-dimensional anatomy. CT will demonstrate subtle avulsion fractures, while MRI will demonstrate the ligamentous elements of the injury.*

Lisfranc injuries, involving the tarsometatarsal (TMT) joints, represent a spectrum from subtle ligamentous sprain to frank fracture–dislocation. These injuries are often missed on initial radiographs but carry significant morbidity if untreated.

The Lisfranc ligament is a key component and extends between the medial cuneiform and the second metatarsal bases. It comprises dorsal, interosseous, and plantar bands (Fig. 8.11) [21].

Radiographic features include widening of the interval between the first and second metatarsal bases (> 2 mm) and misalignment of the medial cuneiform with the second metatarsal. Frequently disruption of the ligament complex is associated with avulsion fractures from the cuneiform and metatarsal base. Weight-bearing radiographs may better demonstrate osseous malalignment.

MRI is usually the modality of choice, particularly because of its ability to demonstrate purely ligamentous injuries. MRI will demonstrate discontinuity or edema of the Lisfranc ligament complex and associated bone marrow changes in case of fracture [21]. It is important to recognize that subtle fractures can be challenging to see on radiographs and MRI, and CT may be useful to clarify the picture (Fig. 8.12).

8.4.3.3 Stress and Insufficiency Fractures

Stress fractures of the foot are common in athletes, military recruits, and individuals exposed to repetitive loading. Insufficiency fractures occur when normal stress is applied to weakened bone, such as in osteoporosis, metabolic bone disease, or chronic steroid use.

The metatarsals are particularly prone to stress injury, especially the second and third shafts. Radiographs may initially be normal but later reveal periosteal reaction and cortical thickening.

Table 8.5 Types of fifth metatarsal base fracture

Type	Location	Description
Zone 1 (tuberosity avulsion fractures)	Proximal tuberosity	Often due to avulsion by the peroneus brevis tendon or lateral band of the plantar fascia Typically heal uneventfully with conservative treatment
Zone 2 (Jones fractures)	Metaphyseal–diaphyseal junction, extending into the fourth–fifth metatarsal articulation	Prone to delayed union or nonunion due to limited blood supply to the region Often require surgical fixation in active individuals
Zone 3	Diaphysis of the metatarsal, within 1.5 cm of the tuberosity	Mechanism involves the plantarflexed and inverted foot Stress fractures can be seen here

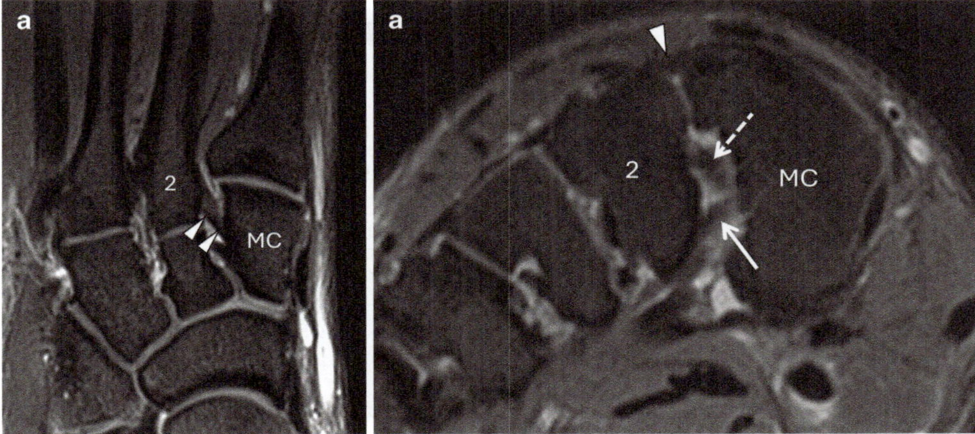

Fig. 8.11 MRI showing the normal Lisfranc ligament complex. Proton density fat-suppressed (**a**) axial (long-axis) image demonstrates the plantar component of the ligament complex extending obliquely between the medial cuneiform and the base of the second metatarsal while (**b**) coronal (short-axis) image shows parts of the dorsal (*arrowheads*), interosseous (*broken arrow*), and plantar bands (*solid arrow*) of the ligament complex. *MC, medial cuneiform. 2: Second metatarsal*

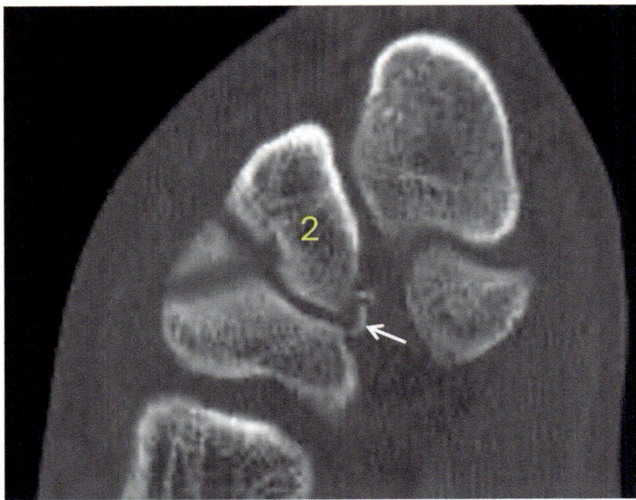

Fig. 8.12 Axial (short-axis) CT through the second metatarsal base (*2*) in a patient who sustained a Lisfranc fracture–dislocation demonstrates a small avulsion fracture at the insertion of the plantar component of the Lisfranc ligament (*arrow*)

MRI is the most sensitive modality for early diagnosis, detecting bone marrow edema before radiographic changes appear. On MRI, a stress fracture demonstrates a linear low-signal line within a region of marrow edema. CT, while less sensitive in early stages, is occasionally useful for defining fracture morphology and healing response. Dual energy CT (DECT) is becoming increasingly available for the detection of bone edema and is proving accurate in the diagnosis of stress injuries in the foot, able to identify stress reactions and accurately delineate any fracture line [22].

Other common sites include the navicular, talus, calcaneus, and sesamoids. Navicular stress fractures, common in track and field athletes, are particularly important due to the risk of nonunion, related to the bone's limited vascular supply. These fractures can be extremely subtle on radiographs. If the radiograph is normal and symptoms suggest a navicular stress fracture, cross-sectional imaging with MRI and/or CT is needed to avoid delayed diagnosis.

8.4.3.4 Sesamoid Fractures

Fractures of the hallux sesamoids may result from acute trauma or repetitive stress. Distinguishing an acute fracture from a bipartite sesamoid is essential. Acute fractures show irregular, noncorticated margins, whereas bipartite sesamoids display smooth, well-corticated margins with rounded edges. Another useful distinction is that the fracture fragments of a fractured sesamoid will appear as if they would fit back together, whereas the components of a bipartite sesamoid tend not to. MRI is useful in ambiguous cases, as acute fractures demonstrate adjacent marrow edema and soft tissue swelling, while bipartite sesamoids do not.

8.4.4 Soft Tissue Injury

The soft tissue structures of the foot are complex and highly specialized, providing both dynamic and static support, allowing precise locomotion, and protecting osseous structures from injury. Soft tissue pathology can arise from acute trauma, chronic overuse, inflammatory conditions, or degenerative processes. Imaging evaluation is critical, as many injuries are subtle and may not be apparent on radiographs. Ultrasound and MRI are the primary modalities for detailed assessment.

8.4.4.1 Plantar Fascia

The plantar fascia is a thick fibrous aponeurosis arising from the calcaneal tuberosity and extending to the metatarsal heads. It comprises three distinct bands:

- *Medial band* originates alongside the central band, covering the abductor hallucis.
- *Central band* is the largest and functionally most important, covering the flexor digitorum brevis and dividing into bands toward the metatarsal heads. It is most commonly affected in plantar fasciitis.
- *Lateral band* covers the abductor digiti minimi and inserts onto the base of the fifth metatarsal.

Plantar fasciitis is the most common source of plantar heel pain, frequently affecting runners, dancers, and individuals with obesity. On ultrasound, there is thickening (>4 mm) of the plantar fascia with hypoechoic change and loss of the fibrillar pattern (Fig. 8.6a). MRI also demonstrates thickening of the plantar fascia with increased T1 and T2 signal intensity (Fig. 8.6b). Adjacent bone marrow edema or soft tissue edema may be present in severe or chronic cases. Partial or full-thickness tears can occur, particularly in advanced disease. Patients with lateral band involvement can present with pain at the base of the fifth metatarsal where the lateral band inserts, which may mimic peroneus brevis tendon disease.

The plantar fascia enthesis is also a common site of involvement in *seronegative spondyloarthropathy*, necessitating careful correlation with clinical and laboratory findings.

Plantar fibromatosis is characterized by nodular thickening along the fascia, often bilateral and genetically linked to conditions such as Dupuytren's disease. MRI demonstrates well-circumscribed nodules with low-to-intermediate signal intensity on T1 and T2, while ultrasound shows hypoechoic nodules with preserved fibrillar architecture.

8.4.4.2 Tendons

Key Point

As well as movement tendons play an important role in supporting the arches of the foot. Sesamoid bones are found in the tendons of the foot and fracture to a sesamoid bone should highlight the likelihood of associated tendon disruption.

The long tendons of the foot arise from musculature in the lower leg and more commonly give symptoms at the ankle. However, the flexor hallucis longus (FHL) and flexor digitorum longus (FDL) pass through the sole of the foot crossing at the *knot of Henry*. Tenosynovitis may occur here, visible as fluid within the tendon sheaths on ultrasound or MRI. It is important to note that the normal FHL tendon sheath communicates with the ankle joint, which may allow physiological fluid, or even osteochondral debris from the ankle joint to track into the foot.

The *tibialis posterior (TP)* inserts on the navicular and medial cuneiform, with an accessory navicular present in some individuals. Tendinosis and tearing can occur at the insertion, giving rise to medial midfoot pain. Ultrasound here can be challenging due to the complex nature of the insertion, but MRI shows tendon thickening, signal alteration, and potentially associated marrow edema at the insertion.

The *peroneus longus* tendon courses round the cuboid on the lateral side of the foot, inserting on the plantar aspect of the first metatarsal. The os peroneum, located within the tendon, may be subject to fracture or chronic injury (painful os peroneum syndrome, POPS). Ruptures near the os peroneum can displace the ossicle proximally. The *peroneus brevis* inserts on the base of the fifth metatarsal. Distal tears or tendinopathy may cause lateral foot pain.

On the dorsum of the foot rupture of the tibialis anterior is an important diagnosis to make given the important role the tendon plays in gait. Despite its relative rarity, it is still the third most commonly ruptured tendon in the lower limb after the Achilles and Patellar tendons [23]. The tibialis anterior inserts onto the medial cuneiform and base of the first metatarsal which can give it a bifid appearance which may mimic a split tear and requires careful imaging interpretation [24, 25].

8.4.4.3 Sinus Tarsi Syndrome

The sinus tarsi, found between the talus and calcaneus, contains fat, vessels, nerve endings, and the talocalcaneal ligaments. Sinus tarsi syndrome presents with lateral foot pain, commonly following ankle inversion injuries. MRI shows edema, fibrotic tissue, or ligamentous disruption within the sinus tarsi. Chronic cases may result in subtalar osteoarthritis.

8.4.4.4 Plantar Plate and Turf Toe Injuries

The plantar plates, composed of fibrocartilage, reinforce the plantar aspect of the MTP joints. There is a more complex structure to the plantar mechanism at the first toe which includes the medial and lateral sesamoid bones as well as the plantar plate. Here hyperextension injury to the plantar articular structures is known as turf toe. Radiographs may reveal avulsion fractures from the sesamoid bones or the proximal phalangeal base. Ultrasound allows dynamic evaluation and visualization of partial or full-thickness tears. MRI will demonstrate plantar plate disruption (Fig. 8.13), bone marrow edema, and associated soft tissue injuries [26, 27].

The second through to fifth MTP joints also contain plantar plates. Chronic injury here leads to toe deformities such as clawing. Both MRI and ultrasound are effective, with dynamic imaging particularly helpful in differentiating partial from complete tears.

8.4.4.5 Nerve Entrapment

The foot contains multiple cutaneous nerves, which may be entrapped by bony prominences, accessory muscles, or masses. Imaging evaluation with MRI and ultrasound allows direct visualization of nerves, surrounding soft tissues, and compression sites. The most common entrapments include the following:

- *Morton neuroma*: Very common resulting in perineural fibrosis of the interdigital nerve, usually between the second and third or third and fourth metatarsal heads. There may be associated bursitis. Ultrasound shows a hypoechoic mass; MRI demonstrates T2 hyperintense nerve enlargement.
- *Tarsal tunnel syndrome*: Posterior tibial nerve entrapment under the flexor retinaculum on the medial ankle and hindfoot. It may involve lateral or medial plantar branches. Ganglia cysts and accessory muscles are common causes. US and MRI may show the cause of the nerve compression. They may also demonstrate nerve enlargement, edema, or atrophy of supplied muscles.
- *Baxter neuropathy*: The inferior calcaneal nerve or Baxter nerve is the first branch of the lateral plantar nerve. Entrapment, which may be seen particularly in runners and those with flat foot deformity, causes heel pain. The nerve also provides the motor supply to abductor digiti minimi which may show atrophy.

Less commonly, sural, superficial peroneal, and deep peroneal nerve entrapment may occur, often related to trauma or footwear.

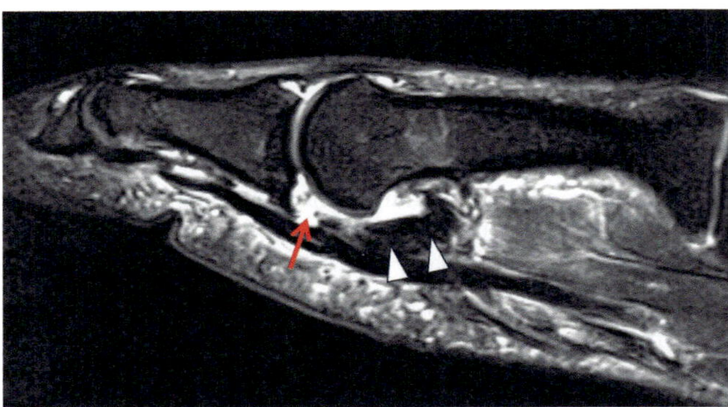

Fig. 8.13 Turf Toe. T2-weighted MRI with fat suppression shows a tear of the plantar plate in a patient in its insertion onto the proximal phalangeal base (*arrow*). The plantar plate is retracted and bunched up (*arrowheads*)

8.5 Further Practical MRI Pearls for Radiologists

8.5.1 Bone Marrow Edema-Like Signal

Bone marrow edema appears T1 hypointense and hyperintense on fat-suppressed fluid-sensitive sequences. It reflects mechanical stress, fracture (Fig. 8.14), contusion, arthropathy, infection, or postoperative change [28]. In infection, marrow abnormalities often extend beyond articular margins and are associated with cortical destruction and soft tissue findings [28]. In younger patients with focal edema and nocturnal pain, consider osteoid osteoma [28] (Fig. 8.15).

8.5.2 Osteochondral Lesions

Osteochondral lesions (Fig. 8.2). most often involve the talar dome and are typically trauma-related. MRI establishes stability; a fluid rim between fragment and bed indicates instability [29]. Medial lesions are usually deeper and posterior; lateral lesions are more anterior and shallow. Reports should include size, cartilage integrity, fragment viability, marrow changes, and secondary findings such as effusion or loose bodies [29].

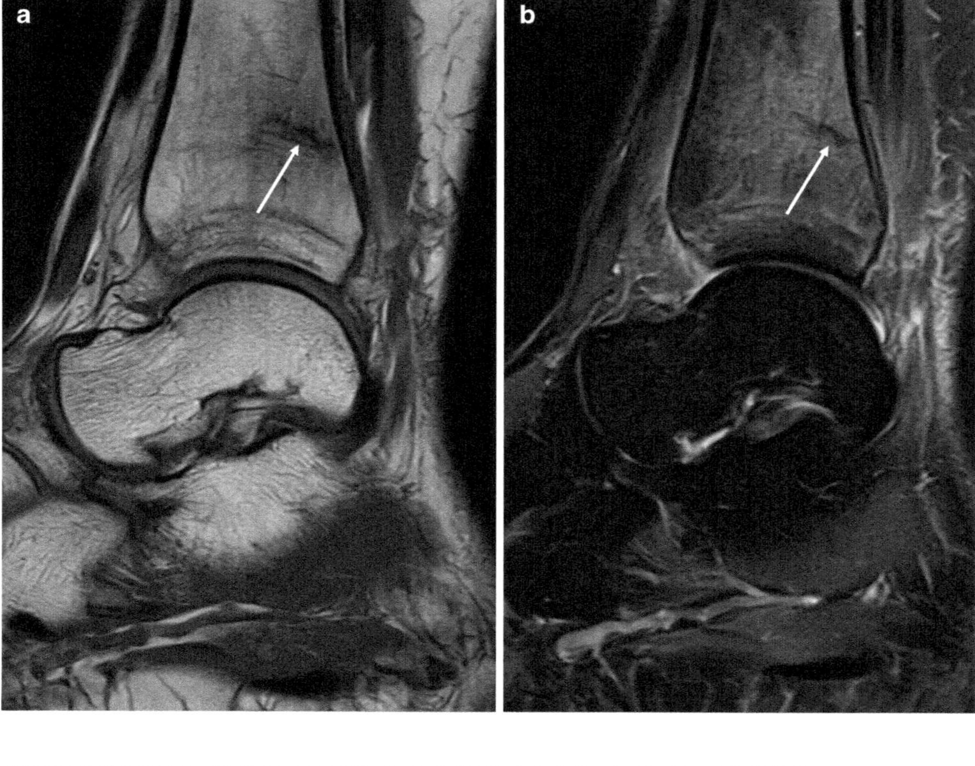

Fig. 8.14 Stress fracture in the tibia: (**a**) Sagittal T1-weighted MRI demonstrates a fracture line in keeping with the diagnosis of a stress fracture. (**b**) A sagittal STIR image shows associated bone marrow edema-like abnormality; the fracture line is less conspicuous

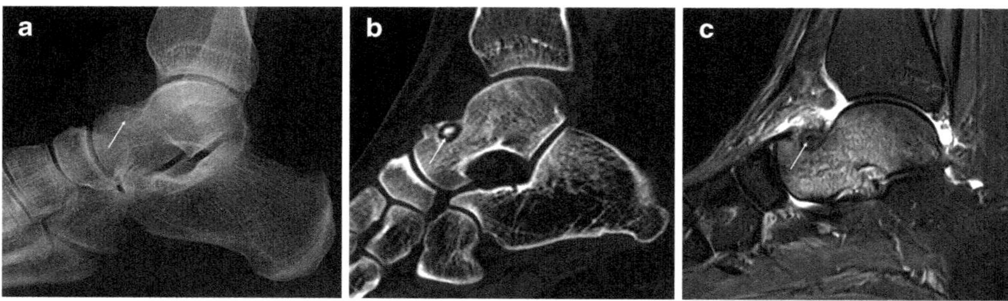

Fig. 8.15 Osteoid osteoma of the talus. (**a**) Sagittal STIR MRI shows extensive bone marrow edema in the talus but not in the surrounding bones (tibia, navicular, and calcaneus bone). There is an effusion in the ankle joint. The osteoid osteoma nidus is visible on the MRI (*arrow*) and clearly shown on (**b**) CT. However, the nidus is hardly visible on (**c**) the lateral radiograph (*arrow*)

8.5.3 Tumors and Tumor-Like Lesions

Benign tumor-like conditions predominate in the ankle and hindfoot. Ganglion cysts are most frequent, appearing T2 hyperintense with thin rim enhancement. Other T2-hyperintense but enhancing masses include neurogenic and glomus tumors and synovial sarcomas [30]. T2-hypointense lesions include tenosynovial giant cell tumor and plantar fibromatosis; gout and rheumatoid nodules may also be relatively low on T2 due to paramagnetic or fibrous content. Assessment should emphasize anatomic relationships, margins, enhancement pattern, and systemic disease associations.

8.6 Summary

Foot pathology spans a broad spectrum, from traumatic fractures to overuse injuries and nerve entrapments. Conventional radiographs remain the initial diagnostic modality, particularly for fractures and alignment abnormalities. However, these must be supplemented by CT, MRI, and ultrasound as indicated, for accurate diagnosis and optimal patient management.

MRI protocols must be tailored to the clinical question and region of interest. MRI along with US provides superior evaluation of ligaments, tendons, and tumor-like conditions. MRI is also suited for assessing marrow abnormalities and osteochondral lesions.

Recognition of normal anatomical variants, detailed understanding of soft tissue anatomy, and familiarity with common pathological patterns are critical for radiologists and clinicians alike. This chapter provides a framework for evaluating foot and ankle pathology, ensuring precise, reproducible, and clinically relevant imaging interpretation.

Take-Home Messages

- *Multimodality imaging is essential* for accurate diagnosis of foot and ankle pathology, with radiographs, CT, MRI, and ultrasound each playing a complementary role based on clinical context.
- *Knowledge of normal variants and congenital abnormalities* is crucial to avoid misdiagnosis and to correctly interpret complex anatomical findings.
- *Understanding the mechanism of injury to the ankle joint* helps in interpreting equivocal ligament and tendon abnormalities.
- *Soft tissue injuries and subtle fractures of the foot are frequently underdiagnosed* and require a high index of suspicion and appropriate use of cross-sectional imaging for early detection and effective management.

Conflict of Interest I/We declare no competing interests as defined by Springer Nature or other interests that might be perceived to influence results and/or discussion reported in this manuscript.

References

1. Saltzman CL, El-Khoury GY. The hindfoot alignment view. Foot Ankle Int. 1995;16:572–6.
2. Siddiqui NA, Galizia MS, Almusa E, et al. Evaluation of the tarsometatarsal joint using conventional radiography, CT, and MR imaging. Radiographics. 2014;34:514–31.
3. Weishaupt D, Treiber K, Kundert H-P, et al. Morton neuroma: MR imaging in prone, supine, and upright weight-bearing body positions. Radiology. 2003;226:849–56.
4. Guermazi A, Tannoury C, Kompel AJ, et al. Improving radiographic fracture recognition performance and efficiency using artificial intelligence. Radiology. 2022;302:627–36.
5. Lauge-Hansen N. Fractures of the ankle: II. Combined experimental-surgical and experimental-roentgenologic investigations. Arch Surg. 1950;60:957–85.
6. Weber BG. Malleolarfrakturen. Schweiz Med Wochenschr. 1967;97:790–2.
7. Duc SR, Mengiardi B, Pfirrmann CW, et al. Improved visualization of collateral ligaments of the ankle: multiplanar reconstructions based on standard 2D turbo spin-echo MR images. Eur Radiol. 2007;17:1162–71.
8. Hermans JJ, Ginai AZ, Wentink N, et al. The additional value of an oblique image plane for MRI of the anterior and posterior distal tibiofibular syndesmosis. Skeletal Radiol. 2011;40:75–83.
9. Mengiardi B, Pinto C, Zanetti M. Medial collateral ligament complex of the ankle: MR imaging anatomy and findings in medial instability. Semin Musculoskelet Radiol. 2016;20:091–103.
10. Mengiardi B, Pinto C, Zanetti M. Spring ligament complex and posterior tibial tendon: MR anatomy and findings in acquired adult flatfoot deformity. Semin Musculoskelet Radiol. 2016;20:104–15.
11. Taljanovic MS, Alcala JN, Gimber LH, et al. High-resolution US and MR imaging of peroneal tendon injuries. Radiographics. 2015;35:179–99.
12. Erickson SJ, Prost R, Timins M. The "magic angle" effect: background physics and clinical relevance. Radiology. 1993;188:23–5.
13. Mengiardi B, Pfirrmann CW, Schöttle PB, et al. Magic angle effect in MR imaging of ankle tendons: influence of foot positioning on prevalence and site in asymptomatic subjects and cadaveric tendons. Eur Radiol. 2006;16:2197–206.
14. Dombek MF, Lamm BM, Saltrick K, et al. Peroneal tendon tears: a retrospective review. J Foot Ankle Surg. 2003;42:250–8.
15. Schweitzer ME, Karasick D. MR imaging of disorders of the Achilles tendon. Am J Roentgenol. 2000;175:613–25.
16. Berkowitz J, Kier R, Rudicel S. Plantar fasciitis: MR imaging. Radiology. 1991;179:665–7.
17. Marth AA, Feuerriegel GC, Marcus RP, et al. How accurate is MRI for diagnosing tarsal coalitions? A retrospective diagnostic accuracy study. Eur Radiol. 2024;34:3493–502.
18. Lawrence DA, Rolen MF, Haims AH, et al. Tarsal coalitions: radiographic, CT, and MR imaging findings. HSS J. 2014;10:153–66.
19. Newman JS, Newberg AH. Congenital tarsal coalition: multimodality evaluation with emphasis on CT and MR imaging. Radiographics. 2000;20:321–32.
20. Beddard L, Roslee C, Kelsall N. Acute and stress fractures of the metatarsals in athletes. Orthop Trauma. 2024;38:46–50.
21. Castro M, Melão L, Canella C, et al. Lisfranc joint ligamentous complex: MRI with anatomic correlation in cadavers. Am J Roentgenol. 2010;195:W447–55.
22. Foti G, Sanfilippo L, Longo C, et al. Diagnostic accuracy of dual-energy CT for bone stress injury of the lower limb. Radiology. 2024;313:e232415.
23. Vosoughi AR, Heyes G, Molloy AP, et al. Management of tibialis anterior tendon rupture: recommendations based on the literature review. Foot Ankle Surg. 2020;26:487–93.
24. Karauda P, Podgorski M, Paulsen F, et al. Anatomical variations of the tibialis anterior tendon. Clin Anat. 2021;34:397–404.
25. Varghese A, Bianchi S. Ultrasound of tibialis anterior muscle and tendon: anatomy, technique of examination, normal and pathologic appearance. J Ultrasound. 2014;17:113–23.
26. Nery C, Baumfeld D, Umans H, et al. MR imaging of the plantar plate: normal anatomy, turf toe, and other injuries. Magn Reson Imaging Clin N Am. 2017;25:127–44.
27. Crain JM, Phancao J-P, Stidham K. MR imaging of turf toe. Magn Reson Imaging Clin N Am. 2008;16:93–103.
28. Rios AM, Rosenberg ZS, Bencardino JT, et al. Bone marrow edema patterns in the ankle and hindfoot: distinguishing MRI features. Am J Roentgenol. 2011;197:W720–9.
29. De Smet AA, Fisher DR, Graf B, et al. Osteochondritis dissecans of the knee: value of MR imaging in determining lesion stability and the presence of articular cartilage defects. Am J Roentgenol. 1990;155:549–53.
30. Murphey MD, Rhee JH, Lewis RB, et al. Pigmented villonodular synovitis: radiologic-pathologic correlation. Radiographics. 2008;28:1493–518.

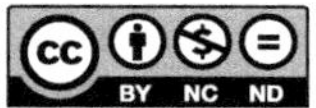
BY NC ND

9 Postoperative Imaging of Joints

Erin F. Alaia and Christoph Schäffeler

Learning Objectives:
- To discuss postoperative imaging of common shoulder, elbow, hip, knee, and ankle procedures, and to identify common complications and potential pitfalls.
- To discuss common complications following arthroplasty.

9.1 Shoulder

9.1.1 Imaging After Rotator Cuff (RC) Repair

RC reconstruction aims to restore tendon integrity by reattaching them to the humerus, typically with fixation by arthroscopic suture anchors (SAs). The transosseous-equivalent method uses two rows of SAs with lateral suture bridging for added stability [1]. Alternative techniques, such as open transosseous suturing or arthroscopic single- and double-row fixation with various SA types, may be chosen based on tear size, patient age, or can be found on images after surgery performed further back in time.

Shoulder radiography (AP and Neer views) helps assess humeral head alignment, SA placement, and detects osteolysis or joint degeneration. Progressive superior decentration suggests RC repair failure. Post-reconstruction MRI often shows variable T2 signal of the tendon due to metal artifact, fibrosis, or granulation tissue; elevated T2 signal is seen in over 90% of cases, usually normalizing within 3–12 months but sometimes persisting for years [2]. On MRI, the tendon may present thinner initially, and comparison with preoperative tendon images assists in interpretation [3]. Bone preparation and SA placement at the tuberosities during surgery may result in bone marrow edema (BME) like signal. Susceptibility artifacts are observed when metal anchors are implemented. Bioabsorbable SAs undergo hydrolysis, beginning with a peripheral fluid-equivalent film that progresses centrally and are replaced by bone tissue within roughly 2 years.

Impaired tendon integrity is the most reliable criterion for a retear (Fig. 9.1) [4]. Signs of a re-tear include progressive atrophy and fatty infiltration of muscle, fluid-filled tendon gaps, loss of continuity to the anchor site, and tendon retraction [1, 5]. The Sugaya classification on RC integrity is useful for evaluating postoperative tendons (Table 9.1) [6].

Standard MRI identifies full-thickness re-tears with a sensitivity of 91% and specificity of 84%. For partial tears, both sensitivity and specificity are 83% [7]. Studies on MR arthrography have found a sensitivity between 86% and 100%, and specificity from 59% to 100% [8, 9]. Although MR arthrography (MR-A) is preferred for assessing postoperative RC integrity, contrast medium passing from the joint into the subacromial space does not reliably indicate a RC retear. Even after successful repair, the RC is typically not watertight, as seen in the preoperative intact RC.

Additional postoperative complications associated with RC reconstruction include anchor loosening, material failure, shoulder stiffness with adhesive capsulitis, and infection.

Key Point
MR arthrography is the preferred imaging method to evaluate the shoulder after rotator cuff repair.

E. F. Alaia (✉)
Department of Radiology, NYU Langone Health, New York, NY, USA
e-mail: Erin.Fitzgerald@nyulangone.org

C. Schäffeler
Department of Radiology, Cantonal Hospital Grisons, Chur, Switzerland

J. Hodler et al. (eds.), *Musculoskeletal Diseases 2026-2029*, IDKD Springer Series, https://doi.org/10.1007/978-3-032-17040-8_9

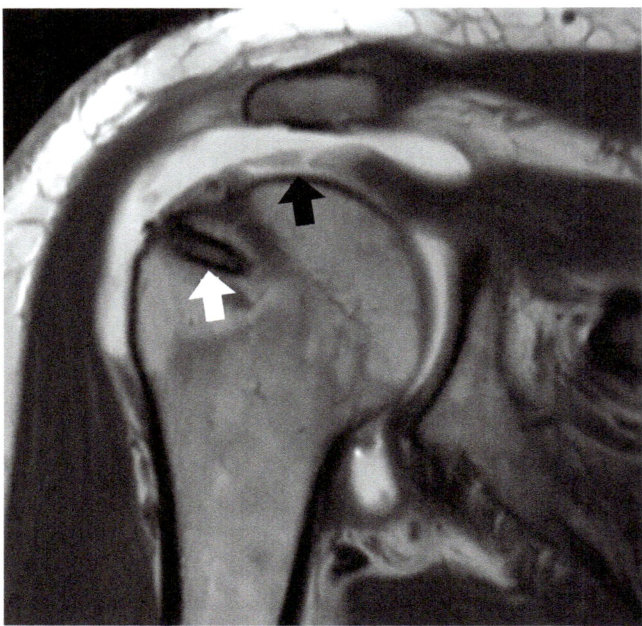

Fig. 9.1 Coronal T1-weighted MR arthrogram of the right shoulder after transosseous-equivalent supraspinatus reconstruction, with non-metallic suture anchor (white arrow). The black arrow shows a full-thickness re-tear of the posterior tendon

Table 9.1 Classification of postoperative rotator cuff integrity on T2-weighted MR images according to Sugaya [6]

Type I	Sufficient thickness compared with normal cuff; homogenous low signal intensity
Type II	Sufficient thickness compared with normal cuff; partial high-intensity area
Type III	Insufficient thickness – less than half the thickness compared with normal cuff, no discontinuity ➔ partial-thickness delaminated tear
Type IV	Minor discontinuity on 1 or 2 slices on both oblique coronal and sagittal images ➔ small full-thickness tear
Type V	Major discontinuity on >2 slices on both oblique coronal and sagittal images ➔ medium- or large full-thickness tear

9.1.2 Imaging After Surgery for Irreparable Rotator Cuff Tears

Extensive RC tears with muscle atrophy, fatty infiltration, and tendon retraction may lead to poor outcomes of tendon reconstruction. Reverse total shoulder arthroplasty (RTSA) is increasingly used in older patients to restore shoulder function by shifting the humeral center of rotation medially, enhancing deltoid tension, and allowing better movement and joint stability through a semi-constrained design [10]. However, greater reliance on deltoid-induced shoulder movement with impaired bone quality in this patient group increases the risk of acromion and scapular spine stress fractures, and careful review of follow-up radiographs, including axillary views, is essential [11].

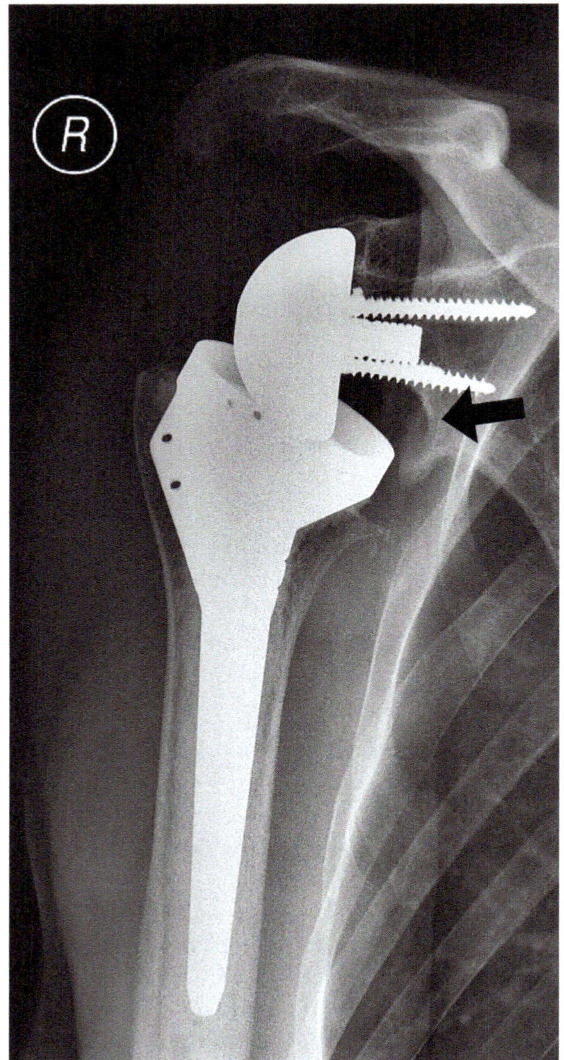

Fig. 9.2 Anteroposterior radiograph after reverse total shoulder arthroplasty shows advanced osteolysis at the inferior glenoid (arrow), consistent with scapular notching grade 4

Dislocation is the most common early complication after RTSA [12]. The progressive appearance of radiolucent lines greater than 2 mm adjacent to implants, as well as migration of components, are indications of loosening. Progressive radiolucency, periosteal reaction, or bone resorption may also be associated with infection. In situations where infection is suspected, MRI has the potential to identify sinus tracts, fluid collections, or lamellar synovitis [13]. Following RTSA, scapular notching, defined by osteolysis of the inferior glenoid neck near the metaglene of the prosthesis, is a common observation [14]. The Sirveaux classification categorizes the severity of scapular notching; lower degrees are generally regarded as benign. However, progression of scapular notching may contribute to glenoid component loosening and clinical failure of the prosthesis (Fig. 9.2).

RTSA should be avoided in patients <60 years of age presenting with irreparable RC tears and minimal arthrosis. Accordingly, a range of restorative procedures have been developed, including tendon transfer, bridging techniques, and superior capsular reconstruction (SCR).

SCR restores the shoulder's superior capsule using an acellular dermal or fascia lata graft, fixed via SA between glenoid and greater tuberosity. On MRI, the graft should be a low-signal band, at least 3 mm thick. Superior migration of the humeral head up to 5 mm may be normal but decentering over 10 mm indicates graft failure. Detachment of the graft from the humeral insertion is pathologic. Visible suture holes within 5 mm of the graft insertion are normal [15].

Tendon transfers (latissimus dorsi, lower trapezius for posterosuperior tears; pectoralis major for anterosuperior defects) improve function and pain, but osteoarthritis often progresses. Main complications include fluid-filled gaps representing tears, or avulsions. Latissimus dorsi transfer can lead to denervation edema of muscle if nerves are affected [16].

Interpositional grafts – biceps tendon, fascia lata, allografts, synthetics – are used to bridge irreparable tendon gaps and improved outcomes are reported [16].

Subacromial spacers can be used to manage irreparable RC tears by preventing humeral head elevation and helping center it in the glenoid, enabling the deltoid muscle to elevate the shoulder. The saline-inflated degradable balloon should dissolve within 2–12 months [16].

9.1.3 Imaging After Anatomic Stabilization

Particularly in young and active individuals there is a preference for early stabilizing surgery over conservative management. If glenoid bone loss is less than 10–20% and the labrum and anterior band of the inferior glenohumeral ligament (aIGHL) are present, anatomical repair of the anteroinferior labroligamentous complex (LLC) is possible.

Bankart repairs are typically performed arthroscopically. The LLC is mobilized, and the anterior glenoid rim is prepared. Three or more SAs, polyether ether ketone (PEEK), or bio-absorbable, are placed at the glenoid rim in the 3–5 o'clock position. The usage of metallic SAs is considered obsolete. Correct SA placement, especially the lowest one, is essential for adjusting aIGHL tension. Small bone fragments usually don't hinder soft tissue repairs, but larger Bankart fragments may require fixation with SAs or plates. Off-track Hill-Sachs defects may need allograft reconstruction or remplissage [17].

After Bankart repair, continuity from the glenoid to the humerus via the repaired labrum and aIGHL should be seen. Postoperative labra appear plump and rounded. Minor fraying or fluid entry is common, but significant fluid between the labrum and glenoid should not be present. BME and visible bioabsorbable anchors are expected findings depending on the timing of imaging. Capsulorrhaphy results in a thickened anterior capsule, and changes in aIGHL thickness are possible, with maintained continuity being crucial [18].

Failures are most often due to new trauma, technical errors (e.g., poor SA placement), rehabilitation issues, underestimated bone loss, labral defect expansion, or tissue hyperlaxity. On MRI, recurrent tears show fluid penetration at the labrum-glenoid interface. MR-A offers high sensitivity (100%) and specificity (85%) for detecting a re-tear [19]. Non-contrast MRI is somewhat less sensitive (80%). Granulation tissue may obscure retears, but abduction/external rotation (ABER) MR-A has the potential to enhance detection [18].

9.1.4 Imaging After Non-anatomic Stabilization

The most common non-anatomic shoulder stabilization method is coracoid transfer, either after Bristow (coracoid tip) or more commonly Latarjet (entire horizontal coracoid), including the conjoined tendon (Fig. 9.3) [20]. The coracoid

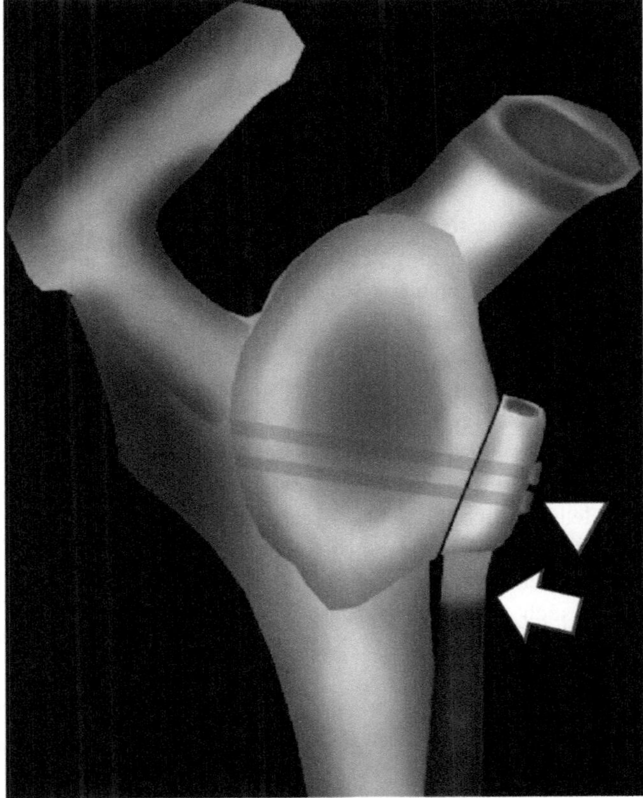

Fig. 9.3 Illustration of a normal Latarjet procedure, demonstrating the block of transferred coracoid bone augmenting the anteroinferior glenoid (arrowhead), with the intact conjoint tendon sling (arrow) acting as a dynamic stabilizer

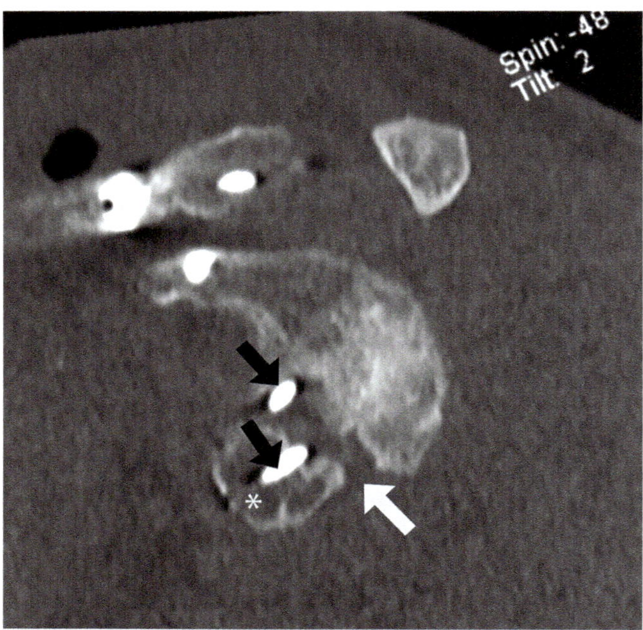

Fig. 9.4 Sagittal CT reformation of the shoulder after Latarjet procedure fixed with two screws (black arrows). There is marked osteolysis of the transferred coracoid bone block (asterisk) and evidence of non-union (white arrow)

bone block is fixed to the anteroinferior glenoid, producing a hammock effect that stabilizes the joint, particularly during ABER. This technique also augments significant glenoid bone defects and can be a primary or secondary treatment. Clinical outcomes are generally good, with low recurrence rates (3–9%).

Poor preparation, fixation, or healing can cause non-union, screw loosening, and fracture, detectable mainly by CT (Fig. 9.4). Bone block fractures (0–7%) often result from technical mishaps due to thin coracoid cortex or stress. Proper placement of the bone block (anteroinferior glenoid, flush with articular surface) and screws (perpendicular) is vital. Malposition risks non-union, instability, stiffness, osteolysis, osteoarthritis, or nerve/vessel injury [21].

Changes in biomechanics or reduced vascularization may lead to upper bone block resorption exposing the screw that can damage cartilage or irritate the subscapularis tendon. Infection occurs rarely (1–6%), usually subclinical. Signs such as screw loosening, non-union, or osteolysis warrant suspicion.

Key Point
Non-union and screw fracture are the most common complications after coracoid transfer.

9.2 Elbow

9.2.1 Imaging After Tendon Repair

Tendon repair procedures involving the biceps, triceps, common flexor (CF), and extensor (CE) tendon attachments are indicated for tears that are symptomatic or mechanically significant. Repair of medial and lateral tendon attachments generally utilizes sutures placed through drilled bone tunnels or secured with SAs. Triceps and biceps repair typically require larger bioabsorbable SAs, metallic buttons, or interference screws. The position of metallic buttons and other radiopaque material should be evaluated on radiographs.

Evaluation of postoperative MRI should focus on tendon integrity, possible loosening or migration of SAs and screws, and the quality of suture attachment to the tendon. On MRI, sutures appear as curvilinear low-signal structures linked to the anchor. Focal fluid signal at the tendon insertion and exposure of the SA site may suggest recurrent tendon tear or repair breakdown. Additionally, new tears may develop distant from the original implantation area. Cortical button fixation, particularly used for distal biceps tendon repair, may lead to heterotopic ossifications or even radioulnar synostosis.

Radiographs or CT can show implant loosening by the presence of lucency around a metallic SA or expansion of the SA site when a bioabsorbable implant is present. MRI findings of fluid signal surrounding the implant need careful interpretation for potential loosening or failure, particularly in bioabsorbable material. Displacement of an SA from the implant tunnel indicates repair failure.

A further complication of CE or CF tendon surgery includes potential injury to underlying ligaments, which may result in joint instability. At the medial epicondyle, injury to the ulnar nerve (UN) or the medial antebrachial cutaneous nerve is possible, and postoperative scar tissue can contribute to nerve impingement.

9.2.2 Imaging After Cubital Tunnel Release

Cubital tunnel (CuT) release or UN transposition is performed for ulnar compressive neuropathy caused by nerve impingement in the CuT. A retinaculum overlies the tunnel, which sits at the posteromedial elbow. Osteophytes, synovial proliferation, variant muscles, or triceps bundles can narrow this space, and injury is common due to its superficial position [22].

Surgery involves releasing the retinaculum and moving the UN anterior to the medial epicondyle. The procedure may involve simple decompression or nerve transposition (subcutaneous, intramuscular, or submuscular) [23]. Muscle coverage or the growth of scar tissue may cause further impingement. The medial antebrachial cutaneous nerve can be injured, causing medial forearm and olecranon skin numbness or pain.

The postoperative appearance following CuT release varies with surgical technique. In simple decompression, the UN may appear prominent with increased T2 signal and mild edema, while thickening or thinning of the CuT retinaculum can be seen [24]. Additional medial epicondylectomy often shows mild BME and increased signal at the CF tendon's origin. After anterior transposition, the UN courses anteriorly in the subcutaneous fat or deep to the flexor-pronator muscles in submuscular decompression. Signal changes, edema, and muscle atrophy are common. Failure of decompression may result from incomplete release, nerve instability, kinking, seroma, hematoma, or perineural fibrosis (Fig. 9.5) [24]. Key aspects for assessment should include course of the UN, caliber, signal, fascicular architecture, and perineural fat, although suspicious findings do not reliably predict symptom recurrence [25]. Focal changes of the UN at the retinaculum suggest incomplete decompression. If medial epicondylectomy is performed, partial tearing of the CF tendon may occur. Injury to the ulnar collateral ligament (UCL), especially after anterior transposition, should also be considered when evaluating persistent symptoms.

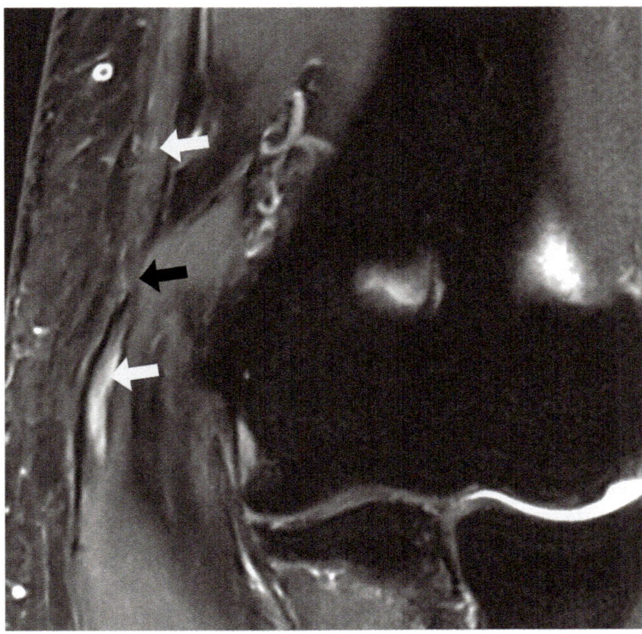

Fig. 9.5 Intermediate-weighted fat-suppressed coronal MR image of the elbow after transposition of the ulnar nerve. The ulnar nerve (white arrows) shows normal signal intensity proximal and increased signal distal with compression at the subfascial reentry (black arow)

Key Point

Assessment after ulnar nerve transposition should include course of the nerve, caliber, signal, fascicular architecture, and perineural fat fibrosis.

In overhead athletes, repeated valgus stress frequently causes injury to the UCL. The Tommy John procedure, which involves excising the damaged UCL and replacing it with a graft, is widely recognized among American baseball pitchers [23]. Typically, an autograft harvested from the palmaris longus tendon is utilized, although allografts are also an option. The graft is secured in a figure-of-eight pattern at the medial joint using intraosseous anchor material at the proximal ulna and medial epicondyle [22]. Additional UN transposition is commonly performed. Reports indicate that reconstruction failure often occurs at the proximal insertion site [26]. Characteristic indicators of graft disruption include visible discontinuity and evidence of joint fluid traversing from the medial recess of the joint into the adjacent soft tissues. MR-A of the elbow is considered particularly effective for identifying the leakage of joint fluid [27].

Repair of lateral elbow ligaments, particularly the lateral-ulnar collateral ligament (LUCL), is uncommon and generally follows significant trauma, such as elbow dislocation. Most traumatic tears occur at the proximal attachment and can usually be repaired using bioabsorbable SAs if conservative treatment fails. The resorption rate varies depending on composition. As bioabsorbable anchors and sutures are radiolucent, migration or loosening is best detected with ultrasound (US) or MRI. Properly placed SAs should not protrude from the bone; this would indicate possible failure. SA detachment or uncovered anchor sites can also be seen on MRI and suggest repair breakdown.

For chronic posterolateral instability due to LUCL tears, reconstruction with a tendon graft, like the Tommy John procedure, may be performed to restore stability [23].

9.3 Hip

9.3.1 Imaging After Labral Debridement or Repair

Arthroscopic hip surgery is commonly utilized for the treatment of symptomatic labral tears. The labrum may be debrided to remove any unstable flaps, degenerated labral tissue, or nondisplaced tears not amenable to repair, with the goal of preserving the maximal amount of labral tissue.

Following debridement, the labrum may appear attenuated on MRI, with loss of the native triangular morphology. If labral repair is performed, SAs will appear along the acetabular roof repair site [28, 29].

A labral re-tear may be diagnosed if surfacing fluid signal or injected gadolinium contrast is observed within the substance of the labrum or at the chondrolabral junction. Displaced labral tissue, unstable labral flap fragments, or displaced suture anchors may also indicate re-tear [28]. A labral re-tear may demonstrate formation of a paralabral cyst or distortion of labral tissue beyond what would be expected following debridement [29]. Correlation with preoperative imaging allows for a more confident diagnosis of labral re-tear if surfacing signal is seen in a new location when compared to the preoperative MRI [29].

9.3.2 Imaging After Femoroacetabular Impingement (FAI) Surgery

Arthroscopic surgery for FAI commonly includes resection of a femoral cam lesion. Femoral cam lesions appear as a bony protuberance or decreased offset at the femoral head-neck junction, producing an elevated alpha angle on preoperative imaging. Femoral cam lesions are treated with resection, or osteochondroplasty, which may produce a concave contour at the femoral-head neck junction (Fig. 9.6) [28]. Following femoral osteochondroplasty, the femoral alpha angle is expected to decrease when compared to the preoperative MRI, and subchondral signal alterations, such as edema-like signal and cystic change, may be observed [30]. The treated femoral cam lesion should be assessed for a possible complication of incomplete resection [28].

FAI surgery also commonly includes resection of an acetabular pincer lesion, an area of acetabular over-coverage which may appear global or focal (i.e., cranial retroversion) on preoperative imaging. Pincer lesions are treated with acetabuloplasty or acetabular rim resection [28]. Following pincer resection, the acetabular osseous margin may be attenuated or irregular, and subchondral marrow signal alterations and cystic change may be observed [30].

9.3.3 Imaging of the Post-operative Hip Joint Capsule

The hip joint capsule frequently demonstrates alterations following arthroscopic surgery. The hip joint capsule may demonstrate an anterior defect. Adhesions may form along the anterior femoral neck, appearing as an abnormally broad area of contact between capsular tissue and the anterior femoral neck margin. Additionally, the normal paralabral sulcus, located between the labrum and hip joint capsule, may be completely effaced, or display band-like adhesions between the labrum and joint capsule [31].

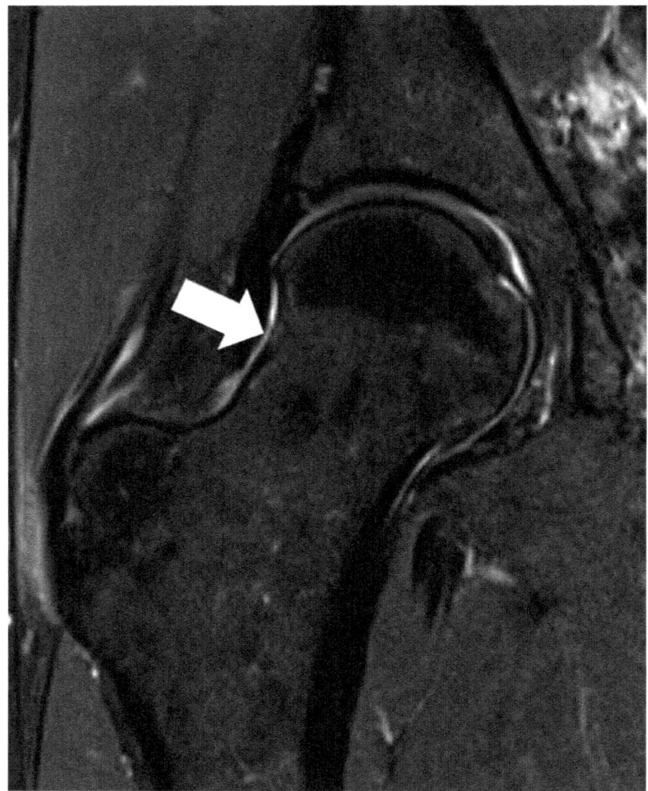

Fig. 9.6 Coronal proton density fat-suppressed image showing typical postoperative changes of femoral cam resection, with femoral osteochondroplasty producing a concave defect at the femoral head-neck junction (arrow)

9.4 Knee

9.4.1 Imaging After Meniscectomy or Meniscal Repair

The most common treatment options for a torn meniscus include meniscal repair and partial meniscectomy. Evolving treatment algorithms support an increased interest in repair and preservation of meniscal tissue whenever possible [32]. The decision to proceed with partial meniscectomy versus meniscal repair is influenced by tear location and morphology. Branches of the geniculate artery perforate the outer third of the meniscus, creating an environment that promotes healing of meniscal tissue, while the inner third of the meniscus is relatively avascular. Due to poorer healing potential, tears involving the inner third of the meniscus were classically treated with partial meniscectomy alone, but evolving treatments now support the repair of tears involving the avascular zone in selected patients [32].

Following partial meniscectomy, the meniscus may appear more deficient and irregular in contour when compared to native tissue. Degenerative intra-meniscal signal may reach an articular surface following partial meniscal resection, simulating a re-tear. Similarly, the repaired meniscus may demonstrate surfacing signal representing granulation tissue that should not be mistaken for re-tear. Thus, the criteria used to diagnose tear of the native meniscus cannot be used in the postoperative setting [33].

In the postoperative meniscus, the preoperative MRI and the operative report, when available, are essential tools to an accurate imaging diagnosis. Surfacing signal, a displaced flap of meniscal tissue, or new contour abnormality in a location remote from a treated tear based on preoperative imaging or the arthroscopic report can be reported as a new tear. In the area of prior treatment, a meniscal re-tear can be diagnosed if surfacing fluid-like signal or surfacing intra-articular contrast (in MR arthrography) is observed (Fig. 9.7), if there is a flap of displaced meniscal tissue, or if there is an irregular meniscal contour [33]. Development of a new parameniscal cyst may be a useful feature supporting the diagnosis of meniscal re-tear.

Meniscal root tears are commonly addressed with a transtibial root repair, in which sutures are passed through root tissue and shuttled through a tibial tunnel to reduce the meniscus to its osseous attachment. On the postoperative MRI, a transtibial root repair may demonstrate intermediate signal but meniscal tissue should remain in continuity. A root re-tear will demonstrate partial or complete discontinuity with fluid-like signal abnormality at the defect site [34]. The ipsilateral joint compartment should be inspected for new bone marrow edema-like signal, subchondral fracture, or progression of osteoarthritis.

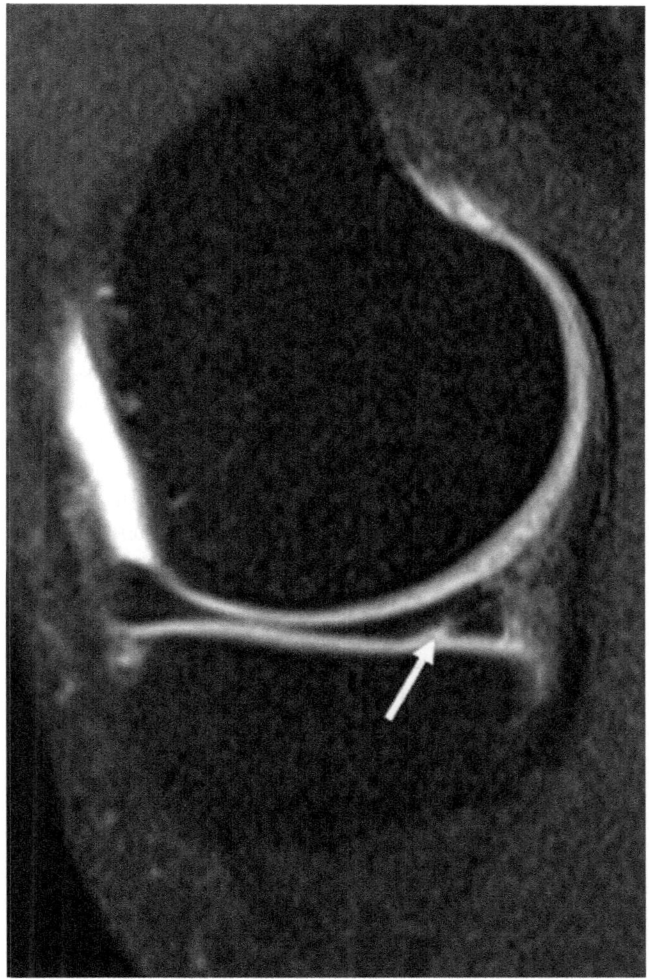

Fig. 9.7 Sagittal T1 fat-suppressed MR arthrogram image in a patient with prior meniscal repair shows surfacing imbibition of intra-articular contrast within the medial meniscal posterior horn (arrow), compatible with meniscal re-tear

9.4.2 Imaging After Anterior Cruciate Ligament (ACL) Reconstruction

Tears of the ACL are most commonly addressed with graft reconstruction in order to stabilize the knee and to prevent or delay the progression of osteoarthritis. Graft selection is impacted by surgeon preference and patient age and lifestyle factors. A bone-patellar tendon-bone autograft is commonly used, harvesting the central third of the patellar tendon with contiguous bone plugs harvested from the inferior patella and the tibial tuberosity. Alternate graft choices may include a hamstring or quadriceps tendon graft, or a bone-patellar tendon-bone allograft [35].

Graft isometry is critical for optimized graft function and longevity, and the graft is commonly transfixed with hardware such as interference screws or an endobutton to maintain isometry during the process of incorporation. The inferior margin of the femoral tunnel is positioned at the intersection of Blumensaat's line and the posterior cortex of the femur in the sagittal plane, and in the coronal plane has an opening along the posterior superolateral intercondylar notch. The tibial tunnel is oriented parallel to the Blumensaat line, with the tunnel opening positioned posterior to the intersection of Blumensaat's line with the tibia [35]. The normal graft undergoes a process of ligamentization, in which the tendon graft biomechanically functions as a ligament and as a result of this new environment undergoes histologic changes of a ligament. Graft ligamentization on MRI may appear as high graft signal on fluid-sensitive images up to 4 years postoperatively [36]. Multi-strand grafts, such as the hamstring, may demonstrate fluid signal oriented parallel to graft fibers [35]. These normal evolving findings of an ACL graft should not be mistaken for graft failure or tear.

An anterior malposition of the tibial tunnel may cause the graft to become impinged by the roof of the intercondylar notch, a complication known as roof impingement. On MRI, the tibial tunnel will appear anterior in position, and the graft may appear kinked, focally high in signal, and may display partial or complete rupture if left untreated [35].

Focal or diffuse arthrofibrosis may occur and will present clinically with limited extension. The more common process of focal arthrofibrosis, known as the "cyclops lesion", appears on MRI as a rounded area of soft tissue within the intercondylar notch adjacent to the opening of the tibial tunnel. The less common diffuse form demonstrates band-like soft tissue which may extend around the graft, into the suprapatellar recess, Hoffa's fat, and along the joint capsule [35].

Tear of the ACL graft requires a multiplanar evaluation for graft integrity. On MRI, a graft tear will demonstrate fiber discontinuity, graft attenuation, and high graft signal on fluid-sensitive images (Fig. 9.8). The torn graft may appear abnormally redundant or horizontal in orientation, and in the chronic setting may be completely resorbed. Kissing contusions of the lateral femoral condyle and the posterior lateral tibial plateau, resulting from a pivot-shift injury mechanism, are the most useful secondary features supporting a diagnosis of graft tear. Other features supportive of graft tear include anterior tibial translation and uncovering of the posterior horn of the lateral meniscus [37].

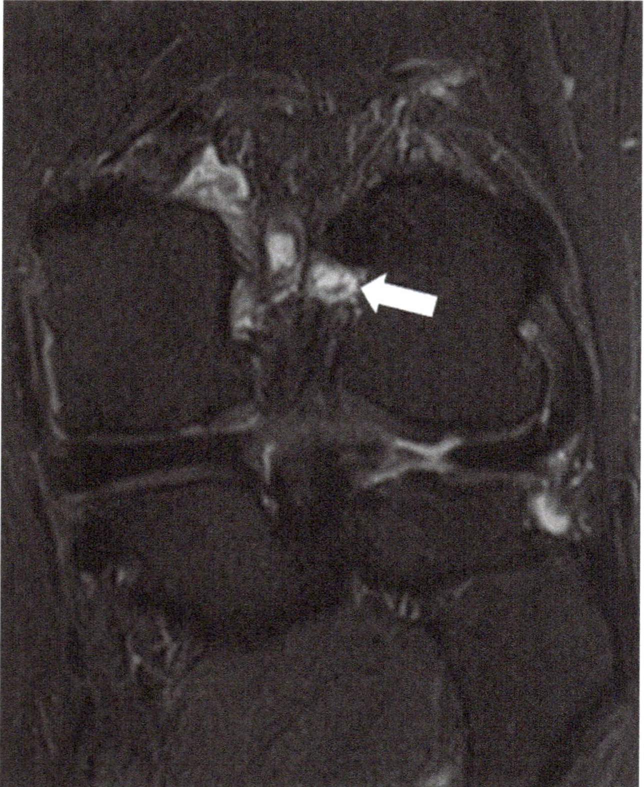

Fig. 9.8 Coronal proton density fat-suppressed image showing a complete ACL graft tear, with fluid-filled gap (arrow) at the interface of the proximal graft and the femoral tunnel

> **Key Point**
> During the normal process of ligamentization, the ACL graft may appear high in signal, findings which should not be misinterpreted as graft failure.

9.4.3 Imaging After Cartilage Repair

Cartilage intrinsically has poor regenerative capacity owing to a combination of poor vascularity and a limited number of chondrocytes. Surgical repair, therefore, may be indicated to repair cartilage or restore the osteochondral unit. The most common surgical options include chondroplasty, marrow stimulation, osteochondral autograft transfer (OATS), osteochondral allograft implantation, and cell-based repair.

Chondroplasty is an effective and low-cost option in which chondral-based lesions are debrided and smoothed [38]. The postoperative MRI may show resection of chondral flap lesions and a more attenuated and smoothed appearance of the articular surface. Marrow stimulation is most commonly performed with microfracture, reserved for small (<2 cm^2) chondral-based lesions. Microfracture involves the penetration of subchondral bone, allowing pluripotent stem cells to migrate to the articular surface and form fibrocartilage, biomechanically inferior to normal hyaline cartilage, which in combination with subchondral bone plate trauma results in poor long-term outcomes [38]. Cell-based restoration, most commonly with autologous chondrocyte implantation (ACI), is a 2-stage procedure used for chondral lesions ≥ 2 cm^2. In the primary surgery, chondrocytes are harvested from a relatively non-weight-bearing articular surface of the knee and are cultured ex vivo. Chondrocytes are then implanted back into the knee via a collagen membrane in the second-stage surgery [38].

Small (≤ 3 cm^2) osteochondral lesions may be addressed with OATS, in which a small osteochondral plug is transferred from a lesser weight-bearing portion of the knee and transferred to the site of osteochondral injury. OATS has the advantage of an autograft transfer, promoting early integration and transfer of hyaline cartilage, with a potential disadvantage of morbidity at the donor site, limiting the procedure to the treatment of small lesions [38]. Larger osteochondral lesions (≥ 2 cm^2) are typically treated with osteochondral allograft transplantation, allowing for durable restoration of an osteochondral injury with hyaline cartilage [38].

The Magnetic Resonance Observation of Cartilage Repair Tissue (MOCART) 2.0 Atlas is commonly used for research of chondral repair tissue [39]. Clinically, the MOCART Atlas may be useful in guiding the search pattern and descriptors for chondral repair tissue. The MOCART scoring system assesses the structure of chondral repair tissue, including the volume of defect infill, the integration of repair tissue with native cartilage, as well as the surface, structure, and signal of repair tissue. The structure of subchondral bone is assessed for defects or bony overgrowth, and the subchondral marrow is assessed for edema-like signal, cystic change, or osteonecrosis [39]. It is important to consider the time interval from surgery and longitudinal findings when assessing chondral repair tissue on MRI. For example, autologous chondrocyte implantation and microfracture are expected to show incomplete infill in the early postoperative state, with complete infill after approximately 1–2 years. Bone marrow edema-like signal may be observed in the postoperative state but should gradually resolve [40].

9.5 Ankle

9.5.1 Achilles Tendon

In cases of acute Achilles tendon (AT) rupture, surgical intervention is recommended if there is inadequate approximation of the tendon edges during passive plantar flexion. Reconstruction is achieved through a direct end-to-end anastomosis via various suture patterns [41]. To achieve increased AT strength or for chronic tears and significantly retracted tendon stumps, augmentation and reconstruction procedures are often necessary [42]. These procedures are commonly performed using local tendon autografts, such as the gracilis, peroneus brevis, or flexor hallucis longus tendons. The postoperative appearance of the AT varies depending on the timing of examination. A residual gap at the anastomosis, which appears T2 hyperintense due to vascular ingrowth and granulation tissue, may be present for up to 4 weeks. This tissue is typically replaced by fibrous tissue over 6–14 weeks, resulting in a reduction of the T2 signal at the anastomosis. However, T2 heterogeneity can persist for up to 12 months following suturing [43]. Generally, the postoperative AT remains noticeably thickened (about 10 cm in diameter) compared to a native healthy tendon; however, in the long-term, MRI should demonstrate hypointensity on all imaging sequences [41, 42].

Delayed healing is a common problem after open repair and affects 2–10% of patients. This is related to limited blood supply to the AT and often to underlying comorbidities of patients, which may impair wound healing. In cases of incomplete healing or intrasubstantial degeneration, MRI may show linear intermediate signal intensity within the non-insertional fibers.

After AT repair, there is an increased risk of tendon re-rupture due to reduced tendon strength, although the incidence of re-rupture is reported to be less than 5% [42]. US and MRI reliably can detect re-rupture following the same signs as native AT injury: presence of a tendon gap filled with fluid or hematoma and tendon retraction.

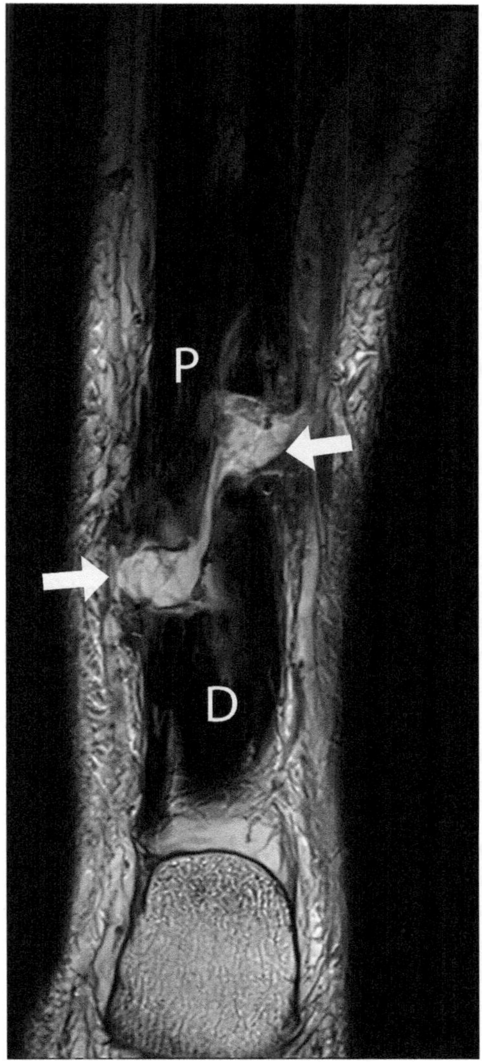

Fig. 9.9 Coronal T2-weighted MR image of the Achilles tendon in a 35-year-old male in recovery after shortening Z-plasty and recent misstep. Note the fluid accumulation (arrows) between the separated proximal (P) and distal (D) Achilles tendon parts consistent with suture breakdown

Previous AT injuries may cause either lengthening, which reduces force transmission, or more frequently, shortening with limited mobility. To lengthen the tendon, a Z-plasty involves making Z-shaped incisions that allow extension as the tissue heals. For shortening, tendon tissue is removed via a Z-shaped tenotomy and subsequent reattachment (Fig. 9.9).

9.5.2 Peroneal Tendons

Surgical intervention is required for significant tears or dislocation of the peroneal tendons, more common the peroneus brevis tendon (PBT). When possible, the tendon can be preserved through debridement, but tenodesis of the

PBT to the peroneus longus is often needed, either proximally or distally in relation to the fibular tip. If both tendons are irreparable, they should be replaced with either the flexor hallucis or digitorum longus tendon; bridging procedures with auto- or allografts are possible [44]. Dislocations may require extensive procedures such as superior peroneal retinaculum reconstruction, fibular osteotomy, posterior fibular groove deepening, or complete rerouting of the peroneal tendons [45].

In addition to early complications such as infection and hematoma, patients may experience specific late complications including recurrent tendon degeneration, tears, dislocations, and the formation of peritendinous adhesions. In the postoperative period, dynamic US is an effective modality for assessing the mobility of the repaired tendon, particularly when adhesions are suspected. Typically, increased echogenicity is observed following surgery, attributable to the presence of sutures, granulation tissue, and scar development. Indicators of tendon re-rupture include the absence of tendon visualization, tendon retraction, and disruption of suture integrity. The criteria for re-rupture are likewise applicable to MRI [41]. However, MRI offers enhanced visualization of the surgical intervention and facilitates the evaluation of tendon healing. Elevated T2 signal is considered within normal limits for up to 12 months postoperatively; by approximately 24 months, the postoperative tendon should typically demonstrate homogeneous T2 hypointense appearance [46]. Indicators of delayed healing or recurrent degeneration include persistent or newly developed alterations in tendon diameter and T2 signal intensity after this period.

9.5.3 Posterior Tibial Tendon (PTT) and Flatfoot Deformity

In advanced cases of pes planovalgus, surgical management includes PTT repair, midfoot and hindfoot osteotomy along with spring ligament repair and flexor digitorum longus (FDL) tendon transfer to support a compromised PTT. However, there is currently no consensus on the optimal surgical technique, and postoperative imaging outcomes can differ based on the chosen method [47].

For FDL tendon transfer procedures, the distal attachment site depends on the integrity of the plantar slip of the PTT. If the plantar slip remains intact, the FDL is typically sutured directly to the distal PTT; otherwise, anchoring to the navicular bone is preferred. This technique often involves passing the FDL tendon through a bone tunnel in the navicular tuberosity, transferring it from the plantar to the dorsal aspect, and securing it either by anchoring or tendon-to-tendon repair [45].

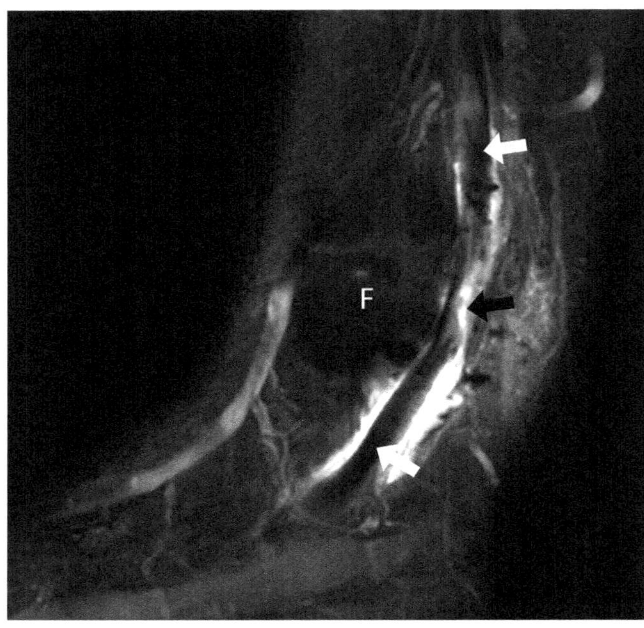

Fig. 9.10 Sagittal intermediate-weighted MR images after posterior tibial tendon (white arrows) repair. Note focal substantial thinning of the tendon (black arrow), representing a partial re-tear

Postoperative imaging is valuable for detecting complications associated with FDL tendon transfer, such as avulsion of the transferred tendon leading to recurrence of pes planus deformity. Other issues include tendinosis of the FDL or residual PTT, which may present clinically as pain and swelling and may be related to suture material reaction [45]. MRI can demonstrate tendon thinning or thickening, increased T2 signal, and peritendinous fibrosis (Fig. 9.10). Differentiating between normal postsurgical changes and symptomatic tendinosis can be difficult. US may provide greater sensitivity in certain instances by precisely localizing tenderness and revealing hyperemia via Doppler imaging, commonly seen in symptomatic individuals [48].

9.5.4 Collateral Ligament Reconstruction

The lateral ligaments of the ankle are commonly injured, with conservative treatment typically being effective. Surgical intervention may be considered when chronic instability of the ankle joint is identified. There are anatomical and non-anatomical stabilization procedures; however, current practice does not generally recommend non-anatomical approaches. Anatomical procedures encompass direct ligament repair, anatomical reconstruction, and ligamentoplasty using grafts. The Broström technique and its modifications are currently regarded as standard surgical options for stabilizing the lateral ankle joint. However, radiologists may still observe non-anatomical procedures such as the Watson-

Jones, Evans, and Chrisman-Snook techniques when interpreting imaging studies [49]. These procedures commonly utilize the peroneus brevis tendon, which is routed through various osseous tunnels to provide stabilization, depending on the specific technique used.

Injuries to the medial collateral ligament of the ankle are generally managed through conservative treatment methods. Should these prove insufficient, surgical interventions may be considered. Anatomical repair is feasible when the ligament tissue quality is adequate, in instances of significant tissue damage, grafting techniques may be employed.

Recurrent trauma occurs and can injure a reconstructed ligament, leading to instability. Imaging findings for rerupture are like those of primary injuries [42]. Arthrofibrosis of the ankle joint, a late complication seen as fibrotic capsule thickening (up to 6 mm), initially shows intermediate T2 signal and later appears homogeneously hypointense on T2-weighted MRI scans [50]. Ankle instability increases the risk of premature osteoarthrosis; thus, careful postoperative imaging evaluation of the tibiotalar and subtalar joints is necessary [41].

9.6 MRI of Hip and Knee Arthroplasty Complications

9.6.1 Fracture and Stress Reaction

On MRI, periprosthetic stress reaction may demonstrate bone marrow and/or cortical edema and periostitis, without a fracture line. A low-signal fracture line traversing the cortex or the medullary canal will confirm the presence of a periprosthetic fracture. Periprosthetic hip fractures most commonly occur along the femoral shaft, while periprosthetic knee fractures most commonly occur within the patella, followed by the supracondylar femur, and least commonly the tibia. Normal edema-like signal along the medullary canal resulting from surgical reaming or apparent high signal resulting from susceptibility artifact are important mimics and should not be overcalled as stress reaction [51, 52].

9.6.2 Aseptic Loosening

Solid osseous fixation is required for optimal function and durability of arthroplasties, achieved through the bony trabecular ingrowth onto porous-coated non-cemented arthroplasty systems or bone cementation in a cemented prosthesis. Mechanical stress resulting from micromotion along the interface of host bone and the arthroplasty or cement allows for synoviocyte migration along these interfaces, forming a synovial or fibrous membrane, and activating osteoclasts to resorb bone. This fibrous membrane will appear as a thin (1–2 mm) intermediate to high-signal interface between the bone and arthroplasty or cement, with a more pronounced (>2 mm) interface indicating bone resorption. A diagnosis of aseptic loosening can be made in cases of circumferential resorption, and may show secondary features of implant subsidence, rotation, or displacement [51, 52].

9.6.3 Polyethylene Wear and Osteolysis

Progressive wear of a polyethylene liner is a slowly evolving process which results from the shedding of polyethylene particles which are phagocytosed by macrophages and incite an inflammatory reaction, which in turn activates osteoclasts to resorb bone. On MRI, the inflamed synovium will appear thickened and proliferated with internal debris and pseudocapsular expansion. Osteolysis will appear as geographic, often rounded areas of intermediate signal abnormality along the arthroplasty interface [51]. Osteolysis may occasionally result in substantial bone loss which may complicate future revision arthroplasties [53].

9.6.4 Adverse Local Tissue Reaction

Adverse local tissue reaction is an inclusive term for the adverse consequences of hip arthroplasty metal components. Metal arthroplasty components may provoke an immune response similar to a type 4 hypersensitivity reaction. In the most advanced presentation, patients may present with aseptic lymphocytic vasculitis-associated lesion (ALVAL), which may potentially lead to aggressive destruction of the periprosthetic soft tissues requiring an early revision arthroplasty [53]. MRI in patients with adverse tissue reaction will demonstrate the presence of an expanded pseudocapsule with frequent pseudocapsular dehiscence, with the formation of bulky periprosthetic mass-like synovial debris, or "pseudotumors" which may compress or compromise regional nerves and tendons (Fig. 9.11) [51].

Metallosis in hip arthroplasty systems may occur in response to the shedding of metallic debris, which on MRI will demonstrate synovitis with low-signal metallic debris which may locally erode periprosthetic bone and may be taken up by regional lymph nodes which may appear low in signal [51].

9.6.5 Infection

In addition to clinical and laboratory markers, MRI is a useful diagnostic tool in the workup of suspected prosthetic joint injection. Prosthetic joint infections will demonstrate the presence of a joint effusion with synovitis and may have

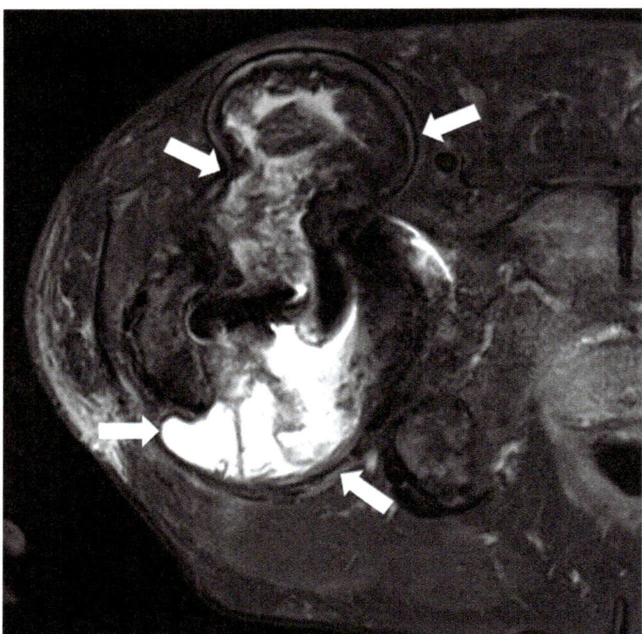

Fig. 9.11 Axial STIR image in a patient with a total hip arthroplasty complicated by adverse local tissue reaction with anterior and posterior pseudocapsular dehiscence and bulky pseudotumor formation (arrows)

a layered, or lamellated appearance of the synovial lining. Ancillary features which support the presence of a prosthetic joint infection include a sinus tract leading to the skin surface, periprosthetic fluid collections, regional soft tissue edema, and enlarged, reactive inguinal lymph nodes. Patients with coexistent osteomyelitis will demonstrate confluent low T1 marrow signal changes. A diagnostic aspiration is required to definitively confirm or rule out the presence of periprosthetic infection [51].

Key Point
Presence of a joint effusion, sinus tracts, periprosthetic edema and fluid collections, and enlarged lymph nodes are features supporting a diagnosis of prosthetic joint infection.

9.6.6 Imaging of Hip-Specific Arthroplasty Complications

Hip arthroplasties may result in iliopsoas tendinopathy, impingement, or iliopsoas bursitis, which may be the result of the compression of an oversized or proud acetabular cup. The gluteal tendons may demonstrate evidence of tendinosis, tears, or trochanteric bursal fluid. Nerve injury may occur due to intraoperative transection or ischemia or due to local compression which may result from heterotopic bone, hematoma, malpositioned arthroplasty hardware, or bulky pseudotumor formation. Nerve injury may also occur after an arthroplasty dislocation event [51].

9.6.7 Imaging of Knee-Specific Arthroplasty Complications

Patellar clunk is a complication unique to knee arthroplasties, appearing on MRI as a mass-like formation of fibrous tissue in the region of the quadriceps fat pad. This fibrous tissue produces a clunk sensation as it moves into the intercondylar notch in flexion and is displaced in extension. Other observed complications of knee arthroplasty include tendinosis or tear of the patellar or quadriceps tendon [52].

9.7 Concluding Remarks

This comprehensive review discussed common surgeries and complications of major joints, including the shoulder, elbow, hip, knee, and ankle, as well as common complications following arthroplasty. Postoperative imaging should be interpreted with an understanding of the procedure performed with comparison to preoperative, intraoperative, and postoperative imaging. In addition to common complications, it is imperative to appreciate acceptable imaging findings in the postoperative state which should not be misinterpreted as abnormality or surgical failure.

Take Home Messages

- Accurate interpretation of postoperative imaging requires a clear understanding of the surgery performed, with review of the operative report or consultation with the referring surgeon if needed.
- When available, imaging should be read in the context of any available preoperative imaging, intraoperative imaging, and earlier postoperative imaging.
- Common complications of and acceptable postoperative imaging findings of each surgery should be recognized.

Conflict of Interest I/We declare no competing interests as defined by Springer Nature or other interests that might be perceived to influence results and/or discussion reported in this manuscript.

References

1. Duquin TR, Buyea C, Bisson LJ. Which method of rotator cuff repair leads to the highest rate of structural healing? A systematic review. Am J Sports Med. 2010;38(4):835–41.
2. Spielmann AL, Forster BB, Kokan P, Hawkins RH, Janzen DL. Shoulder after rotator cuff repair: MR imaging findings

in asymptomatic individuals—initial experience. Radiology. 1999;213(3):705–8.
3. Crim J, Burks R, Manaster BJ, Hanrahan C, Hung M, Greis P. Temporal evolution of MRI findings after arthroscopic rotator cuff repair. AJR Am J Roentgenol. 2010;195(6):1361–6.
4. Saccomanno MF, Cazzato G, Fodale M, Sircana G, Milano G. Magnetic resonance imaging criteria for the assessment of the rotator cuff after repair: a systematic review. Knee Surg Sports Traumatol Arthrosc. 2015;23(2):423–42.
5. Goutallier D, Postel JM, Bernageau J, Lavau L, Voisin MC. Fatty muscle degeneration in cuff ruptures. Pre- and postoperative evaluation by CT scan. Clin Orthop Relat Res. 1994;304:78–83.
6. Sugaya H, Maeda K, Matsuki K, Moriishi J. Functional and structural outcome after arthroscopic full-thickness rotator cuff repair: single-row versus dual-row fixation. Arthroscopy. 2005;21(11):1307–16.
7. Magee T, Shapiro M, Hewell G, Williams D. Complications of rotator cuff surgery in which bioabsorbable anchors are used. AJR Am J Roentgenol. 2003;181(5):1227–31.
8. Duc SR, Mengiardi B, Pfirrmann CW, Jost B, Hodler J, Zanetti M. Diagnostic performance of MR arthrography after rotator cuff repair. AJR Am J Roentgenol. 2006;186(1):237–41.
9. Tudisco C, Bisicchia S, Savarese E, Fiori R, Bartolucci DA, Masala S, et al. Single-row vs. double-row arthroscopic rotator cuff repair: clinical and 3 tesla MR arthrography results. BMC Musculoskelet Disord. 2013;14:43.
10. Rugg CM, Coughlan MJ, Lansdown DA. Reverse Total shoulder arthroplasty: biomechanics and indications. Curr Rev Musculoskelet Med. 2019;12(4):542–53.
11. Levy JC, Anderson C, Samson A. Classification of postoperative acromial fractures following reverse shoulder arthroplasty. J Bone Joint Surg Am. 2013;95(15):e104.
12. Boileau P. Complications and revision of reverse total shoulder arthroplasty. Orthop Traumatol Surg Res. 2016;102(1 Suppl):S33–43.
13. Lee DH, Choi YS, Potter HG, Endo Y, Sivakumaran T, Lim TK, et al. Reverse total shoulder arthroplasty: an imaging overview. Skeletal Radiol. 2020;49(1):19–30.
14. Sirveaux F, Favard L, Oudet D, Huquet D, Walch G, Mole D. Grammont inverted total shoulder arthroplasty in the treatment of glenohumeral osteoarthritis with massive rupture of the cuff. Results of a multicentre study of 80 shoulders. J Bone Joint Surg Br. 2004;86(3):388–95.
15. Samim M, Walsh P, Gyftopoulos S, Meislin R, Beltran LS. Postoperative MRI of massive rotator cuff tears. AJR Am J Roentgenol. 2018;211(1):146–54.
16. Cvetanovich GL, Waterman BR, Verma NN, Romeo AA. Management of the irreparable rotator cuff tear. J Am Acad Orthop Surg. 2019;27(24):909–17.
17. Boileau P, McClelland WB Jr, O'Shea K, Vargas P, Pinedo M, Old J, et al. Arthroscopic Hill-Sachs Remplissage with Bankart repair: strategy and technique. JBJS Essent Surg Tech. 2014;4(1):e4.
18. Sugimoto H, Suzuki K, Mihara K, Kubota H, Tsutsui H. MR arthrography of shoulders after suture-anchor Bankart repair. Radiology. 2002;224(1):105–11.
19. Magee T. Imaging of the post-operative shoulder: does injection of iodinated contrast in addition to MR contrast during arthrography improve diagnostic accuracy and patient throughput? Skeletal Radiol. 2018;47(9):1253–61.
20. Latarjet M. Treatment of recurrent dislocation of the shoulder. Lyon Chir. 1954;49(8):994–7.
21. Métais P. Failure of coracoid bone-block. Orthop Traumatol Surg Res. 2021;107(1s):102782.
22. Lo L, Ashimolowo T, Beltran LS. Postoperative MR imaging of the elbow. Magn Reson Imaging Clin N Am. 2022;30(4):629–43.
23. Deely DM, Morrison WB. Imaging the postoperative elbow. Semin Musculoskelet Radiol. 2021;25(4):628–36.
24. Rhodes NG, Howe BM, Frick MA, Moran SL. MR imaging of the postsurgical cubital tunnel: an imaging review of the cubital tunnel, cubital tunnel syndrome, and associated surgical techniques. Skeletal Radiol. 2019;48(10):1541–54.
25. Bucknor MD, Stevens KJ, Steinbach LS. Elbow imaging in sport: sports imaging series. Radiology. 2016;280(1):328.
26. Daniels SP, Mintz DN, Endo Y, Dines JS, Sneag DB. Imaging of the post-operative medial elbow in the overhead thrower: common and abnormal findings after ulnar collateral ligament reconstruction and ulnar nerve transposition. Skeletal Radiol. 2019;48(12):1843–60.
27. Wear SA, Thornton DD, Schwartz ML, Weissmann RC 3rd, Cain EL, Andrews JR. MRI of the reconstructed ulnar collateral ligament. AJR Am J Roentgenol. 2011;197(5):1198–204.
28. Kassarjian A, Isern-Kebschull J, Tomas X. Postoperative hip MR imaging. Magn Reson Imaging Clin N Am. 2022;30(4):673–88.
29. Blankenbaker DG, De Smet AA, Keene JS. MR arthrographic appearance of the postoperative acetabular labrum in patients with suspected recurrent labral tears. AJR Am J Roentgenol. 2011;197(6):W1118–22.
30. Foreman SC, Zhang AL, Neumann J, von Schacky CE, Souza RB, Majumdar S, et al. Postoperative MRI findings and associated pain changes after arthroscopic surgery for Femoroacetabular impingement. AJR Am J Roentgenol. 2020;214(1):177–84.
31. Kim CO, Dietrich TJ, Zingg PO, Dora C, Pfirrmann CWA, Sutter R. Arthroscopic hip surgery: frequency of postoperative MR Arthrographic findings in asymptomatic and symptomatic patients. Radiology. 2017;283(3):779–88.
32. Bansal S, Floyd ER, Aikman E, Elrod P, Burkey K, et al. Meniscal repair: the current state and recent advances in augmentation. J Orthop Res. 2021;39(7):1368–82.
33. Kijowski R, Rosas H, Williams A, Liu F. MRI characteristics of torn and untorn post-operative menisci. Skeletal Radiol. 2017;46(10):1353–60.
34. Palisch AR, Winters RR, Willis MH, Bray CD, Shybut TB. Posterior root meniscal tears: preoperative, intraoperative, and postoperative imaging for transtibial pullout repair. Radiographics. 2016;36(6):1792–806.
35. Meyers AB, Haims AH, Menn K, Moukaddam H. Imaging of anterior cruciate ligament repair and its complications. AJR Am J Roentgenol. 2010;194(2):476–84.
36. Saupe N, White LM, Chiavaras MM, Essue J, Weller I, Kunz M, et al. Anterior cruciate ligament reconstruction grafts: MR imaging features at long-term follow-up—correlation with functional and clinical evaluation. Radiology. 2008;249(2):581–90.
37. Bencardino JT, Beltran J, Feldman MI, Rose DJ. MR imaging of complications of anterior cruciate ligament graft reconstruction. Radiographics. 2009;29(7):2115–26.
38. Dekker TJ, Aman ZS, DePhillipo NN, Dickens JF, Anz AW, LaPrade RF. Chondral lesions of the knee: an evidence-based approach. J Bone Joint Surg Am. 2021;103(7):629–45.
39. Schreiner MM, Raudner M, Marlovits S, Bohndorf K, Weber M, Zalaudek M, et al. The MOCART (magnetic resonance observation of cartilage repair tissue) 2.0 knee score and atlas. Cartilage. 2021;13(1_suppl):571S–87S.
40. Liu YW, Tran MD, Skalski MR, Patel DB, White EA, Tomasian A, et al. MR imaging of cartilage repair surgery of the knee. Clin Imaging. 2019;58:129–39.

41. Merkle AN, Moon DK, Selan JN, Lowry MKJ. Postoperative imaging of the ankle: ligament and tendon reconstruction. Semin Musculoskelet Radiol. 2025;29(1):93–111.
42. Shrestha R, Sill AP, Haug LP, Patel KA, Kile TA, Fox MG. Postoperative ankle imaging, 2022. Semin Musculoskelet Radiol. 2022;26(3):203–15.
43. Fujikawa A, Kyoto Y, Kawaguchi M, Naoi Y, Ukegawa Y. Achilles tendon after percutaneous surgical repair: serial MRI observation of uncomplicated healing. AJR Am J Roentgenol. 2007;189(5):1169–74.
44. Stamatis ED, Karaoglanis GC. Salvage options for peroneal tendon ruptures. Foot Ankle Clin. 2014;19(1):87–95.
45. Abou Diwan R, Badr S, Boulil Y, Demondion X, Maynou C, Cotten A. Presurgical perspective and postsurgical evaluation of non-Achilles tendons of the ankle and retinaculum. Semin Musculoskelet Radiol. 2022;26(6):670–83.
46. Vega J, Batista JP, Golano P, Dalmau A, Viladot R. Tendoscopic groove deepening for chronic subluxation of the peroneal tendons. Foot Ankle Int. 2013;34(6):832–40.
47. Jesse MK, Hunt KJ, Strickland C. Postoperative imaging of the ankle. AJR Am J Roentgenol. 2018;211(3):496–505.
48. Dimmick S, Chhabra A, Grujic L, Linklater JM. Acquired flat foot deformity: postoperative imaging. Semin Musculoskelet Radiol. 2012;16(3):217–32.
49. Perez A, Vega J, Llopis E, Cerezal L. Presurgical perspective and postsurgical evaluation of instability and microinstability secondary to ankle ligaments injury. Semin Musculoskelet Radiol. 2022;26(6):644–55.
50. Velasco BT, Patel SS, Broughton KK, Frumberg DB, Kwon JY, Miller CP. Arthrofibrosis of the ankle. Foot Ankle Orthop. 2020;5(4):2473011420970463.
51. Fritz J, Lurie B, Miller TT, Potter HG. MR imaging of hip arthroplasty implants. Radiographics. 2014;34(4):E106–32.
52. Fritz J, Lurie B, Potter HG. MR imaging of knee arthroplasty implants. Radiographics. 2015;35(5):1483–501.
53. Burge AJ. Update on MR imaging of hip arthroplasty. Magn Reson Imaging Clin N Am. 2025;33(1):155–65.

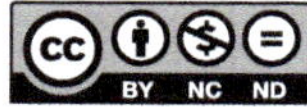

Musculoskeletal Tumors: Current State and Future Directions of MRI, Artificial Intelligence, and Structured Reporting Systems

10

Hillary W. Garner and Mark D. Murphey

Learning Objectives
- Describe important imaging features that allow optimal characterization and local staging of bone and soft tissue masses.
- Describe the current roles, limitations, and future directions of artificial intelligence (AI) tools into musculoskeletal oncologic imaging workflows.
- Describe the current state of structured reporting systems for bone and soft tissue lesions.

10.1 Introduction

The role of imaging in evaluating soft tissue, bone, and bone marrow tumors remains central to patient care. Most primary bone tumors and soft tissue lesions are benign, but distinguishing malignant from benign lesions is critical, as certain types of soft tissue and bone sarcomas are aggressive and associated with 5-year mortality rates exceeding 30% [1, 2]. Although radiographs, ultrasound, computed tomography (CT), and positron emission tomography (PET)/CT each have important roles, magnetic resonance imaging (MRI) remains the gold standard for tumor characterization. The readily apparent MRI features, including tumor size, margin, internal signal complexity, and surrounding tissue involvement, are currently the primary imaging parameters used for diagnosis and initial management in clinical practice. Functional MRI techniques may also be used to supplement morphologic tumor assessment. Beyond initial tumor characterization, MRI is also essential for staging, monitoring response to therapy, and detecting recurrence. However, there can be overlap in MRI characteristics among malignant, benign, and nonneoplastic lesions in both the initial presentation and posttreatment settings.

In recent years, advances in artificial intelligence (AI) and structured reporting have demonstrated increasing potential in the diagnostic, prognostic, and operational value of imaging in multidisciplinary decision-making. In this chapter, we expand on the current state of MRI characterization as well as future directions in the development and integration of advanced AI tools and structured reporting.

10.2 Current State

Bone Lesions When characterizing bone lesions on MRI, several structural features should be analyzed to help distinguish benign from malignant. The size, lesion margin, zone of transition, pattern of periosteal reaction, and soft tissue involvement are important discriminators. Benign lesions tend to have well-defined margins, often with a thin rim of sclerosis, and a narrow zone of transition that can be easily traced. Conversely, malignant lesions often show poorly defined margins with a wide transition zone and greater perilesional marrow edema. Regarding periosteal reaction patterns, benign processes more often show simple, smooth, and/or solid periosteal reaction, whereas malignant lesions are more likely to show interrupted, lamellated, spiculated, sunburst, or Codman's triangle-type reactions. Of note, radiography and CT provide a more accurate assessment of the periosteum and should be compared to the MRI whenever possible. The adjacent cortex, physis, joint, and surrounding soft tissues should also be carefully inspected as transit through or into these tissue planes favors malignancy [3] (Fig. 10.1). Functional MRI characteristics, such as those defined by diffusion-weighted or dynamic perfusion imag-

H. W. Garner (✉)
Department of Radiology, Mayo Clinic, Jacksonville, FL, USA
e-mail: garner.hillary@mayo.edu

M. D. Murphey
ACR Institute for Radiologic Pathology (AIRP), Silver Spring, MD, USA

Department of Radiology and Nuclear Medicine, Uniformed Services University of the Health Sciences, Bethesda, MD, USA
e-mail: mmurphey@acr.org

J. Hodler et al. (eds.), *Musculoskeletal Diseases 2026-2029*, IDKD Springer Series,
https://doi.org/10.1007/978-3-032-17040-8_10

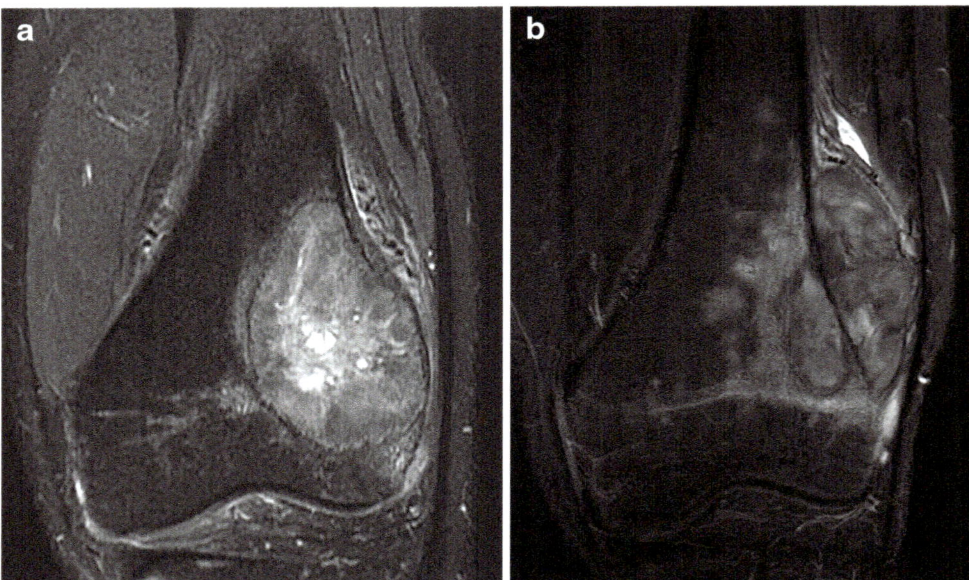

Fig. 10.1 Example of an intermediate (locally aggressive) giant cell tumor of bone (**a**) and of a malignant osteosarcoma (**b**) in the distal femur, both displayed on coronal fluid-sensitive images to highlight features that are key to report during MRI interpretation. The giant cell tumor of bone (**a**) shows a narrow zone of transition with a well-defined margin manifested by the continuous thin dark traceable line around the lesion and mild perilesional edema. There is no cortical destruction or soft tissue mass. Conversely, the osteosarcoma (**b**) shows more ill-defined and irregular margins with a wider zone of transition, greater perilesional edema, and a large soft tissue mass

ing, have also demonstrated value in distinguishing benign from malignant bone lesions. Benign lesions typically do not restrict diffusion and have higher apparent diffusion coefficient values compared to malignant lesions. Similarly, benign lesions usually demonstrate slower enhancement and washout on dynamic perfusion imaging compared to malignant lesions [4].

Soft Tissue Lesions For soft tissue masses, salient MRI features that help discriminate benign from malignant include size (larger lesions being more suspicious), depth relative to fascia (deep lesions are more likely malignant), and signal complexity (malignant lesions are usually heterogenous). Other features that favor malignancy are lobulated or irregular contours, nonuniform enhancement patterns, presence of necrosis or hemorrhage, and invasion of adjacent structures (neurovascular bundles, bone, joints). When morphologic characteristics are not diagnostic, application of functional diffusion and perfusion imaging techniques can add value in the differentiation of lesions. As with benign bone lesions, benign soft tissue lesions usually demonstrate higher apparent diffusion coefficient values and slower enhancement and washout compared to malignant lesions [5]. While no individual MRI feature is definitive, considering multiple imaging characteristics in combination improves diagnostic accuracy. A thorough evaluation of each morphologic feature (and functional feature when performed) is therefore critical to ensure high-quality patient care.

Key Point
MRI remains the gold standard for characterizing musculoskeletal tumors.

10.3 Future Directions – Artificial Intelligence Applications

Deep Learning (DL) Reconstruction AI-based DL reconstruction and acceleration MRI techniques have shown greater than 50% reduction in acquisition time without compromising image quality in many musculoskeletal (MSK) imaging settings, particularly joint imaging [6]. One small study focused specifically on MSK tumors found that DL reconstruction of T2-weighted sequences improved image noise, contrast, and sharpness with associated enhanced lesion detectability and diagnostic confidence [7]. Beyond the benefits of improved efficiency and productivity, these advancements have also boosted patient comfort and experience. This is particularly relevant in MSK oncologic MRI, where patients typically undergo more extensive pre- and post-contrast imaging compared to non-oncologic protocols (Fig. 10.2). DL technology options from several vendors have received clearance in the European Union and the United States and are now commercially available. Therefore, adoption into routine clinical protocols is growing and expected to become standard practice in the coming years.

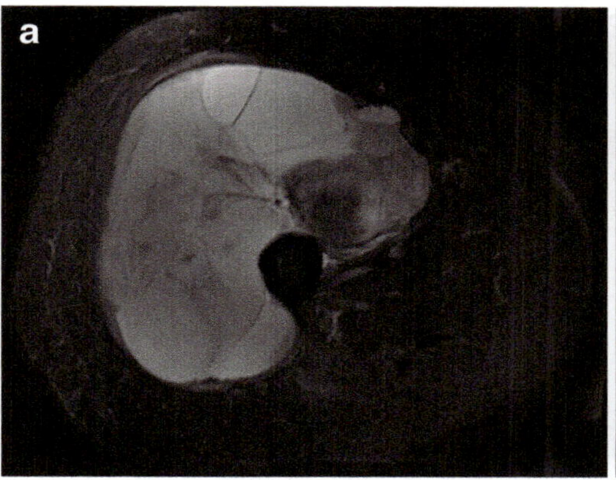

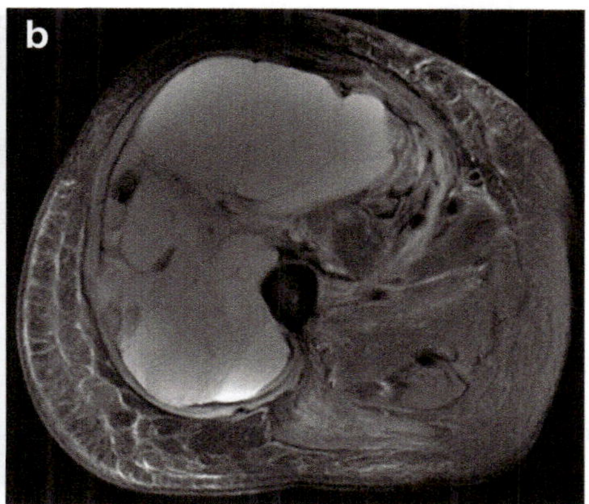

Fig. 10.2 Example of two axial T2 fat-saturated images performed in the same patient with myxofibrosarcoma of the right thigh on the same 3 T MRI scanner 3 months apart. The images were obtained during an MRI of the entire right femur as part of a tumor protocol without and with contrast. The earlier study was performed *without* deep learning reconstruction and the T2 fat-saturated sequence of the entire femur had an acquisition time of 16 min 47 s (**a**). The latter study was performed *with* deep learning reconstruction and the T2 fat-saturated sequence of the entire femur had an acquisition time of 9 min 34 s (**b**). Total time savings for the study using deep learning reconstruction over 5 sequences was 34 min 20 s with no appreciable loss in image quality. Of note, the latter study was performed following completion of neoadjuvant radiation with associated posttreatment change in the tumor and surrounding tissues

Segmentation Integrating reliable AI-based automated tumor segmentation into daily workflow is highly appealing to radiologists, as it can help reduce known subjective variability in both the orientation and measurement of tumor diameter or volume across observers and within the same observer. Furthermore, traditional size-based criteria for assessing treatment response are considered suboptimal compared to newer imaging metrics, such as those derived from diffusion-weighted and perfusion imaging [8], which diminishes the clinical value of time spent on manual size measurements. Although investigative momentum of automated segmentation models for bone tumors has outpaced the momentum for soft tissue tumors, employment of larger datasets and external validation is becoming increasingly common in both areas, bringing clinical integration closer to reality.

- *Bone Tumors:* A growing body of research has investigated AI-based automated segmentation of bone tumors across a range of imaging modalities, including MRI [9]. The employed deep learning models can combine segmentation with lesion detection and benign-versus-malignant classification, which is an approach that aligns well with a radiologist's diagnosis and management recommendation perspective. Given that accurate segmentation is key to modern bone tumor analysis, there is a strong imperative to pursue automation. The path toward practice assimilation will depend on the development of well-validated multi-institutional studies that can demonstrate both performance and generalizability.
- *Soft Tissue Tumors:* Although automated segmentation has shown promising results in bone tumors, the generalizability of a fully automated algorithm for soft tissue tumors is less certain due to the broad array of soft tissue tumor types and varying MRI tumor protocol parameters. A recent multi-center Dutch study posed a solution using a minimally interactive tumor segmentation algorithm where the user clicks two points near the extreme margins in three dimensions, similar to the standard practice of measuring the diameter of the lesion in three planes. To better reflect the heterogeneity of soft tissue tumor types and MRI protocols, the algorithm was trained and internally validated on CT and MRI studies of a public dataset of 9 different tumor types in various anatomical locations and externally validated on a different public dataset of five tumor types not encountered during training [10]. Their results demonstrated stronger generalizability compared to automatic segmentation and up to 94%-time savings compared to manual segmentation. Although minimally interactive segmentation methods will require broader validation, the progress already made points to greater reproducibility and confidence when comparing volumetrics and other tumor radiomic data before and after neoadjuvant therapy.

Key Point

Deep learning reconstruction and automated segmentation can significantly reduce time investment and enhance reproducibility in tumor evaluation.

Radiomics The term radiomics was first described in the early 2010s as the process of extracting and analyzing a large number of quantitative features from radiological images, with the goal of correlating these data with clinical outcomes [11]. It represents the imaging biomarker equivalent of genomic or proteomic biomarkers. For example, quantitative texture and shape features derived from MRI can assist in distinguishing benign from malignant lesions, predicting tumor histology and grade, assessing treatment response, and estimating overall survival [12].

Key Point
Overlaps in imaging features among benign and malignant lesions can limit diagnostic accuracy – radiomics has the potential to better distinguish lesions and predict malignant lesion treatment response.

Since 2015, interest in radiomics has grown rapidly. As of recent estimates, 3874 institutions across 89 countries or regions have contributed to published radiomics research, with the majority located in East Asia, North America, and Western Europe [13]. Due to this surge in activity, the Radiomics Quality Score (RQS) was introduced in 2017 to provide a standardized framework for evaluating the methodological rigor and clinical translatability of radiomics studies [14]. In addition, the Image Biomarker Standardization Initiative (IBSI) was launched to enable research teams to collaboratively standardize feature definitions, reference values [15], and convolutional filters [16]. While such standardizations are essential, further progress will depend on the use of larger datasets, consistent external validation, and the development and sharing of open-source algorithms. Given these challenges, broad clinical integration is likely several years away.

10.4 Structured Reporting

Structured reporting in radiology offers significant value by establishing a standardized framework for documenting and communicating imaging findings. This structured approach promotes greater clarity, consistency, and completeness in radiologic interpretations, reducing variability and minimizing the risk of omitted information. By using predefined templates and terminology, structured reporting ensures that key diagnostic elements are systematically addressed, enhancing the interpretive quality and comparability of reports.

Moreover, structured reporting facilitates more efficient and effective communication between radiologists and referring clinicians. The uniform use of language and report organization improves interpretability, reduces ambiguity, and supports more confident clinical decision-making (Fig. 10.3—Bone and Fig. 10.4—Soft Tissue). Standardized lexicons, such as those developed by professional societies, help unify descriptive terms across different reports and institutions, promoting interoperability and reducing misinterpretation.

Another important advantage of structured reporting is its ability to integrate management recommendations directly with imaging findings. This linkage not only guides referring providers but also supports adherence to evidence-based guidelines. Additionally, structured data formats enable automated extraction of information for research, quality assurance, registries, and auditing purposes, which makes large-scale data analysis more feasible and accurate.

In the setting of musculoskeletal tumors, structured reporting using a standardized Reporting and Data Systems (RADS) format was introduced for whole-body MRI in multiple myeloma in 2019 [17] and is now incorporated into myeloma clinical trials and is being used by many academic research centers. Both retrospective [18] and prospective [19] validation studies support the establishment of whole-body MRI and MY-RADS as a standard of care.

More recently, several RADS tailored specifically to bone lesions have been developed and published. These include the American College of Radiology (ACR) Bone-RADS for radiographs [20], the Society of Skeletal Radiology (SSR) Bone-RADS for CT and MRI [21], and the Bone Tumor Imaging (BTI)-RADS [22] for CT and MRI.

The largest external validation study of the ACR radiograph-based Bone-RADS on 778 patients [23] confirmed high performance for identifying malignant bone tumors, but relatively low specificity and low interreader consensus for certain radiographic features. In contrast, when the same ACR radiographic system was applied to CT on a retrospective cohort of 273 bone tumors, interreader consensus between 2 musculoskeletal radiologists was almost perfect [24]. In short, while the ACR Bone-RADS shows promise for both radiographic and CT evaluation, additional validation and refinement are necessary.

External investigations on the SSR CT-based Bone-RADS [25] led to refinements of the decision tree algorithm, resulting in improved specificity, accuracy, and interreader reliability of the system without compromising sensitivity [26]. Subsequently, the external performance of the refined SSR algorithms was retrospectively studied for both MSK and non-MSK radiologists using three local and two public databases on 328 cases for CT [27] and 275 cases for MRI [28]. Overall, both the CT and MRI validation studies showed that the algorithms are useful for identifying bone lesions that require further workup, but their reliability for non-MSK radiologists was only moderate.

Similarly, a recent 2.0 version of the BTI-RADS algorithm and risk stratification system using machine learning for CT and MRI was developed and applied to 1113 patients across multiple centers in Western Europe. This updated ver-

Fig. 10.3 Example of a structured MRI report for a bone lesion

EXAM: MRI [ANATOMICAL SITE] WITHOUT + WITH CONTRAST

Technique: Multiplanar multisequence MR imaging of the [anatomical site] was performed before and after the uneventful intravenous administration of [x] mL of [contrast agent].

History: [xx]-year-old male/female with history of pain in the [anatomical site] for [xx] months. Radiographs demonstrated a geographic lucent lesion in the [anatomical site].

Comparisons: Radiographs dated [date].

FINDINGS:

Long axis site (epiphysis/metaphysis/diaphysis/flat bone):
Short axis site (intramedullary/cortical/surface):

Lesion characteristics:

Location:

Long axis site (epiphysis/metaphysis/diaphysis/flat bone):
Short axis site (intramedullary/cortical/surface):

Size:
Margin (well-defined/lobular/ill-defined):
Morphology and T1/T2 signal characteristics:
Enhancement characteristics (avid/heterogeneous/central/peripheral):
Most aggressive portion for biopsy target:
Necrosis (None vs <50% vs >50%):
Radiographic appearance (mineralization/cortical involvement):

Status of surrounding tissues:

Endosteal/cortical involvement:
Periosteal reaction:
Soft tissue involvement:
Joint involvement:
Other:

Other findings:

Staging information:

Longest diameter of tumor (T):
Lymph node (L): may be unknown at time of MRI; report expected date of staging CT
Metastasis (M): may be unknown at time of MRI; report expected date of staging CT
Necrosis:

FINAL IMPRESSION:

Most likely Diagnosis:
Differential Diagnosis:

MANAGEMENT RECOMMENDATION:

*Not applicable items above can be reported as such or removed from the template

sion showed improvements in sensitivity, specificity, and accuracy compared to the original, and allows for automated estimation of malignancy risk [29]. Importantly, the 2.0 version is currently accessible for educational purposes to all radiologists online [https://bti-rads.cic-it-nancy.fr/]. On this site, the user can enter data related to the bone lesion and will then be provided a BTI score and a percentile probability of malignancy, which is explained using a SHAP (SHapley Additive exPlanations) decision plot.

Structured reporting for soft tissue lesions has also been developed (ST-RADS) [30], but external validation has been relatively limited. The ACR is currently supporting a "work in progress" of a new version, Soft-Tissue RADS, with broader multi-institutional collaboration. This revised framework was recently published [31], and validation studies are ongoing.

> **Key Point**
> Structured reporting systems (e.g., MY-RADS) provide standardized frameworks for imaging interpretation, which support consistency, data extraction, and communication.

EXAM: MRI [ANATOMICAL SITE] WITHOUT + WITH CONTRAST

Technique: Multiplanar multisequence MR imaging of the [anatomical site] was performed before and after the uneventful intravenous administration of [x] mLof [contrast agent].

History: [xx]-year-old male/femalewith history of a slow-growing painless mass in the [anatomical site]. The patient has no other health concerns.

Comparisons: Ultrasound/Radiograph of the [anatomical site] obtained [date].

FINDINGS:

Lesion characteristics:

- Location:
  - Anatomical site:
  - Tissue depth/location (subcutaneous,fascial,intra-/intermuscular,intraarticular, multifocal):
- Size:
- Margin (circumscribed/irregular):
- Morphology and T1/T2 signal characteristics:
- Enhancement characteristics (avid/heterogeneous/central/peripheral):
- Most aggressive portion for biopsy target:
- Necrosis (None vs <50% vs >50%):
- Radiographic appearance (mineralization/cortical involvement):
- Sonographic appearance (solid vs cystic/echogenicity/vascularity):

Status of surrounding tissues:

- Edema (peritumoral/fascial):
- Hemorrhage:
- Neurovascular involvement:
- Bone involvement:
- Joint involvement:
- Other:

Other findings:

Staging information:

- Longest diameter of tumor (T):
- Lymph node (L): may be unknown at time of MRI; report expected date of staging CT
- Metastasis (M): may be unknown at time of MRI; report expected date of staging CT
- Necrosis:

FINAL IMPRESSION:

- Most likely Diagnosis:
- Differential Diagnosis:

MANAGEMENT RECOMMENDATION:

*Not applicable items above can be reported as such or removed from the template

Fig. 10.4 Example of a structured MRI report for a soft tissue mass

Despite the promise of these structured reporting systems, their clinical integration is likely to be delayed until further validation, particularly prospective studies demonstrating clinical value for non-MSK radiologists, is achieved. Furthermore, broader education and greater engagement of non-radiologist clinicians involved in musculoskeletal tumor care will also be critical. Nonetheless, the anticipated benefits of improved diagnostic accuracy, enhanced patient care, and streamlined data collection underscore the importance for continued development, validation, and eventual integration of structured reporting tools into clinical practice.

Key Point

Cliniacal integration of these advanced tools is promising but contingent upon further prospective validation, methodological transparency, and broader clinician education.

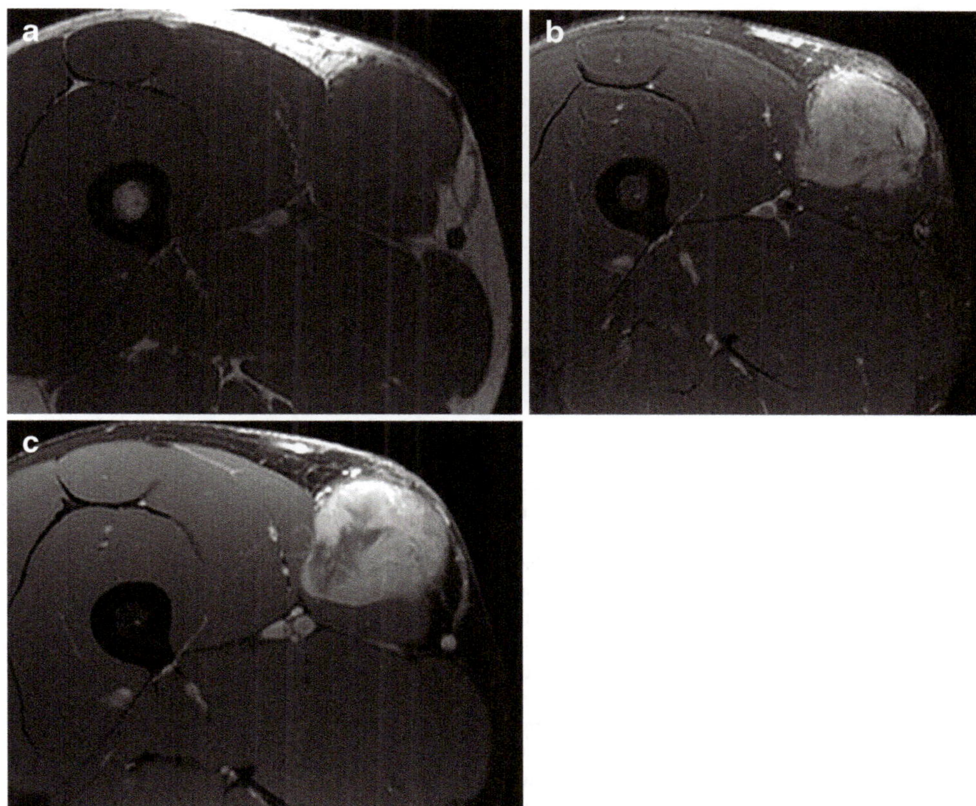

Fig. 10.5 Axial T1-weighted (**a**), T2-weighted fat-saturated (**b**), and T1-weighted fat-saturated postcontrast (**c**) MR images of the right thigh demonstrate a highly suspicious soft tissue mass. The structured report (**d**) includes a description of the index of suspicion and a clear recommendation for management, similar to what is being incorporated into the RADS for soft tissue lesions. The final diagnosis was synovial sarcoma

While we wait for these systems to become more widely adopted, it remains important for radiologists to actively evaluate and report the presence or absence of key imaging features that surgeons and other treating physicians need to know for treatment planning. Specifically, a description of the mass's relationship to surrounding structures, such as neurovascular bundles or joints, is essential. Also, offering a clear management recommendation is an essential part of a radiologist's contribution when evaluating a new bone or soft tissue mass, as it directly influences the clinical decision-making process (Fig. 10.5).

10.5 Concluding Remarks

MRI is the gold standard for initial characterization, local staging, and assessment of treatment response. Advancements in artificial intelligence, radiomics, and structured reporting are further transforming the imaging landscape for musculoskeletal tumors. Specifically, AI-powered deep learning reconstruction, segmentation, and radiomics are poised to enhance diagnostic precision, efficiency, and consistency. Structured reporting systems demonstrate the potential for standardizing evaluations and improving communication across clinical teams, ultimately improving patient outcomes and streamlining oncologic care. However, challenges remain in the form of methodological variability, generalizability, and the need for prospective validation. Continued multidisciplinary collaboration, broader clinical education, and high-quality research will be essential for the successful integration of these tools into routine clinical practice.

Take Home Messages

- MRI is the gold standard for musculoskeletal tumor characterization. Although no single MRI feature can definitively distinguish benign from malignant, identification and combined analysis of multiple structural and functional imaging characteristics improves diagnostic accuracy and guides appropriate patient management.
- Artificial intelligence tools including radiomics have the potential to further amplify diagnostic accuracy in musculoskeletal tumor imaging, but their clinical impact depends on improved methodological standards and robust validation.
- Structured reporting systems enhance diagnostic consistency and communication, but wider adoption requires robust external validation, education, clinical buy-in, and integration into multidisciplinary workflows.

Fig. 10.5 (continued)

d

EXAM: MRI RIGHT FEMUR WITHOUT + WITH CONTRAST

Technique: Multiplanar multisequence MR imaging of the right femur was performed before and after the uneventful intravenous administration of 10 mL of Gadavist.

History: Male in his 20's with history of a slow-growing painless mass at the medial aspect of the left mid thigh. The patient has no other health concerns.

Comparisons: No available comparison.

FINDINGS:
Lesion characteristics:
- Location:
  - Anatomical site: Right thigh
  - Tissue depth/location: Subcutaneous fat with invasion through the deep fascia into the sartorius and vastus lateralis muscles
- Size (AP, TR, CC): 4.9 x 5.0 x 6.4 cm
- Margin (circumscribed/irregular): Irregular
- Morphology and T1/T2 signal characteristics: Solid mass with slightly hyperintense T1 signal relative to muscle and heterogeneous hyperintense T2 signal
- Enhancement characteristics (avid/heterogeneous/central/peripheral): Avid heterogeneous central
- Most aggressive portion for biopsy target: Central portion
- Necrosis (None vs <50% vs >50%): <50%
- Radiographic appearance (mineralization/cortical involvement): Not performed
- Sonographic appearance (solid vs cystic/echogenicity/vascularity): Not performed

Status of surrounding tissues:
- Edema (peritumoral/fascial): Mild peritumoral edema
- Hemorrhage: None
- Neurovascular involvement: None, 5 mm-wide plane at closest proximity
- Bone involvement: None
- Joint involvement: None
- Other: Invades through deep fascia into sartorius and vastus lateralis muscles (crosses compartments)

Other findings: No osseous abnormality. Other myotendinous structures are normal. No adenopathy.

Staging information:
- Longest diameter of tumor (T): 6.4 cm
- Lymph node (L): staging PET/CT scheduled in 4 days
- Metastasis (M): staging PET/CT scheduled in 4 days
- Necrosis: Yes

FINAL IMPRESSION: Soft tissue mass in the right thigh, which is highly suspicious for malignancy
- Most likely Diagnosis: Synovial sarcoma
- Differential Diagnosis: Synovial sarcoma, undifferentiated pleomorphic sarcoma, extraskeletal Ewing's sarcoma

MANAGEMENT RECOMMENDATION: Referral to sarcoma treatment center for further evaluation and work-up. Ultrasound-guided biopsy and staging studies are ideally performed at a specialized sarcoma center to ensure optimal diagnostic accuracy and treatment planning.

- Ongoing collaboration between radiologists, data scientists, and clinicians is crucial to advancing these technologies from research to real-world clinical practice.

Conflict of Interest I/We declare no competing interests as defined by Springer Nature or other interests that might be perceived to influence results and/or discussion reported in this manuscript.

References

1. Maretty-Nielsen K, Aggerholm-Pedersen N, Keller J, Safwat A, Baerentzen S, Pedersen AB. Relative mortality in soft tissue sarcoma patients: a Danish population-based cohort study. BMC Cancer. 2014;14:682.
2. National Cancer Institute. Surveillance, Epidemiology, and End Results (SEER) Program. SEER*Stat Database: Incidence – SEER Research Data, 9 Registries, Nov 2022 Sub (1975–2020). Update 2022. https://seer.cancer.gov. Accessed 28 Sept 2025
3. Nascimento D, Suchard G, Hatem M, de Abreu A. The role of magnetic resonance imaging in the evaluation of bone tumours and tumour-like lesions. Insights Imaging. 2014;5(4):419–40.
4. Debs P, Ahlawat S, Fayad LM. Bone tumors: state-of-the-art imaging. Skeletal Radiol. 2024;53(9):1783–98.
5. Dodin G, Salleron J, Jendoubi S, Abou Arab W, Sirveaux F, Blum A, Gondim Teixeira PA. Added-value of advanced magnetic resonance imaging to conventional morphologic analysis for the differentiation between benign and malignant non-fatty soft-tissue tumors. Eur Radiol. 2021;31(3):1536–47.
6. Vosshenrich J, Koerzdoerfer G, Fritz J. Modern acceleration in musculoskeletal MRI: applications, implications, and challenges. Skeletal Radiol. 2024;53(9):1799–813.
7. Wessling D, Herrmann J, Afat S, Nickel D, Othman AE, Almansour H, Gassenmaier S. Reduction in acquisition time and improvement in image quality in T2-weighted MR imaging of musculoskeletal tumors of the extremities using a novel deep learning-based reconstruction technique in a turbo spin Echo (TSE) sequence. Tomography. 2022;8(4):1759–69.
8. Valenzuela RF, Duran-Sierra E, Antony M, et al. Building a presurgical multiparametric-MRI-based morphologic, qualitative, semiquantitative, first and high-order radiomic predictive treatment response model for undifferentiated pleomorphic sarcoma to replace RECIST. Cancer Imaging. 2025;25(1):56.
9. Rich JM, Bhardwaj LN, Shah A, et al. Deep learning image segmentation approaches for malignant bone lesions: a systematic review and meta-analysis. Front Radiol. 2023;3:1241651.
10. Spaanderman DJ, Starmans MPA, van Erp GCM, et al. Minimally interactive segmentation of soft-tissue tumors on CT and MRI using deep learning. Eur Radiol. 2025;35(5):2736–45.
11. Lambin P, Rios-Velazquez E, Leijenaar R, Carvalho S, van Stiphout RG, Granton P, Zegers CM, Gillies R, Boellard R, Dekker A, Aerts HJ. Radiomics: extracting more information from medical images using advanced feature analysis. Eur J Cancer. 2012;48(4):441–6.
12. Crombé A, Spinnato P, Italiano A, Brisse HJ, Feydy A, Fadli D, Kind M. Radiomics and artificial intelligence for soft-tissue sarcomas: current status and perspectives. Diagn Interv Imaging. 2023;104(12):567–83.
13. Zhang P, Wei L, Nie Z, Hu P, Zheng J, Lv J, Cui T, Liu C, Lan X. Research on the developments of artificial intelligence in radiomics for oncology over the past decade: a bibliometric and visualized analysis. Discov Oncol. 2025;16(1):763.
14. Lambin P, Leijenaar RTH, Deist TM, et al. Radiomics: the bridge between medical imaging and personalized medicine. Nat Rev Clin Oncol. 2017;14:749–62.
15. Zwanenburg A, Vallières M, Abdalah MA, et al. The image biomarker standardization initiative: standardized quantitative radiomics for high-throughput image-based phenotyping. Radiology. 2020;295(2):328–38.
16. Whybra P, Zwanenburg A, Andrearczyk V, et al. The image biomarker standardization initiative: standardized convolutional filters for reproducible radiomics and enhanced clinical insights. Radiology. 2024;310(2):e231319.
17. Messiou C, Hillengass J, Delorme S, et al. Guidelines for acquisition, interpretation, and reporting of whole-body MRI in myeloma: myeloma response assessment and diagnosis system (MY-RADS). Radiology. 2019;291(1):5–13.
18. Belotti A, Ribolla R, Crippa C, et al. Predictive role of sustained imaging MRD negativity assessed by diffusion-weighted whole-body MRI in multiple myeloma. Am J Hematol. 2023;98(9):E230–2.
19. Messiou C, Porta N, Koh DM. Whole body MRI by MY-RADS for imaging response assessment in multiple myeloma. Blood Cancer J. 2025;15(1):122.
20. Caracciolo JT, Ali S, Chang CY, et al. Bone tumor risk stratification and management system: a consensus guideline from the ACR bone reporting and data system committee. J Am Coll Radiol. 2023;20(10):1044–58. https://doi.org/10.1016/j.jacr.2023.07.017. Epub 2023 Oct 17. Erratum in: J Am Coll Radiol. 2024 May;21(5):700
21. Chang CY, Garner HW, Ahlawat S, et al. Society of Skeletal Radiology- white paper. Guidelines for the diagnostic management of incidental solitary bone lesions on CT and MRI in adults: bone reporting and data system (bone-RADS). Skeletal Radiol. 2022;51(9):1743–64.
22. Ribeiro GJ, Gillet R, Hossu G, et al. Solitary bone tumor imaging reporting and data system (BTI-RADS): initial assessment of a systematic imaging evaluation and comprehensive reporting method. Eur Radiol. 2021;31(10):7637–52.
23. Park SY, Yoon MA, Lee MH, Lee SH, Chung HW. Validation of American College of Radiology Bone Reporting and Data System (bone-RADS) version 2023 for diagnosis of malignant tumors of appendicular bone on conventional radiographs. Eur J Radiol. 2025;183:111861.
24. Ramadan ZA, Elmorsy AH, Taman SE, Denewar FA. Inter-observer and intra-observer agreement of bone reporting and data system (bone-RADS) in the interpretation of bone tumors on computed tomography. Clin Imaging. 2025;117:110367.
25. Park C, Azhideh A, Pooyan A, et al. Diagnostic performance and inter-reader reliability of bone reporting and data system (bone-RADS) on computed tomography. Skeletal Radiol. 2025;54(2):209–17. https://doi.org/10.1007/s00256-024-04721-4.
26. Haseli S, Park C, Azhideh A, Karande G, Chalian M. Performance and reliability comparison: original vs. revised bone reporting and data system (bone-RADS). Skeletal Radiol. 2025;54(8):1681–8.
27. Xing Y, Ding D, Dai S, et al. Bone reporting and data system on CT (bone-RADS-CT): a validation study by four readers on 328 cases from three local and two public databases. Insights Imaging. 2025;16(1):174.
28. Xing Y, Hu Y, Liu X, et al. Bone reporting and data system on MRI (bone-RADS-MRI): a validation study by four readers on 275 cases from three local and two public databases. Insights Imaging. 2025;16(1):155.
29. Lemore A, Vogt N, Oster J, et al. Enhanced CT and MRI focal bone tumor classification with machine learning-based stratification: a multicenter retrospective study. Radiology. 2025;315(1):e232834.

30. Chhabra A, Ashikyan O, Ratakonda R, et al. Soft-tissue tumor reporting and data system (ST-RADS): MRI reporting guideline with multi-institutional validation study of musculoskeletal extremity Tumors. J Tumor Res. 2022;8:179.
31. Chhabra A, Garner HW, Rehman M, et al. Soft tissue-RADS: an ACR work-in-progress framework for standardized reporting of soft-tissue lesions on MRI. Am J Roentgenol. 2025 Nov 26. https://doi.org/10.2214/AJR.25.34013.

IDKD: Arthritis—Focus on Peripheral Joints

11

Soterios Gyftopoulos and Lennart Jans

Learning Objectives

1. To review the common terminology used to describe peripheral arthritis on imaging
2. To discuss how osteoarthritis and deposition diseases such as gout and calcium pyrophosphate deposition are best characterized on imaging
3. To define the most important imaging findings in inflammatory arthritis, including rheumatoid arthritis and psoriatic arthritis

11.1 Introduction

The peripheral joints of the human body allow for the movements vital for daily function. When these joints cannot function appropriately, this negatively impacts the individual both from a physical and psychological perspective. Imaging plays an important role in the care spectrum for patients who suffer from conditions affecting the peripheral joints, commonly referred to as peripheral arthritis. The diagnosis of a specific condition can lead to the most appropriate treatment, which includes medication and/or activity modifications, and symptom and functional improvement.

The objective of this chapter is to provide an overview of common conditions that affect the peripheral joints and the role that imaging plays in their diagnosis. We will begin with a description of key terminology to describe the imaging findings for the most common conditions. Then, we will provide comprehensive overviews of each condition.

11.2 Key Terminology

The classic finding for a degenerative joint process is the osteophyte, which is new bony production at the site of cartilage breakdown [1]. An osteophyte can be found both along the margin and central aspect of the joint. Marginal osteophytes are typically found in the setting of joint space narrowing and subchondral changes, including sclerosis and cyst formation. In most synovial lined joints, this constellation of findings is referred to as osteoarthritis or osteoarthrosis [we will use "osteoarthritis" for the remainder of the review for consistency]. When found at specific joints, such as the radiocarpal or second and third metacarpophalangeal joints, these findings may represent calcium pyrophosphate dihydrate (CPPD) arthropathy especially if there are associated chondrocalcinosis and large subchondral cysts [1].

The classic finding of an inflammatory joint process is the marginal bone erosion, which is an intraarticular osseous defect found along the edge of an inflamed synovium lined joint. The inflamed synovium erodes this portion of the bone, while sparing the subchondral bone which is protected by the overlying hyaline cartilage [2].

Enthesophyte formation is bony production at the site where a tendon or ligament attaches to bone, typically resulting from inflammation referred to as enthesitis. As opposed to osteophytes, which are typically bulky in appearance, enthesophytes have a finer/thinner appearance on imaging. Periostitis represents new bone formation along the margins of a joint, typically seen in the setting of spondyloarthritis such as psoriatic arthritis [2].

The pattern of joint space narrowing can help differentiate between disease processes. Uniform joint space narrowing is typical of an inflammatory arthropathy as the inflammation typically involves all the joint's synovium, resulting in a more balanced loss of hyaline cartilage and loss of joint space. Asymmetric joint space spacing is more typical of osteoarthritis, as the underlying degenerative processes typi-

S. Gyftopoulos (✉)
Department: Radiology, NYU Langone Health, New York City, NY, USA
e-mail: Soterios.Gyftopoulos@nyulangone.org

L. Jans
Department: Radiology, Ghent University Hospital, Ghent, Belgium
e-mail: LENNART.JANS@UGent.be

J. Hodler et al. (eds.), *Musculoskeletal Diseases 2026-2029*, IDKD Springer Series,
https://doi.org/10.1007/978-3-032-17040-8_11

cally result in an uneven loss of cartilage along the articular surfaces that occurs gradually over time.

11.3 Degenerative Diseases

11.3.1 Osteoarthritis

11.3.1.1 Background

Osteoarthritis (OA) is the most common disease process affecting the peripheral joints in the body. It can be divided into two main categories based on underlying causative factors: primary and secondary. Primary OA (also referred to as generalized or typical) is considered a chronic process caused by repetitive microtrauma to the cartilage lining the joints. Several other factors such as body habitus, ethnicity, gender, genetics, and nutrition are also considered contributing factors to its development [3].

Joint involvement in primary OA progresses in a somewhat predictable manner and will depend on patient specific factors including activity rates and body habitus. Osteoarthritis can be seen in the acromioclavicular joint as early as the fourth decade of life. As the patient ages, osteoarthritis can be present in multiple joints including the thumb basal joint (first carpometacarpal joint); distal interphalangeal joints of the hand, hips, and knees; and first metatarsophalangeal joint.

Secondary OA (also referred to as atypical) refers to degenerative disease with a known underlying cause, including trauma, congenital/developmental factors such as hip dysplasia, metabolic disease such as hemochromatosis, and endocrine disorders such as acromegaly [3]. Important factors that should cause you to consider this type of osteoarthritis include degenerative changes in uncommon locations, unusual severity of the degenerative findings given patient age, and presence in young patients. Trauma is the most common cause of secondary osteoarthritis and can occur after a one-time traumatic event or recurrent, chronic injury that can be seen in athletes who place repetitive stress on specific areas of their body.

> **Key Point**
> Primary osteoarthritis (OA) (also referred to as generalized or typical) is considered a chronic process caused by repetitive microtrauma to the cartilage lining the joints. Secondary OA (also referred to as atypical) refers to degenerative disease with a known underlying cause, including trauma and congenital/developmental factors such as hip dysplasia.

CPPD arthropathy is another common cause of atypical osteoarthritis, although some consider it a separate entity. This will be discussed in a separate section in this review. Another cause that you should consider is early neuropathic arthropathy, especially when degenerative changes such as osteophytes, subchondral sclerosis, and joint space narrowing are seen in the midfoot with adjacent vascular calcifications in a patient with diabetes.

11.3.2 Imaging Findings

11.3.2.1 Radiographs

Radiographs are typically the initial screening imaging exam for patients suspected of OA. The most important underlying pathology in OA is the loss of cartilage, which can occur acutely in the setting of trauma or, more commonly, in the chronic setting with gradual loss occurring over time. In either instance, cartilage loss results in joint space narrowing which can be seen on x-ray. Typically, joint space loss is asymmetric, which is an important distinguishing feature from other inflammatory causes of joint space loss which tend to be more uniform in distribution.

Another characteristic imaging finding is the presence of osteophyte formation along the joint margins, adjacent to joint space loss. Osteophytes can also occur along the articular surfaces, called central, but not as often. Subchondral changes, such as sclerosis and cyst formation, also are common in OA, and their extent are directly correlated with the marginal osteophyte presence and size. OA can also contribute to joint malalignment in concert with surrounding supporting capsular/ligament structures, typically in the setting of asymmetric joint space loss and subchondral bone plate collapse.

11.3.2.2 Advanced Imaging

Advanced imaging is not typically used nor needed to make the diagnosis of OA but can demonstrate the typical findings of osteophyte formation, subchondral changes, and joint space loss [4]. MRI's advantage lies in its ability to directly visualize the joint articular cartilage [5]. This, in turn, allows for a more accurate quantification of the degree of cartilage loss which helps with monitoring of disease progression and helps guide treatment decision (Fig. 11.1). This is especially useful when there is mild cartilage loss, which may not result in enough loss in joint space to be evident on radiographs. In addition, MRI better demonstrates the presence and degree of subchondral "edema" like signal and cystic change, which may correlate with patient symptomatology. The main advantage of ultrasound (US) may be its ability to easily and safely guide treatments for OA patients, like steroid and

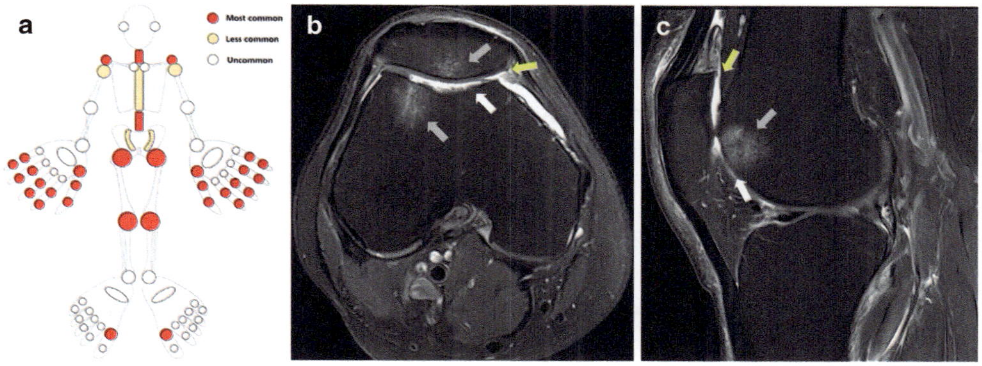

Fig. 11.1 Cartilage loss and subchondral changes. (**a**) Schematic demonstrating the typical distribution of osteoarthritis. Axial (**b**) and sagittal (**c**) fat-suppressed fluid-sensitive MRI images of the right knee demonstrate broad partial-thickness cartilage along the patella (yellow arrows), varying degrees of cartilage loss along the trochlea (white arrows), and underlying subchondral edema like pattern (gray arrows) within the patella and trochlea

hyaluronic acid injections, which can be effective when used in the appropriate patient population.

11.3.2.3 Erosive Osteoarthritis

Erosive osteoarthritis is an OA variant that predominantly involves the hands and has imaging characteristics that can be easily confused with an inflammatory arthropathy. Similar to primary OA, erosive OA involves the interphalangeal joints with imaging findings that include marginal osteophyte formation and subchondral changes. The imaging finding that differentiates it from primary OA and can be confused with an inflammatory arthropathy is the presence of a central erosion along the articular surfaces which produces "wing-like" bone productions along either side of the erosion giving the appearance of seagull wings. Persistent inflammation can eventually result in fusion of the joint space. Radiographs are typically all that is needed to make the diagnosis of erosive OA, while more advanced imaging modalities can also demonstrate the typical osseous findings as well as soft tissue findings such as synovitis and joint effusion which can be seen with active inflammation.

11.3.2.4 Septic Arthritis

Septic arthritis is an important condition that should be considered by the radiologist when they see imaging findings suggesting inflammation involving a single joint [6]. Typical causes include hematogenous spread (most common in pediatric patients), spread from adjacent infections, and direct inoculation (the latter two most common in adults). Predisposing conditions for septic arthritis can vary, including weakened immune systems, IV drug abuse, and recent joint surgery, including placement of arthroplasties.

It is important to consider the imaging findings in the context of the patient's clinical history when considering a diagnosis of septic arthritis. Radiographs are most often normal in the early stages of infection. In early stages of infection, there may be a joint effusion, periarticular demineralization, and/or surrounding soft tissue swelling. Joint space widening can also be seen secondary to joint effusion with severe widening characteristic of atypical infections such as tuberculosis. As the infection advances, these previously noted features become more prominent and may be seen along with osseous erosions and destruction along the articular surfaces.

On advanced imaging such as MRI and ultrasound, similar findings can be seen in addition to more specific soft tissue findings such as synovitis, joint effusions, and periarticular fluid/edema. MRI provides additional information on the presence and extent of associated osteomyelitis or abscess formation and is typically performed with IV contrast to improve accuracy. Ultrasound does not provide the same advantages as MRI for the osseous findings of infection but can provide useful information suggestive of infection including demonstrating joint effusion with internal debris which is more common in septic arthritis compared to noninfected joint collections as well as the presence of abscess formation in the surrounding soft tissues. As the diagnosis of septic arthritis is most commonly established via the analysis of joint fluid, image guidance with either ultrasound or fluoroscopy provides a safe route for arthrocentesis and confirmation of infection.

11.3.2.5 Rapidly Progressive Osteoarthritis

Rapidly progressive osteoarthritis of the hip, also referred to as rapidly progressive idiopathic arthritis (RPIA), is a condition that can mimic an inflammatory or infectious joint-centered process at the hip [7]. While its cause remains unclear, potential predisposing factors include prior trauma, steroid and anesthetic injections, female sex, higher body mass index, and older age. Clinically, patients with RPIA can present with nonspecific hip pain and maintained joint mobility. On imaging, typical findings include rapid loss of joint space and collapse of the hip articular surfaces. Rapid joint space loss has been defined as more than 2 mm in a year or greater than 50% loss of joint space in one year [7]. As is the case with other joint-centered processes, an understanding of the patient's clinical history when reviewing the imaging findings is vital to differentiating this entity from septic arthritis and inflammatory arthritis.

11.4 Inflammatory Arthritis

11.4.1 Rheumatoid Arthritis

11.4.1.1 Background

Rheumatoid arthritis (RA) is a common chronic inflammatory joint disease, which typically involves the small joints of the appendicular skeleton [8]. It is characterized by proliferative synovitis, which leads to cartilage and bone erosions [9]. The disease may also present with extraarticular manifestations such as rheumatoid nodules, pulmonary involvement, vasculitis, and other systemic comorbidities. RA occurs more frequently in women than in men and typically develops gradually, presenting as bilateral polyarthritis that most often affects the hands and feet [9]. Laboratory findings usually show positivity for anticitrullinated peptide antibodies (ACPA) and rheumatoid factor.

11.4.2 Imaging Findings

11.4.2.1 Radiographs

Conventional radiography shows early periarticular joint demineralization, particularly of the carpal bones, the MCP (metacarpophalangeal), and the MTP (metatarsophalangeal) joints. Marginal erosions of the MCP/MTP joints without new bone formation are the hallmark of the disease (Fig. 11.2). In later stages, joint and ligament destruction leads to changes in alignment that include ulnar deviation and volar subluxation of the MCP joints, boutonnière deformity, swan neck deformity, and hammer toe deformity. Pencil-in-cup deformity can also be present, with pencil-like bone resorption of the proximal portion of the joint and cup-like erosion of the distal portion.

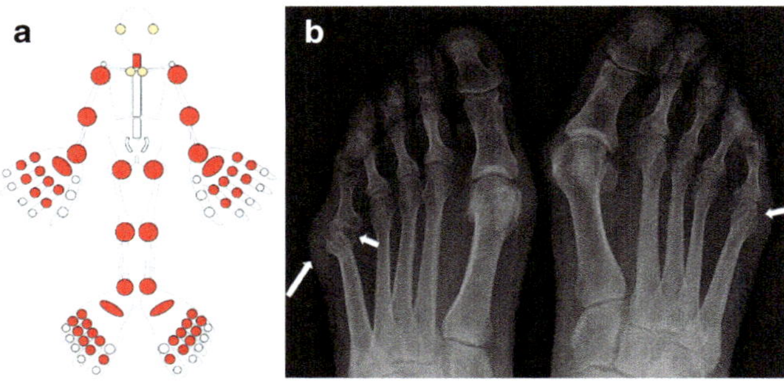

Fig. 11.2 Rheumatoid arthritis. (**a**) Schematic demonstrating the typical distribution of rheumatoid arthritis. (**b**) Radiography of the feet shows marginal erosions of the head of the fifth metatarsal bilaterally (short arrows), with adjacent soft tissue swelling (long arrow)

11.4.2.2 Advanced Imaging

Ultrasound and MRI reveal soft tissue swelling, synovitis, and tenosynovitis in the early stages. MRI depicts bone marrow edema as an early sign of active inflammation. In later stages, MRI shows subchondral erosions, subchondral cysts, and severe bone destruction, evolving to severe joint deformity and even ankylosis [8–10].

> **Key Point**
> Rheumatoid arthritis is a common chronic inflammatory joint disease, which typically involves the small joints of the appendicular skeleton. Radiography shows symmetric periarticular joint demineralization and marginal erosions, particularly of the carpal bones, and the metacarpophalangeal and metatarsophalangeal joints.

11.5 Psoriatic Arthritis

11.5.1 Background

Psoriatic arthritis (PsA) is the most common coexisting condition in patients with psoriasis, affecting between 10% and 30% of them. It presents in five clinical subtypes: polyarticular, oligoarticular involving four or fewer joints, distal, axial, and arthritis mutilans. Clinically, PsA is often associated with skin psoriasis and psoriatic nail changes such as nail pitting and onycholysis [11]. Another hallmark feature is dactylitis, also known as "sausage digit," and the disease typically follows an inflammatory, asymmetric pattern of oligoarthritis or polyarthritis [12]. Arthritis mutilans, ankylosis, joint destruction with luxation, and even acro-osteolysis may occur in severe cases. A key imaging feature of PsA is the presence of slowly progressing erosions in the interphalangeal joints combined with new bone formation [13].

11.5.2 Imaging Findings

11.5.2.1 Radiographs

Imaging of the hands and feet plays a central role in diagnosis and disease monitoring. In the early stages, radiographs

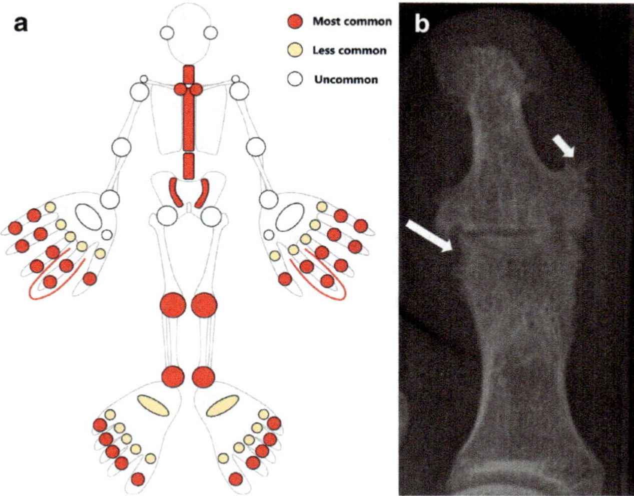

Fig. 11.3 Psoriatic arthritis. (**a**) Schematic demonstrating the typical distribution of psoriatic arthritis. (**b**) Radiography of the thumb shows concomitant marginal erosion (long arrow) and periosteal new bone formation (short arrow)

may appear normal. As the disease progresses, marginal erosions, periostitis, and marginal new bone formation can be observed (Fig. 11.3) [13]. In advanced stages, more severe changes develop, including erosions, joint deformities such as the "pencil-in-cup" appearance, and sclerosis with the characteristic "ivory phalanx." An ivory phalanx is a diffuse sclerosis of the phalanx as a result of concomitant periosteal and endosteal new bone formation.

11.5.2.2 Advanced Imaging

Ultrasound is particularly helpful to assess synovitis and joint effusion of the small joints of the hands and feet. Doppler ultrasound shows active inflammation of the inflamed and thickened synovial tissue [14]. MRI allows for detailed assessment of peripheral joints and can visualize bone marrow oedema as the first sign of inflammation. Contrast-enhanced images allow for differentiation between nonenhancing joint effusion and enhancing synovitis [14].

> **Key Point**
> Psoriatic arthritis (PsA) affects between 10% and 30% of patients with skin psoriasis. A key imaging feature of PsA is the presence of slowly progressing erosions in the interphalangeal joints with concomitant new bone formation.

11.6 Reactive Arthritis

11.6.1 Background

Reactive arthritis is an acute form of arthritis characterized by sterile synovitis in genetically predisposed individuals, typically following a bacterial infection in a distant organ system, most often in the genitourinary or gastrointestinal tract [15]. The disease usually presents as an acute, asymmetrical oligoarthritis, sometimes accompanied by extraarticular manifestations such as conjunctivitis, urethritis, or cervicitis. It most commonly affects individuals between 20 and 40 years of age and typically develops 2–4 weeks but less than 6 weeks, after a triggering infection. The clinical picture often includes oligoarthritis, inflammatory back pain, and uveitis, with around 10% of patients progressing to axial spondyloarthritis [16].

11.6.2 Imaging Findings

11.6.2.1 Radiographs

The radiographic findings of reactive arthritis are nonspecific and include ill-defined erosions, enthesopathy, new bone formation, early periarticular demineralization, and uniform joint space loss. These features, however, only become evident in the late stages of the disease [17].

11.6.2.2 Advanced Imaging

Ultrasound and MRI show changes in the early stages of the disease. Enthesitis (often of the Achilles tendon and plantar fascia), erosions, and bone marrow edema can be present, particularly in the large joints of the lower limbs after a preceding genitourinary or gastrointestinal infection [17].

11.7 Peripheral Spondyloarthritis

Spondyloarthritis (SpA) is a group of chronic inflammatory diseases genetically associated with HLA-B27 [18, 19]. It affects both the axial and peripheral skeleton, with inflammatory pain and enthesitis as key features, and is often accompanied by extramusculoskeletal manifestations such as uveitis, psoriasis, and inflammatory bowel disease. A major distinction is made between axial SpA and peripheral SpA. Axial SpA is characterized by clinical symptoms and imaging findings in the spine and sacroiliac joints, though peripheral sites and joints may also be involved. Peripheral

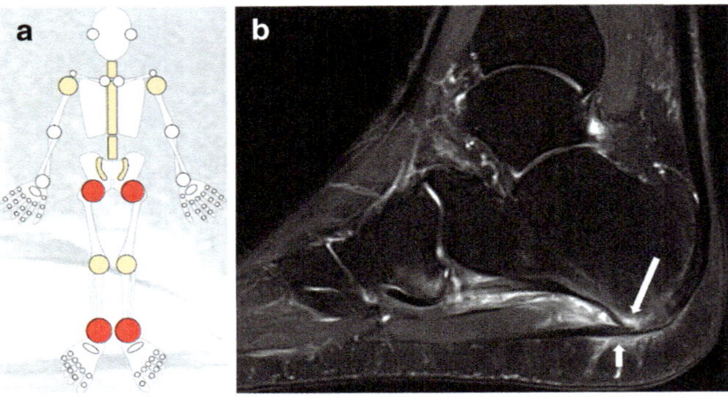

Fig. 11.4 Peripheral spondyloarthritis. (**a**) Schematic demonstrating the typical distribution of peripheral spondyloarthritis. (**b**) Sagittal fat-saturated T2-weighted MRI image shows soft tissue inflammation (short arrow) surrounding the plantar fascia, with bone marrow edema in the calcaneus (long arrow)

SpA (pSpA), on the other hand, mainly affects peripheral joints and tendon insertions, but the axial skeleton may be involved as well [20].

Peripheral SpA typically starts in a asymmetric pattern, with the larger joints of the lower limb most commonly involved; enthesitis and dactylitis are less frequent.

11.7.1 Imaging Findings

11.7.1.1 Radiographs

Peripheral SpA is characterized by erosions and ossification at the entheses of peripheral joints which can be assessed on radiography. Typical sites include the insertion of the Achilles tendon and the origin of the plantar fascia [18].

11.7.1.2 Advanced Imaging

Ultrasound allows for evaluation of effusion and synovitis of small joints; MRI depicts early signs of inflammation [20]. MRI shows active inflammation as enthesitis, bone marrow edema, and soft tissue inflammation that can all be seen as high signal intensity on the fat-suppressed MRI images (Fig. 11.4) [18].

11.8 Deposition Disease

11.8.1 Calcium Pyrophosphate Deposition Disease

11.8.1.1 Background

Calcium pyrophosphate deposition (CPPD) disease is a condition most commonly seen in middle-aged and elderly individuals. CPPD is related to the deposition of calcium pyrophosphate crystals in hyaline cartilage, fibrocartilage, ligaments/capsules, and tendons, commonly referred to as chondrocalcinosis [21]. It will typically present in one of three ways [1, 22]. First, CPPD can present as acute inflammation of a joint secondary to the release of crystals into the joint space. This can mimic gout on clinical presentation and thus has been referred to as pseudogout. Second, CPPD can present as an arthropathy with an imaging appearance similar to OA. Aside from the presence of CPPD in the surrounding soft tissues, the location of the CPPD arthropathy will vary from what is typically seen in OA with common locations such as the radiocarpal joint, second and third metacarpophalangeal joints, and patellofemoral joint. Third, CPPD can be asymptomatic with the only evidence of its presence found on imaging. Common locations for this asymptomatic deposition of CPPD crystals include the triangular fibrocartilage complex and lunate-triquetral ligament at the wrist, acetabular labrum and symphysis pubis at the pelvis, and menisci and gastrocnemius origins at the knee. It is important to note that chondrocalcinosis and CPPD arthropathy can be associated with other metabolic conditions, including hemochromatosis, hyperparathyroidism, and Wilson's disease.

11.8.2 Imaging Findings

11.8.2.1 Radiographs

Radiographs play an important role in the diagnosis and monitoring of CPPD patients. In patients with CPPD arthropathy, the joint space loss is typically asymmetric in nature and a result of cartilage loss. The affected joint space may also have thin calcification deposits along the articular surfaces, related to crystal deposition along the hyaline cartilage, as well as crystals within adjacent fibrocartilage structures, including the labrum and menisci. Subchondral changes and osteophytes can also be seen, although the subchondral cysts are typically larger than what is seen in OA while the osteophytes size does not always correlate with the degree of arthropathy at the joint, which is inconsistent with OA.

Malalignment can also be seen, similar to OA, but there are specific instances that are more specific to CPPD. A common example of this is scapholunate advanced collapsed (SLAC) wrist where there is widening of the scapholunate interval and proximal migration of the capitate in the setting of degenerative changes at the radiocarpal and midcarpal joints (Fig. 11.5).

Acute inflammation related to CPPD deposition (pseudogout) can be suggested on radiographs by the combination of calcium deposition along the margins of a joint space with adjacent soft tissue swelling. It is important to note that acute pseudogout is a clinical diagnosis made by the identification of pyrophosphate crystals in aspirated joint fluid.

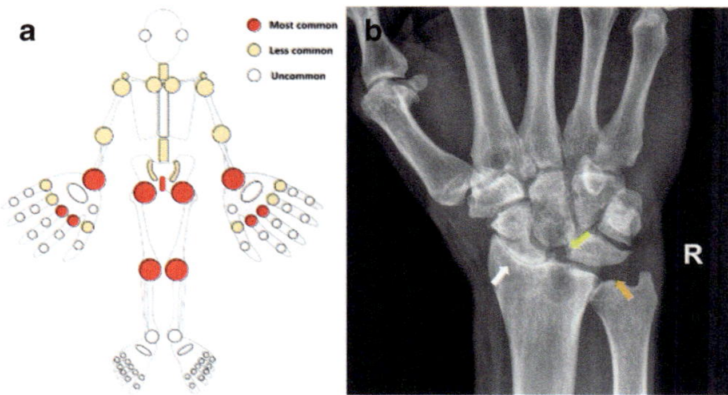

Fig. 11.5 SLAC wrist. (**a**) Schematic demonstrating the typical distribution of calcium pyrophosphate deposition (CPPD). (**b**) PA view of the right wrist demonstrates scapholunate advanced collapse with bone on bone joint space narrowing at the radiocarpal joint (white arrow), scapholunate interval widening (yellow arrow), and chondrocalcinosis along the medial wrist (orange arrow)

11.8.2.2 Advanced Imaging

Advanced imaging modalities play a minor role in the evaluation of CPPD. MRI and ultrasound can be useful when demonstrating the joint effusion and synovitis that can be seen in the setting of pseudogout. Ultrasound is more effective in demonstrating chondrocalcinosis deposition in hyaline cartilage and fibrocartilaginous structures, while MRI is more effective at demonstrating the degenerative changes that are typically found in CPPD arthropathy.

11.9 Gout

11.9.1 Background

Gouty arthritis results from a combination of genetic, dietary, and racial factors and hyperuricemia. Certain patient conditions can also increase the likelihood of gout, including cardiovascular disease, diabetes, decreased renal function, and obesity. Hyperuricemia is a product of either reduced excretion or increased production of uric acid, the end product of purine metabolism. Monosodium urate crystals are created in the setting of hyperuricemia and deposit in a number of different areas in the body, including synovium, tendon sheaths, bursae, joint fluid, and subcutaneous tissues. Hyperuricemia can be asymptomatic, having been seen in approximately one in five individuals [3].

When it becomes symptomatic, it typically presents either acutely or in the chronic setting. The patient with an acute gout episode will report joint swelling and erythema around the affected joint in the setting of marked pain. These acute gout episodes will tend to occur and then dissipate, with the patient remaining asymptomatic in between episodes. In the chronic gout setting, patients will report persistent symptoms secondary to monosodium urate crystal deposition which triggers synovitis, erosions, and joint effusions. The crystals can also form deposits in the surrounding soft tissues, referred to as tophi.

Diagnosis of gout in both settings is most easily made through joint fluid aspiration and the identification of monosodium urate crystal deposition. While there are certain joints that are more commonly affected, like the first metatarsophalangeal joint, gouty arthritis can impact any small or large joint in the body, which has led to the saying "when in doubt, think gout."

> **Key Point**
> While there are certain joints that are more commonly affected, like the first metatarsophalangeal joint, gouty arthritis can impact any small or large joint in the body, which has led to the saying "when in doubt, think gout."

11.9.2 Imaging Findings

11.9.2.1 Radiographs

Radiographs can play an important role in the diagnosis and monitoring of gout, especially in the chronic setting. The classic finding is a "punched-out" round erosion with thin sclerotic margins and overhanging edges. The erosions do not have a typical location along the joint, as they can be seen both at the margins and centrally along the articular surfaces as well as along cortices adjacent to tophi (Fig. 11.6). As opposed to other conditions we have discussed, the joint space is typically maintained even in advanced cases. Tophi can present as focal somewhat irregular soft tissue masses with variable increased density secondary to microcalcifications that accumulate in patients with renal disease. In advanced cases, there can be extensive destruction of the joint spaces and bones leading to marked joint malalignment.

11.9.2.2 Advanced Imaging

Advanced imaging can be helpful in making the diagnosis of gout, especially in acute cases or in scenarios where the involvement is more soft tissue based, such as with the involvement of tendons/tendon sheaths or bursae. Dual energy CT imaging can be an extremely useful diagnostic tool given its ability to identify and differentiate monosodium urate crystal deposition from other forms of mineralization [23]. MRI and ultrasound can nicely demonstrate the presence of joint effusions and synovitis in the setting of joint-centered acute gout and tenosynovitis and bursitis when the surrounding synovial lined structures are involved. The erosions seen with gout and tophi can also be diagnosed with these imaging modalities, although the tophi may not appear as characteristic as they do on radiographs.

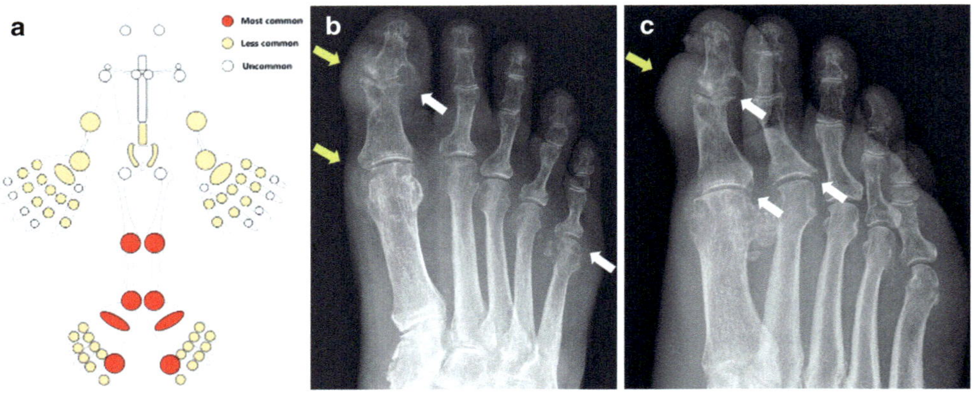

Fig. 11.6 Gout. (**a**) Schematic demonstrating the typical distribution of gout. (**b**) AP and (**c**) oblique views of the right forefoot demonstrate soft tissue tophi (yellow arrows) along the great toe and erosions with sclerotic margins scattered throughout the forefoot (white arrows) consistent with gout. Character schematic—peripheral arthritis: Fig X. Target-site approach of peripheral arthritis. *EOA* erosive osteoarthritis, *OA* osteoarthritis, *PsA* psoriatic arthritis, *RA* rheumatoid arthritis, *HADD* hydroxy apatite deposition disease, *CPPD* calcium pyrophosphate deposition disease

11.10 Conclusion

Imaging is central to the diagnosis, clinical management, and follow-up of peripheral arthritis. MRI and ultrasound enable early detection of inflammatory changes, whereas radiography remains the cornerstone for assessment of structural bone and joint damage. Ongoing collaboration between radiologists and rheumatologists is paramount to ensure that the imaging findings are translated into early diagnosis and treatment, to avoid irreversible joint damage.

Take-Home Messages

1. Peripheral arthritis is a common condition that has an important impact on a patient's physical and mental well-being. Imaging is central to diagnosis, clinical management, and follow-up.
2. Radiography is the preferred imaging modality for late-stage disease assessment. It demonstrates structural bone and joint damage, crystal deposition, and new bone formation.
3. Ultrasound and MRI demonstrate inflammation in the early stages of peripheral arthritis, allowing for early diagnosis and treatment before irreversible changes occur.

Conflict of Interest I/We declare no competing interests as defined by Springer Nature or other interests that might be perceived to influence results and/or discussion reported in this manuscript.

References

1. Jacobson J, Girish G, Jiang Y, Sabb B. Radiographic evaluation of arthritis: degenerative joint disease and variations. Radiology. 2008;248(3):737–47.
2. Jacobson J, Girish G, Jiang Y, Resnick D. Radiographic evaluation of arthritis: inflammatory condition. Radiology. 2008;248(2):378–89.
3. Grainger A, Resnick C. Arthritis. In: Musculoskeletal diseases 2021–2024: diagnostic imaging. Springer; 2021.
4. Haugen I, Boyesen P, Slatkowsky-Christensen B, Sessenf S, Bijsterbosch J, van der Heijde D, et al. Comparison of features by MRI and radiographs of the interphalangeal finger joints in patients with hand osteoarthritis. Ann Rheum Dis. 2012;71(3):345–50.
5. Zandee van Rilland E, Fritz R, Chaudhari A, Boutin R. Cartilage imaging: MRI of chondral degeneration and injury. Clin Sport Med. 2024;44(3):467–98.
6. Beutler B, Chang C, Chang E. Septic arthritis: current concepts. Semin Musculoskelet Radiol. 2025;29(2):293–301.
7. Boutin R, Pai J, Meehan J, Newman J, Yao L. Rapidly progressive idiopathic arthritis of the hip: incidence and risk factors in a controlled cohort study of 1471 patients after intra-articular corticosteroid injection. Skeletal Radiol. 2021;50(12):2449–57.
8. Llopis E, Kroon HM, Acosta J. Conventional radiology in rheumatoid arthritis. Radiol Clin North Am. 2017;55(5):917–41.
9. Walter W, Samim M. Imaging updates in rheumatoid arthritis. Semin Musculoskelet Radiol. 2025;29(2):156–66.
10. Serban O, Badarinza M, Fodor D. The relevance of ultrasound examination of the foot and ankle in patients with rheumatoid arthritis – a review of the literature. Med Ultrason. 2019;21(2):175–82.
11. Kishimoto M, Deshpande G, Fukuoka K, Kawakami T, Ikegaya N, Kawashima S, et al. Clinical features of psoriatic arthritis. Best Pract Res Clin Rheumatol. 2021;35(2):101670.
12. Ritchlin C, Colbert R, Gladman D. Diagnostic imaging of psoriatic arthritis. Part I: etiopathogenesis, classifications and radiographic features. N Engl J Med. 2017;376(21):2095–6.
13. Sudol-Szopinska I, Matuszewska G, Kwiatkowska B, Pracon G. Diagnostic imaging of psoriatic arthritis. Part I: etiopatho-

genesis, classifications and radiographic features. J Ultrason. 2016;16(64):65–77.

14. Ostergaard M, Eder L, Nysom Christiansen S, Kaeley G. Imaging in the diagnosis and management of peripheral psoriatic arthritis-the clinical utility of magnetic resonance imaging and ultrasonography. Best Pract Res Clin Rheumatol. 2016;30(4):624–37.
15. Garcia-Kutzbacj A, Chacon-Suchite J, Garcia-Ferrer H, Iraheta. Reactive arthritis: update 2018. Clin Rheumatol. 2018;37(4):869–74.
16. Selmi C, Gershwin ME. Diagnosis and classification of reactive arthritis. Autoimmun Rev. 2014;13(4–5):546–9.
17. Klecker R, Weissman B. Imaging features of psoriatic arthritis and Reiter's syndrome. Semin Musculoskelet Radiol. 2003;7(2):115–26.
18. Sieper J, Rudwaleit M, Baraliakos X, Brandt J, Braun J, Burgos-Vargas R, et al. The assessment of SpondyloArthritis international society (ASAS) handbook: a guide to assess spondyloarthritis. Ann Rheum Dis. 2009;68(Suppl 2):ii1–44.
19. Taurog J, Chhabra A, Colbert R. Ankylosing spondylitis and axial spondyloarthritis. N Engl J Med. 2016;374(26):2563–74.
20. Puche-Larrubia M, Clementina López-Medina C, Ziadé N. Peripheral spondyloarthritis: what have we learned? Best Pract Res Clin Rheumatol. 2023;37(3):101862.
21. Kong M, Walters H, Teh J. Updates in deposition arthritis other than gout. Semin Musculoskelet Radiol. 2025;29(2):275–92.
22. Miksanek J, Rosenthal A. Imaging of calcium pyrophosphate deposition disease. Curr Rheumatol Rep. 2015;17(3):20.
23. Nicolaou S, Liang T, Murphy D, Korzan J, Ouellette H, Munk P. Dual-energy CT: a promising new technique for assessment of the musculoskeletal system. Am J Roentgenol. 2012;199(5):S78–86.

12 Metabolic-Endocrine

Miriam A. Bredella and Bruno C. Vande Berg

12.1 Introduction

Metabolic and endocrine pathologies can affect the entire musculoskeletal system, involving not only bone but also muscle, tendons, ligaments, and soft tissues [1, 2]. Dysregulation of these pathways, through hormonal imbalance, genetic predisposition, or environmental and nutritional factors, can result in a wide spectrum of clinical and imaging manifestations. Increasing recognition of the systemic impact of metabolic and endocrine diseases underscores the importance of radiologists in identifying subtle imaging findings that may indicate an underlying metabolic or endocrine disorder [1, 2].

Unlike focal musculoskeletal pathology, metabolic and endocrine disorders often present diffusely, with imaging findings that may be nonspecific or mimic other conditions. For example, thyroid dysfunction alters bone turnover and fracture risk, diabetes mellitus contributes to impaired bone quality and tendon pathology, and adrenal and pituitary disorders lead to secondary osteoporosis and muscle weakness [1, 2]. The role of radiologists extends beyond detection of established complications to early recognition of imaging biomarkers that may guide preventive interventions.

Consequences of delayed diagnosis are significant, including fractures, chronic pain, and functional decline, contributing to morbidity, reduced quality of life, and health system burden worldwide [3]. Early imaging-based recognition of metabolic and endocrine musculoskeletal disease is therefore critical to prevent complications, initiate timely therapy, and reduce long-term disability.

M. A. Bredella (✉)
Department of Radiology, NYU Langone Health and Grossman School of Medicine, New York, NY, USA
e-mail: Miriam.Bredella@nyulangone.org

B. C. Vande Berg
Department of Radiology, Centre hospitalier chrétien CHC, Liège, Belgium
e-mail: bruno.vandeberg@chc.be

This chapter will highlight the effects of systemic metabolic and endocrine disorders on the musculoskeletal system and their imaging appearance and discuss under-recognized conditions such as sarcopenia and medication-induced bone fragility.

Learning Objective

- To recognize the imaging manifestations of systemic metabolic and endocrine disorders on bone, muscle, and soft tissue.
- To identify emerging and under-recognized conditions such as sarcopenia, obesity-related marrow changes, and medication-induced metabolic effects.
- To detect complications of metabolic and endocrine disorders, such as insufficiency fractures.

12.2 Systemic Endocrine Influences on the Musculoskeletal System

Endocrine regulation plays a fundamental role in musculoskeletal homeostasis, influencing bone turnover, muscle metabolism, and soft tissue integrity. Disruption of these pathways may lead to clinically significant imaging findings that radiologists must recognize to ensure timely diagnosis and treatment.

12.2.1 Thyroid Disorders

Both hypothyroidism and hyperthyroidism impact the skeleton and soft tissues, albeit through different mechanisms. Hyperthyroidism accelerates bone turnover, leading to increased cortical porosity, trabecular thinning, and a higher risk of osteoporosis and fragility fractures [1, 2]. Hypothyroidism, conversely, is associated with delayed bone

J. Hodler et al. (eds.), *Musculoskeletal Diseases 2026-2029*, IDKD Springer Series,
https://doi.org/10.1007/978-3-032-17040-8_12

growth in children, impaired bone remodeling in adults, and myopathy presenting as muscle stiffness and pseudohypertrophy [4]. Imaging may demonstrate reduced bone density, degenerative changes, or soft tissue edema, depending on the chronicity and severity of disease [1, 4].

12.2.2 Diabetes Mellitus

Diabetes mellitus is increasingly recognized as a metabolic disease that impairs bone quality beyond effects on bone mineral density (BMD). Hyperglycemia and accumulation of advanced glycation end-products (AGEs) weaken collagen cross-linking, compromising bone strength despite normal BMD values. This contributes to an elevated fracture risk [5]. In addition, diabetic patients frequently develop musculoskeletal complications such as Charcot arthropathy, diffuse idiopathic skeletal hyperostosis (DISH), and crystal arthropathies. Soft tissue manifestations include myopathy (Fig. 12.1), tendinopathy, adhesive capsulitis, and limited joint mobility syndromes such as diabetic cheiroarthropathy ("stiff hand syndrome"), Dupuytren's contracture, and trigger finger which may be identified on radiographs, ultrasound, or MRI [6].

12.2.3 Adrenal Disorders

Excess glucocorticoids, as seen in endogenous Cushing's syndrome or exogenous steroid therapy, exert profound effects on bone and muscle. Cortisol excess promotes osteoclast activity and suppresses osteoblast function, resulting in osteoporosis and a high prevalence of fractures [1]. Imaging may reveal fragility fractures, decreased trabecular attenuation, and myopathy with muscle atrophy or fatty infiltration. By contrast, adrenal insufficiency (Addison's disease) is associated with chronic fatigue, muscle weakness, and nonspecific musculoskeletal complaints, though direct imaging correlates are less striking [2, 7].

12.2.4 Pituitary and Growth Hormone Abnormalities

Pituitary dysfunction can lead to either excess or deficiency of growth hormone, with distinct skeletal consequences. Acromegaly, due to growth hormone excess, produces characteristic imaging features including enlarged hands and feet, thickened calvarium, mandibular prognathism, and degenerative joint disease. Radiographs and MRI may show widened joint spaces, enthesopathy, and soft tissue thickening, especially of the heel pad (Fig. 12.2). Conversely, growth hormone deficiency results in reduced bone mass, smaller skeletal size, and increased risk of osteoporosis [1, 2].

Key Points

- Endocrine disorders affect not only bone but also muscle, tendons, and soft tissues.
- Thyroid dysfunction alters bone turnover and fracture risk.
- Diabetes is associated with impaired bone quality, muscle, and tendon abnormalities.
- Cushing's and other adrenal disorders cause osteoporosis and muscle atrophy.

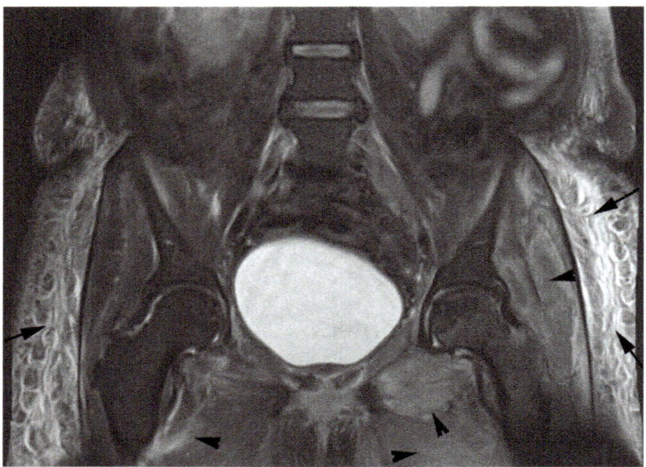

Fig. 12.1 Diabetic myopathy. Coronal fat-suppressed T2-weighted MR image in a 65-year-old woman with type 2 diabetes mellitus shows diffuse edema of the gluteal and adductor musculature (arrowheads), left greater than right. Diffuse subcutaneous edema (arrows) is present

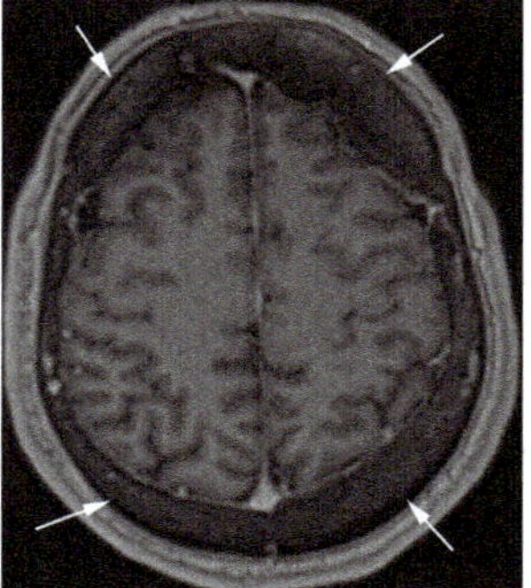

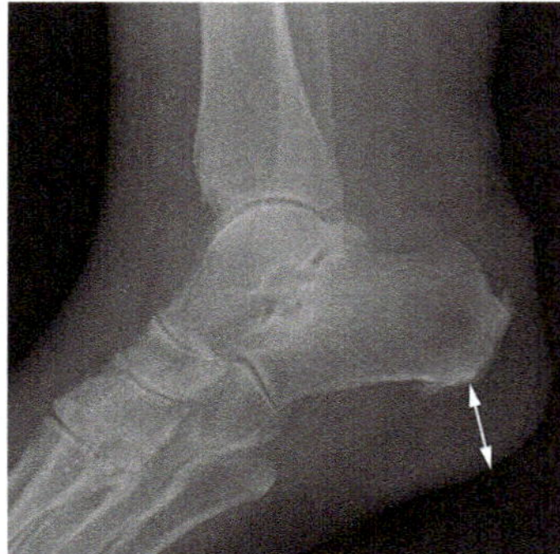

Fig. 12.2 Imaging findings of acromegaly. Axial T1-weighted MR image of the brain shows a thickened calvarium (arrows) (**a**). Lateral radiograph of the ankle shows a thickened heel pad (arrow) (**b**)

12.3 Metabolic Bone and Mineral Disorders

While osteoporosis represents the most prevalent metabolic bone disease, radiologists must also recognize a broader spectrum of metabolic and mineral disorders that manifest with distinctive imaging findings. These conditions, though less common, can carry significant morbidity when not promptly identified.

12.3.1 Hyperparathyroidism

Primary and secondary hyperparathyroidism lead to increased osteoclastic activity, which alters both trabecular and cortical bone. The classic imaging finding is subperiosteal bone resorption particularly along the radial aspects of the middle phalanges of the index and middle fingers or the sacroiliac joints [1]. Additional features include the "salt-and-pepper" skull, bone demineralization, and cystic lesions. Advanced disease may produce brown tumors—osteolytic lesions composed of fibrous tissue and hemosiderin (Fig. 12.3). Soft tissue and vascular calcifications are frequent, especially in the setting of secondary hyperparathyroidism associated with chronic kidney disease. Subtle cases may only demonstrate cortical thinning or equivocal trabecular changes, underscoring the importance of careful imaging review [1].

12.3.2 Vitamin D Abnormalities

Vitamin D deficiency impairs mineralization of osteoid, producing rickets in children and osteomalacia in adults. In adults, imaging may reveal Looser's zones (pseudofractures), diffuse osteopenia, or cortical thinning [1]. In children, imaging may reveal widened growth plates, flared or fractured metaphyses, a bell-shaped thorax, and widening of the anterior rib ends ("rachitic rosary"). Rickets can overlap radiographically with conditions such as hypophosphatasia or renal osteodystrophy [1, 8].

12.3.3 Hypophosphatasia and Phosphate-Wasting Disorders

Hypophosphatasia is a rare genetic disorder characterized by mutations in the ALPL gene, leading to impaired bone mineralization and accumulation of inorganic pyrophosphate [8]. Imaging findings resemble rickets or osteomalacia, with widened growth plates in children, metaphyseal cupping, and recurrent fractures in adults [1, 8]. Similarly, acquired phosphate-wasting disorders (such as tumor-induced osteomalacia) may manifest with insufficiency fractures and diffuse osteopenia, often requiring advanced imaging for diagnosis. MRI may show nonspecific marrow signal changes, but CT or radiographs often provide more definitive clues to mineralization defects.

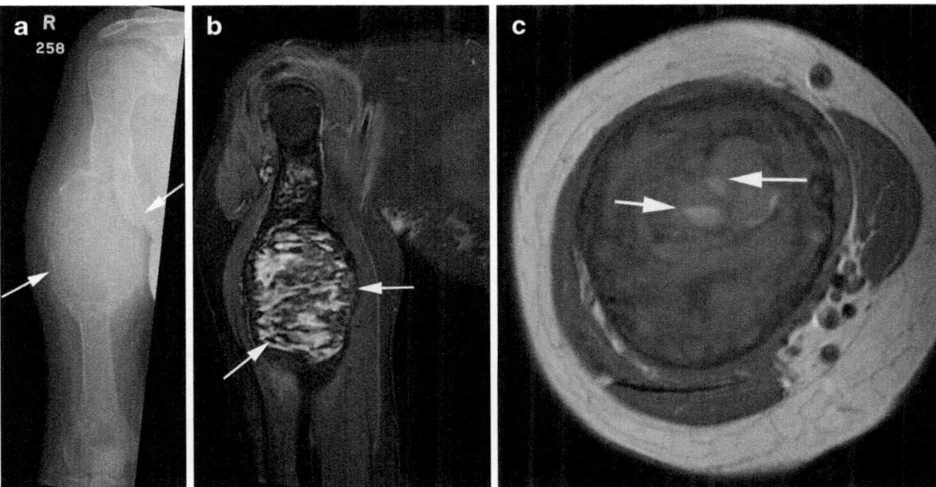

Fig. 12.3 Frontal radiograph in a 41-year-old woman with chronic renal disease shows large lytic lesion in the humeral diaphysis with thinned cortex and internal septations (arrows), consistent with a biopsy-proven brown tumor (**a**). Sagittal fat-suppressed T2-weighted MR image demonstrates solid and cystic components with solid components showing intermediate to hypointense signal intensity (arrows) (**b**). Axial T1-weighted image demonstrates expansion of the humeral diaphysis with fluid-fluid levels (arrows) with internal hyperintense T1 signal (**c**)

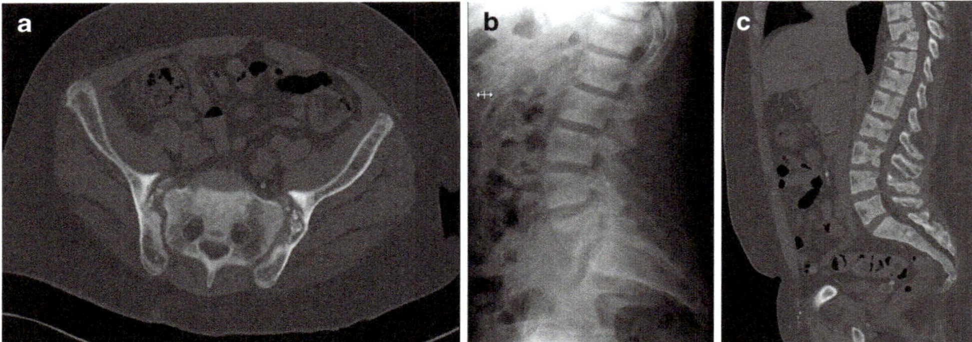

Fig. 12.4 Renal osteodystrophy. Axial CT image of the abdomen in a 62-year-old man with chronic renal disease demonstrates severe resorption and erosions of the sacroiliac joints (**a**). Lateral radiograph shows increased density of the vertebral body endplates with central ill-defined lucency, known as the rugger jersey spine (**b**). Corresponding sagittal CT image shows diffuse sclerosis of the visualized skeleton with ill-defined lucency and compression deformities and pathologic fractures of T9/T10 (**c**)

12.3.4 Renal Osteodystrophy

Renal osteodystrophy is associated with chronic kidney failure and includes osteomalacia, rickets in children, and secondary hyperparathyroidism. The condition often results in increased bone radiodensity, particularly in the axial skeleton. This increase, likely due to the effects of parathyroid hormone, paradoxically leads to weak bones which are prone to fractures. A characteristic "rugger jersey spine" appearance may be seen (Fig. 12.4). Beyond bone, chronic kidney issues can lead to calcium deposits in soft tissues, primarily around large joints, but also potentially in organs, which can be life-threatening [1].

Key Points

- Hyperparathyroidism shows subperiosteal resorption, brown tumors, and vascular/soft tissue calcifications.
- Hypophosphatasia and phosphate-wasting disorders cause rickets-like changes and recurrent fractures.
- Vitamin D deficiency remains globally prevalent and presents with varied imaging patterns in adults and children.

12.4 Emerging and Under-Recognized Conditions

A growing number of endocrine and metabolic factors are now recognized as critical contributors to musculoskeletal health, extending well beyond the classic mineralization disorders. These conditions often have subtle imaging findings but carry major implications for patient outcomes, particularly as populations age and the prevalence of obesity, diabetes, and polypharmacy rises.

12.4.1 Sarcopenia

Sarcopenia refers to progressive loss of muscle mass and function and was once viewed primarily as a consequence of aging. Increasingly, it is considered a systemic metabolic disorder influenced by endocrine pathways, including insulin resistance, sex steroid deficiency, and chronic inflammation. MRI and CT can quantify muscle cross-sectional area and fatty infiltration, which strongly correlate with frailty, falls, and mortality. Muscle cross-sectional area and fatty infiltration assessed using so-called "opportunistic CT" are emerging biomarkers of sarcopenia and fragility [9, 10].

12.4.2 Obesity

Obesity alters bone and marrow composition in ways that extend beyond mechanical loading. Marrow adiposity is elevated in obesity and metabolic syndrome, and increased bone marrow adipose tissue fat has been linked to compromised trabecular microarchitecture and increased fracture risk [11, 12]. Despite higher BMD in many individuals with obesity, fracture susceptibility is paradoxically increased, particularly in the extremities [13]. Imaging may reveal insufficiency fractures or stress injuries in weight-bearing bones, with MRI and CT providing greater sensitivity than radiographs.

12.4.3 Medication-Induced Metabolic Effects

Pharmacologic interventions, while therapeutic, can profoundly alter bone and muscle metabolism. Chronic corticosteroid therapy remains a leading cause of secondary osteoporosis, associated with trabecular bone loss, vertebral compression fractures, and osteonecrosis. Bisphosphonates and denosumab, though highly effective antiresorptives, carry risks of atypical femoral fractures and osteonecrosis of the jaw when used long-term. Statins, widely used to treat hypercholesteremia, can cause myopathy and rarely rhabdomyolysis [14]. Awareness of these medication-induced patterns is essential for accurate image interpretation and clinical management.

Key Points
- Sarcopenia and fatty infiltration of muscle are increasingly recognized as endocrine and metabolic processes.
- Obesity and the metabolic syndrome alter marrow composition and increase stress injury risk.
- Medication-related bone effects (steroids, bisphosphonates, statins) should always be considered when evaluating fractures.

12.5 Complications of Metabolic Bone Disorders

Metabolic bone disorders are a group of diseases with qualitative and/or quantitative changes of the mineralized matrix of the skeleton [15, 16]. These disorders remain usually clinically silent until a fracture occurs. Imaging plays a critical role in the diagnosis of fractures in the setting of metabolic bone disease because of the lack of a typical history and the often-confusing clinical manifestations at presentation [17].

Key points
- Metabolic bone disorders often remain clinically silent unless complications occur.
- Insufficiency fractures represent complications of metabolic bone disease.

12.6 Insufficiency Fractures

Insufficiency fractures are a type of stress fracture that occur in patients with non-tumorous metabolic or endocrine bone disorders and result from normal or moderate increased stress applied on diffusely weakened bones. They differ from fatigue fracture, which are the result of chronic increased repetitive stress on normal bones, by a lack of suggestive clinical history. Of note, the frontier between fatigue and insufficiency fractures can be a matter of debate. As an example, sports-related fatigue fractures may occur in active women with menstrual dysfunction, insufficient energy availability, and low BMD (e.g., the female athlete triad) [18]. Insufficiency fractures may also occur in healthy women during or after pregnancy [19].

12.6.1 What the Radiologists Should Know About Insufficiency Fractures

Insufficiency fractures occur spontaneously without definite triggering events. Therefore, the time of onset is unclear with possible subacute bone changes at the time of imaging. Being due to gravity forces (body weight), insufficiency fractures almost never involve the upper limbs and the non-ankylosed cervical spine due to limited body weight on these body segments. They are merely compression fractures given the vertical orientation of gravity forces. Insufficiency fractures will develop in bones with a high trabecular/cortical bone ratio since trabecular bone is more susceptible to compression fracture than cortical bone [20, 21].

Insufficiency fractures are more common in women and in elderly patients (high prevalence of osteoporosis). However, they occasionally occur in children (rickets, scurvy, familial osteoporosis) and in young adults with or without known metabolic disorders (pregnancy, anorexia nervosa, autism spectrum disorder). These fractures generally heal with supportive measures. Delayed healing may occasionally occur due to systemic (osteomalacia, steroid intake) or local (previous radiation therapy) changes in bone remodeling. Rarely, they may progress to secondary displacement that may require surgical treatment (atypical femoral fracture, vertebral collapse) or may cause early osteoarthritis. Insufficiency fractures rarely recur at the same location, but they may appear later at other locations [1, 20, 21].

12.6.2 What the Radiologists Should Look for in Insufficiency Fractures

At radiography, early diagnosis of insufficiency fractures is challenging and relies on the detection of cortical interruption and bone deformity. These changes can be obvious in vertebral insufficiency fractures but can be barely visible in epiphyseal and small bone fractures [16] (Fig. 12.5). At a subacute stage, fractures may become more conspicuous due to the appearance of callus and periosteal reaction. Trabecular

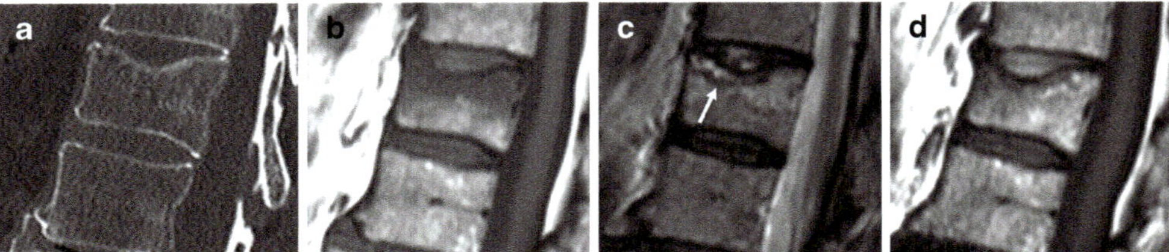

Fig. 12.5 Spontaneous vertebral fracture in a 74-year-old woman with osteoporosis. Sagittal reformatted CT image of the lower thoracic spine demonstrates a deformed vertebral endplate indicating a fracture (**a**). Corresponding T1-weighted (**b**) and T2-weighted (**c**) MR images show bone marrow edema-like signal changes adjacent to the fractured endplate. A low signal intensity line (fracture line) is visible on the T2-weighted image (arrow). Note the lack of sclerosis on CT (**a**). Follow-up MRI obtained 3 months later demonstrates almost complete healing of the fracture (**d**)

callus appears as a sclerotic line usually orientated perpendicular to the weight-bearing trabeculae. CT may better depict these trabecular bone changes and may also highlight subtle soft tissue changes adjacent to the fracture. CT also contributes to the differential diagnosis between acute, subacute, and healed fractures. Soft tissue changes and cortical interruption are present at the acute stage and progressively disappear at the same time as callus mineralizes. Dual-energy CT may increase the confidence with which the fracture is diagnosed given its ability to detect associated bone marrow edema that may remain occult on mono-energetic CT [22].

On MRI, bone marrow edema (BME)-like changes with moderate decrease in signal intensity of fat-sensitive sequences and increased signal intensity on fluid-sensitive sequences are usually a predominant albeit nonspecific imaging finding [21, 23] (Fig. 12.6). Low signal intensity lines within BME-like changes are highly suggestive of trabecular insufficiency fractures. The fracture line is usually thin, irregular, parallel, or curvilinear with respect to the adjacent endplate or epiphyseal contour (Figs. 12.5 and 12.6). It may also be discontinuous or open-ended. The fracture lines may be due to hemorrhage, collapsed trabeculae, granulation tissue with cartilage metaplasia, and callus formation. They may be absent at the very early stage of the fracture. Their conspicuity on the different MR sequences can vary. The presence of fracture lines can facilitate the distinction between stress-reaction and stress fracture. Other imaging features including altered bone shape and periosteal reaction may be observed [21].

In insufficiency fractures of cortical bone, cortical interruption is often barely visible on routine MR images. Focal edema-like changes on the endosteal and periosteal aspects of the cortex may be suggestive of a partial fracture. Focused CT or CT-like MRI sequences may contribute to the detection of linear cortical changes. In chronic partial cortical fractures, edema may be absent [16, 20].

Key Points

- Low-signal intensity lines on MRI or sclerotic lines on radiography/CT, typically oriented perpendicular to the weight-bearing trabeculae, are the most valuable signs of trabecular fractures.
- BME-like change on MRI is an important but nonspecific imaging feature of insufficiency fractures.
- Cortical insufficiency fractures can be missed on MRI.

12.6.3 Topographic Approach of Insufficiency Fractures

12.6.3.1 Spine

Insufficiency fractures in the spine predominantly involve the thoracolumbar junction. The anterior and central midportions of the vertebral bodies are weaker than the posterior elements, which can result in wedge compression or endplate fractures or, less commonly, crush fractures. BME-like changes on MRI involve the upper or lower aspects of the vertebral body and spare the posterior elements and the adjacent vertebral bodies (differential diagnosis from disc-related marrow changes) [16, 20] (Fig. 12.5). Low signal intensity lines are parallel to and located at a few millimeters from the involved vertebral end plate (Fig. 12.5). At the subacute stage, BME-like changes tend to decrease on MRI and bone sclerosis is visible on CT. At the healed stage, bone marrow returns to normal or may show fatty conversion on MRI and returns to normal on CT [24].

12.6.3.2 Pelvic Ring

Insufficiency fractures of the pelvic ring are often multiple and involve the pubic and ischiatic rami, the supraacetabular region, and the sacral ala. Patients with previous radia-

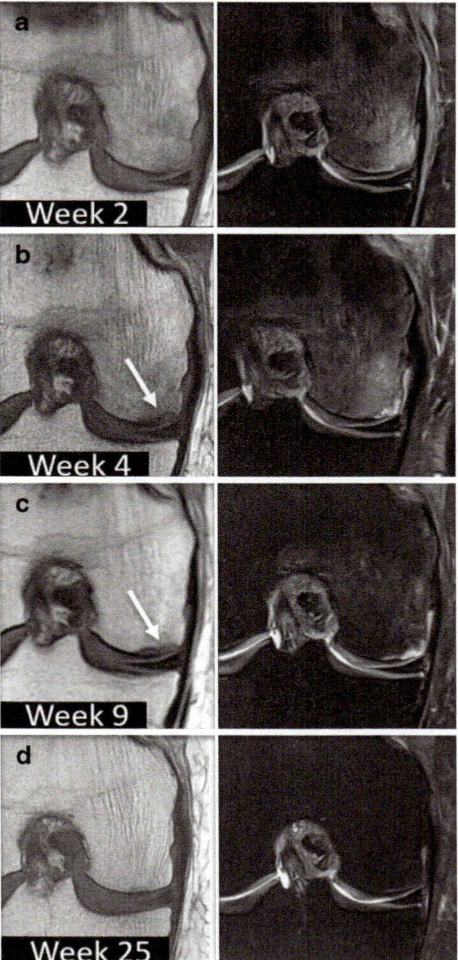

Fig. 12.6 Subchondral insufficiency fracture (SIF) of the right medial femoral condyle in a 61-year-old man with a history of spontaneous knee pain. Two weeks after onset of symptoms, bone marrow edema (BME)-like signal changes involve the medial femoral condyle, near the articular surface (T1- and fat-suppressed proton-density-weighted MR images) (**a**). At the week 4 follow-up MRI, a low signal intensity line (arrow) is detected in the subchondral area within the unaltered BME-like changes (**b**). At the 9-week follow-up MRI, the fracture line becomes more conspicuous on the T1-weighted MR image (arrow) as adjacent BME-like changes have partially regressed (**c**). At the 25-week follow-up MRI, complete healing of the SIF is demonstrated (**d**)

tion therapy or osteomalacia may have multiple pelvic fractures [15, 24] (Fig. 12.7). Radiographs are often non-diagnostic, except in the setting of pubic fractures (cortical fractures). CT may demonstrate cortical interruption or callus formation of trabecular bone (sacrum). MR imaging is the most accurate imaging modality for sacral and supra-acetabular fractures.

12.6.3.3 Femur and Tibia

Early recognition of femoral and tibial insufficiency fractures is important because of the risk for progression to dis-

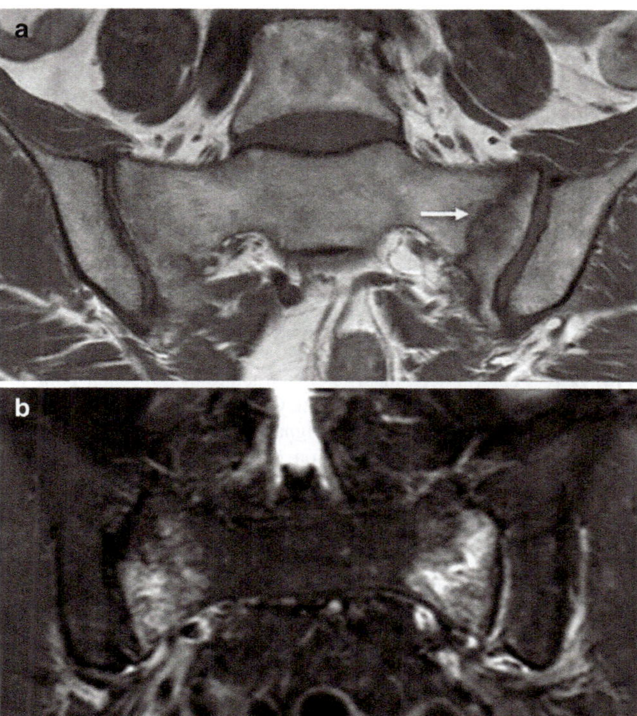

Fig. 12.7 Sacral insufficiency fractures in a 62-year-old woman with osteoporosis. Coronal T1-weighted MR image demonstrates bone marrow edema (BME)-like signal changes in the left sacral ala with a vertical low signal intensity line (arrow) that is parallel to the sacral articular surface. The right side appears almost normal (**a**). Coronal STIR image demonstrates bilateral BME-like changes. On the right side, no line is detected but the BME-like change has the same vertical orientation (**b**)

placed fractures and subsequent complications, particularly in elderly patients. These fractures may involve the femoral neck and proximal femoral diaphysis as well as the epiphyseal regions. Femoral neck fractures involving the trabecular bone are easily detected on MRI due to extensive BME-like changes and low signal intensity lines (Fig. 12.8). Detection of cortical femoral neck fractures can be more challenging [15, 21, 24]. Rarely, cortical insufficiency fractures have a transverse orientation, most frequently in the tibia (Fig. 12.9). They are associated with extensive BME-like edema in the adjacent medullary cavity and soft tissues. Cortical interruption is better recognized on CT compared to MRI.

Atypical insufficiency fractures of the femoral shaft may occur in patients with long-standing osteoporosis with or without bisphosphonate or methotrexate therapy [25] (Fig. 12.10). They may also occur in Paget's disease. These fractures are predominantly transverse in orientation and involve the lateral aspect of the femoral shaft. They can be multiple, bilateral, and clinically silent. On radiographs, atypical femoral fractures demonstrate transverse cortical lucencies involving the lateral aspect of the femur. Associated periosteal new bone

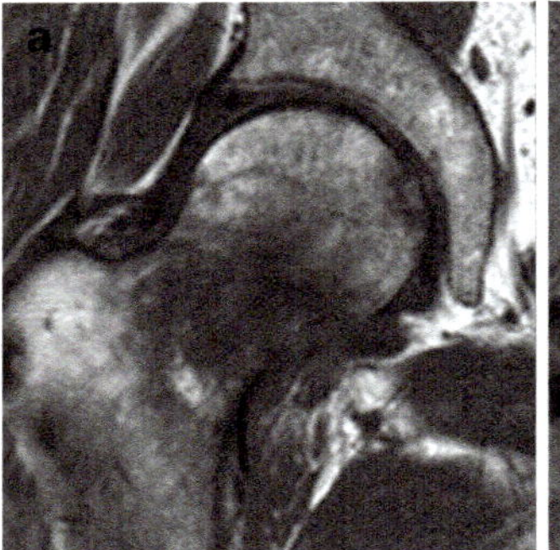

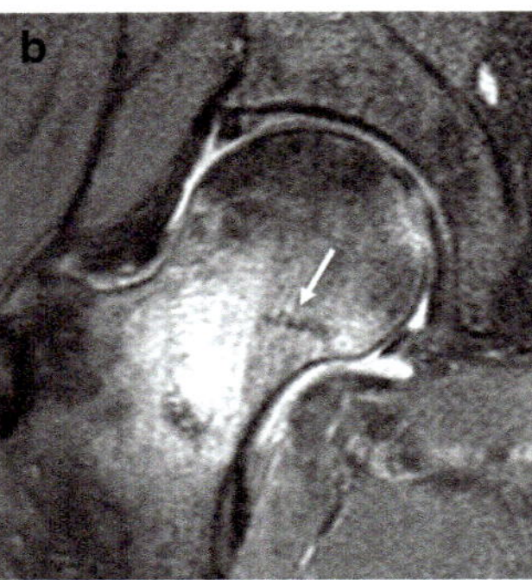

Fig. 12.8 Femoral neck insufficiency fracture of trabecular bone in a 36-year-old man with renal transplant. Coronal T1-weighted MR image demonstrates marked decrease in signal intensity of the femoral neck that may mimic a neoplastic lesion (**a**). On the corresponding fat-suppressed proton-density-weighted MR image, bone marrow edema (BME)-like signal change with ill-defined margins can be seen. The low signal intensity line (arrow) in the center of the lesion is the diagnostic clue for this insufficiency fracture. Note that the line is not visible on the T1-weighted image. Its orientation is perpendicular to the weight-bearing trabeculae (**b**)

formation can be seen leading to a beak appearance. If a complete fracture occurs, the fracture line is typically transverse but may also extend longitudinally. Partial fractures can be detected on radiographs and CT, and can be more difficult to detect on MRI, given the lack of edema. As atypical femoral fractures are often bilateral, imaging of both femurs is recommended. Preventive nailing of involved femurs has been advised to prevent complete fracture [25].

12.6.3.4 Subchondral Insufficiency Fracture (SIF)

Until the early nineties, almost all spontaneous (non-traumatic) subchondral fractures were considered to be due to underlying epiphyseal osteonecrosis or due to transient osteoporosis of the hip. The concept of spontaneous epiphyseal subchondral bone lesions corresponding to non-traumatic fractures (fatigue or insufficiency) is nowadays a widely accepted concept [21] (Fig. 12.6).

SIFs involve convex weight-bearing epiphyses such as the femoral head, the femoral condyles, and metatarsal heads. Concave epiphyses such as the tibial epiphyses are less frequently involved. SIFs are usually occult at radiography, and MRI reveals extensive BME-like changes with low signal intensity lines, located a few millimeters from the subchondral bone plate which is generally not altered. SIF differs from osteoarthritis-associated changes by the presence of normal cartilage overlying the fracture site.

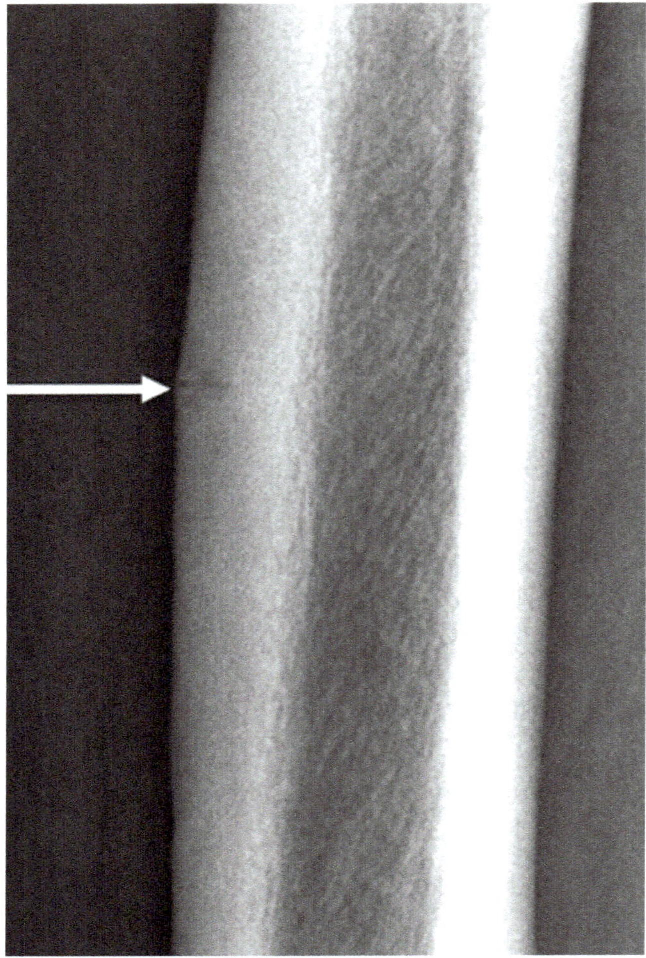

Fig. 12.9 Magnified radiograph of the right femur of an 81-year-old woman with osteoporosis and long-term bisphosphonate therapy. A faint linear lucency (arrow) indicates a partial cortical fracture of the femoral shaft

12.6.4 Outcomes of Insufficiency Fractures

Insufficiency fractures generally heal with appropriate conservative therapy. Bone deformity is usually limited except in vertebral fractures, where wedge-shaped deformity may cause kyphosis and chronic pain. In the spine and pelvic ring, an initially stable fracture can progress to an unstable fracture over time. Awareness of this complication is important for timely diagnosis and early intervention to prevent poor outcomes. In the spine, vertebral body collapse can lead to spinal cord/dural sac compression (Fig. 12.11).

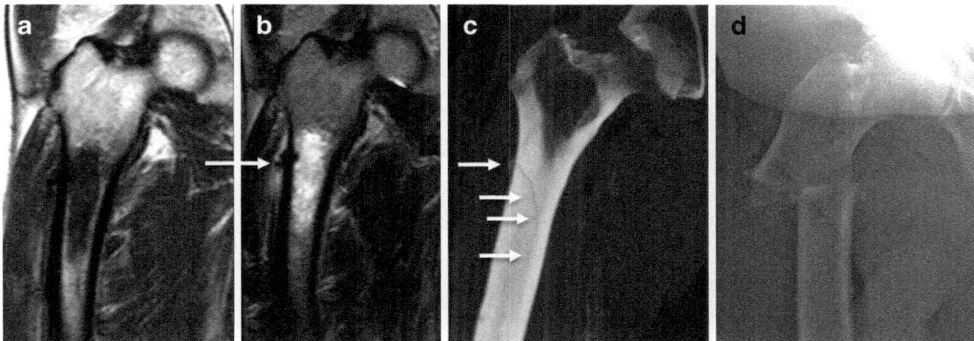

Fig. 12.10 75-year-old man with spontaneous onset of right thigh pain. Coronal T1-weighted (**a**) and T2-weighted (**b**) MR images demonstrate extensive bone marrow edema (BME)-like changes in the femoral shaft suggesting a marrow replacing lesion. Subtle soft tissue change is seen along the lateral aspect of the femur (arrow). Coronal maximum intensity projection reformatted CT image demonstrates a cortical fracture line (arrows) on the lateral and anterior cortex (**c**). Fracture displacement occurred a few weeks later in the absence of specific treatment (**d**)

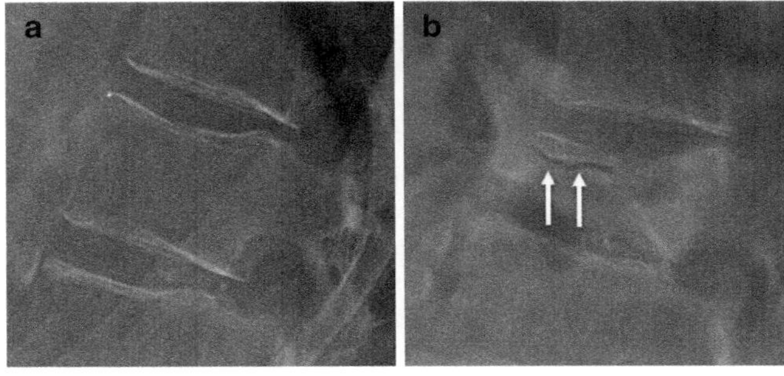

Fig. 12.11 Lateral spine radiographs of an 82-year-old man with spontaneous vertebral fracture at onset of symptoms (**a**) and at 9 months follow-up (**b**). Vertebral body collapse with intravertebral vacuum phenomenon (arrows) (so-called vertebral osteonecrosis) is demonstrated at follow-up with subsequent kyphosis

In the setting of SIF, delayed union with residual osteochondral changes and subsequent osteoarthritis may occur. Clinical outcomes range from residual defects being well tolerated, mainly in elderly patients, to progressive collapse with subsequent early osteoarthritis [21]. SIF has been proposed as a mechanism for the occurrence of rapidly destructive osteoarthritis, although this link remains debated.

In large epiphyses, the distinction between SIF and spontaneous osteonecrosis of the hip and the knee remains a matter of debate. There is a literature shift from spontaneous osteonecrosis to SIF, with the recommendation to abandon the term spontaneous osteonecrosis of the knee (SONK) and hip, given the fact that the etiology of spontaneous osteonecrosis are subchondral fractures [21, 23]. Others suggest that both entities are distinct but should remain under the same umbrella term of SIF because these fractures may have different outcomes [26] (Fig. 12.12). SIFs without signs indicative of necrosis frequently heal, whereas SIFs with signs of osteonecrosis rarely heal.

When facing an isolated epiphyseal BME-like lesion, the radiologist should focus on fluid-sensitive images to look for prognostic indicators [26]:

- An epiphyseal BME-like lesion without additional subchondral change and a normal overlying bone plate and cartilage will heal even in the presence of subchondral low signal lines.
- An epiphyseal BME-like lesion with additional subchondral changes including a thick low signal subchondral area (> 4 mm), cyst-like changes, or significant flattening will not heal and may progress to further collapse.

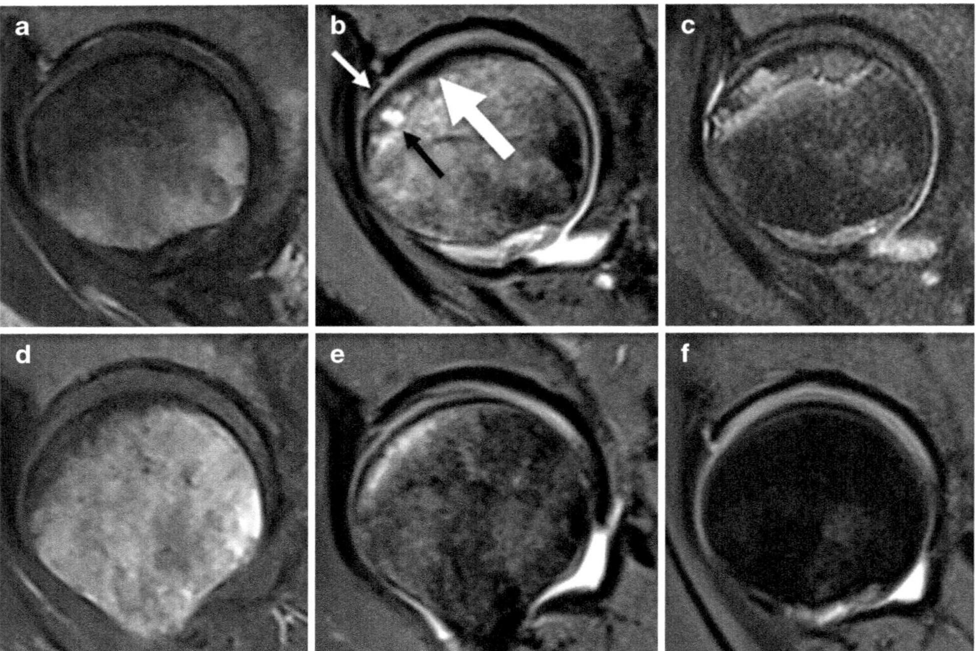

Fig. 12.12 Spontaneous insufficiency fracture (SIF) of the right (**a**–**c**) and left (**d**–**f**) femoral heads(**a**) Sagittal images of the right hip demonstrate BME-like changes in the antero-superior aspect of the femoral head. Additional features such as epiphyseal contour flattening (white arrow), cyst-like changes (black arrow), and low signal subchondral changes (large arrow) indicate SIF with osteonecrosis and a poor prognosis. (**c**) At 6-month follow-up MRI, lack of healing. (**d**) Sagittal T1- and (**e**) fs PD-weighted images of the left hip demonstrate BME-like changes in the antero-superior aspect of the femoral head without additional changes suggestive of a SIF without osteonecrosis with a favorable prognosis. (**f**) Healing is demonstrated at 6-month follow-up MRI

- An epiphyseal BME-like lesion with limited subchondral changes (low signal subchondral area < 3 mm) has an indetermined outcome.
- An epiphyseal BME-like lesion associated with abnormal overlying cartilage has no prognostic significance as the joint outcome depends on the integrity of the cartilage and not on the marrow changes.

12.7 Concluding Remarks

Metabolic and endocrine disorders affecting the musculoskeletal system are characterized by complex interactions involving bone, muscle, tendons, and soft tissues. These conditions often remain clinically silent until complications such as fractures occur. Given the wide-ranging effects of hormonal imbalances, genetic factors, and environmental influences, early detection through imaging is critical. Radiologists play a pivotal role by identifying subtle imaging biomarkers that suggest underlying endocrine or metabolic disorders, enabling timely interventions to avert long-term disability. Imaging, particularly MRI, is essential for assessing diffuse changes and guiding preventive strategies, thereby improving outcomes and quality of life for affected individuals globally.

Take Home Points

- Endocrine and metabolic disorders can significantly impact the musculoskeletal system, affecting bone, muscle, tendons, ligaments, and soft tissues.
- Endocrine and metabolic disorders are often clinically silent until complications occur, such as fractures, arthritis, or myopathy, which can lead to chronic pain and functional decline.
- Radiographs, CT, and MRI all play an important role in diagnosing metabolic and endocrine bone and soft tissue disorders and associated complications.
- Insufficiency fractures of the thoracolumbar spine and lower limb bones are the most frequent complications of metabolic bone disorders, and imaging plays an important role in their diagnosis.
- BME-like changes are a predominant but nonspecific MR feature observed in insufficiency fractures. The presence of low signal intensity lines indicates impaction fracture of the trabeculae. In cortical fractures, cortical discontinuity is best appreciated on CT.
- SIF is an umbrella term covering several conditions with variable spontaneous outcomes ranging from spontaneous healing to advanced collapse. Radiologists should focus on distinctive imaging features that indicate prognosis.

Conflict of Interest I/We declare no competing interests as defined by Springer Nature or other interests that might be perceived to influence results and/or discussion reported in this manuscript.

References

1. Chang CY, Rosenthal DI, Mitchell DM, Handa A, Kattapuram SV, Huang AJ. Imaging findings of metabolic bone disease. Radiographics. 2016;36(6):1871–87. https://doi.org/10.1148/rg.2016160004.
2. Chew FS. Radiologic manifestations in the musculoskeletal system of miscellaneous endocrine disorders. Radiol Clin North Am. 1991;29(1):135–47.
3. Stulberg BN, Watson JT. Management of orthopedic complications of metabolic bone disease. Cleve Clin J Med. 1989;56(7):696–703. https://doi.org/10.3949/ccjm.56.7.696.
4. Sindoni A, Rodolico C, Pappalardo MA, Portaro S, Benvenga S. Hypothyroid myopathy: a peculiar clinical presentation of thyroid failure. Review of the literature. Rev Endocr Metab Disord. 2016;17(4):499–519. https://doi.org/10.1007/s11154-016-9357-0.
5. Upadhyay P, Kumar S. Diabetes and bone health: a comprehensive review of impacts and mechanisms. Diabetes Metab Res Rev. 2025;41(5):e70062. https://doi.org/10.1002/dmrr.70062.
6. Rao A, Gandikota G. Beyond ulcers and osteomyelitis: imaging of less common musculoskeletal complications in diabetes mellitus. Br J Radiol. 2018;91(1088):20170301. https://doi.org/10.1259/bjr.20170301.
7. Leszczynska D, Szatko A, Papierska L, Zgliczynski W, Glinicki P. Musculoskeletal complications of Cushing syndrome. Reumatologia. 2023;61(4):271–82. https://doi.org/10.5114/reum/169889.
8. Sabbagh Y, Carpenter TO, Demay MB. Hypophosphatemia leads to rickets by impairing caspase-mediated apoptosis of hypertrophic chondrocytes. Proc Natl Acad Sci USA. 2005;102(27):9637–42. https://doi.org/10.1073/pnas.0502249102.
9. Amini B, Boyle SP, Boutin RD, Lenchik L. Approaches to assessment of muscle mass and Myosteatosis on computed tomography: a systematic review. J Gerontol A Biol Sci Med Sci. 2019;74(10):1671–8. https://doi.org/10.1093/gerona/glz034.
10. Boutin RD, Yao L, Canter RJ, Lenchik L. Sarcopenia: current concepts and imaging implications. AJR Am J Roentgenol. 2015;205(3):W255–66. https://doi.org/10.2214/AJR.15.14635.
11. Pachon-Pena G, Bredella MA. Bone marrow adipose tissue in metabolic health. Trends Endocrinol Metab. 2022;33(6):401–8. https://doi.org/10.1016/j.tem.2022.03.003.
12. Singhal V, Torre Flores LP, Stanford FC, et al. Differential associations between appendicular and axial marrow adipose tissue with bone microarchitecture in adolescents and young adults with obesity. Bone. 2018;116:203–6. https://doi.org/10.1016/j.bone.2018.08.009.
13. Kessler J, Koebnick C, Smith N, Adams A. Childhood obesity is associated with increased risk of most lower extremity fractures. Clin Orthop Relat Res. 2013;471(4):1199–207. https://doi.org/10.1007/s11999-012-2621-z.
14. Sidhu HS, Venkatanarasimha N, Bhatnagar G, Vardhanabhuti V, Fox BM, Suresh SP. Imaging features of therapeutic drug-induced musculoskeletal abnormalities. Radiographics. 2012;32(1):105–27. https://doi.org/10.1148/rg.321115041.
15. Guglielmi G, Muscarella S, Leone A, Peh WC. Imaging of metabolic bone diseases. Radiol Clin North Am. 2008;46(4):735–54., vi. https://doi.org/10.1016/j.rcl.2008.04.010.
16. Kanis JA. Diagnosis of osteoporosis and assessment of fracture risk. Lancet. 2002;359(9321):1929–36. https://doi.org/10.1016/S0140-6736(02)08761-5.
17. Cummings SR, Melton LJ. Epidemiology and outcomes of osteoporotic fractures. Lancet. 2002;359(9319):1761–7. https://doi.org/10.1016/S0140-6736(02)08657-9.
18. De Souza MJ, Nattiv A, Joy E, et al. 2014 female athlete triad coalition consensus statement on treatment and return to play of the female athlete triad: 1st international conference held in San Francisco, California, may 2012 and 2nd international conference held in Indianapolis, Indiana, may 2013. Br J Sports Med. 2014;48(4):289. https://doi.org/10.1136/bjsports-2013-093218.
19. De Leeuw A, Cherkaoui Jaouad R, Kamoun M, Abidi S, Michelin P, Cotten A. When it is not sacroiliitis. Skeletal Radiol. 2025;54(11):2433–42. https://doi.org/10.1007/s00256-025-04958-7.
20. Cantrell CK, Butler BA. A review on Management of Insufficiency Fractures of the pelvis and acetabulum. Orthop Clin North Am. 2022;53(4):431–43. https://doi.org/10.1016/j.ocl.2022.06.007.
21. Gorbachova T, Amber I, Beckmann NM, et al. Nomenclature of subchondral nonneoplastic bone lesions. AJR Am J Roentgenol. 2019;213(5):963–82. https://doi.org/10.2214/AJR.19.21571.
22. Ghazi Sherbaf F, Sair HI, Shakoor D, et al. DECT in detection of vertebral fracture-associated bone marrow Edema: a systematic review and meta-analysis with emphasis on technical and imaging interpretation parameters. Radiology. 2021;300(1):110–9. https://doi.org/10.1148/radiol.2021203624.

23. Palmer W, Bancroft L, Bonar F, et al. Glossary of terms for musculoskeletal radiology. Skeletal Radiol. 2020;49(Suppl 1):1–33. https://doi.org/10.1007/s00256-020-03465-1.
24. Guglielmi G, Muscarella S, Bazzocchi A. Integrated imaging approach to osteoporosis: state-of-the-art review and update. Radiographics. 2011;31(5):1343–64. https://doi.org/10.1148/rg.315105712.
25. La Rocca VR, Rosenberg ZS, Allison MB, Im SA, Babb J, Peck V. Frequency of incomplete atypical femoral fractures in asymptomatic patients on long-term bisphosphonate therapy. AJR Am J Roentgenol. 2012;198(5):1144–51. https://doi.org/10.2214/AJR.11.7442.
26. Malghem J, Lecouvet F, Vande Berg B, Kirchgesner T, Omoumi P. Subchondral insufficiency fractures, subchondral insufficiency fractures with osteonecrosis, and other apparently spontaneous subchondral bone lesions of the knee-pathogenesis and diagnosis at imaging. Insights Imaging. 2023;14(1):164. https://doi.org/10.1186/s13244-023-01495-6.

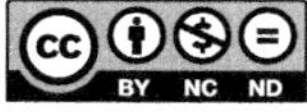

Spine Trauma

13

Mary Kristen Lowry and Connie Y. Chang

Learning Objectives

- **Describe the common fracture patterns and mechanisms of cervical spine injuries**, including odontoid, Hangman, and other C2 fractures, and understand their clinical implications for stability, neurological risk, and management.
- **Explain the principles and application of thoracolumbar spine classification systems**, including TLICS and hybrid AO/TLICS, for assessing fracture morphology, posterior ligamentous complex integrity, and neurological status to guide surgical versus non-surgical management.
- **Identify key descriptive points in fracture assessment**, including location, displacement, angulation, rotation, comminution, articular involvement, and associated soft-tissue injury.
- **Apply standardized fracture classification systems** (Neer, Garden, Schatzker) to specific fractures to improve communication between radiologists and orthopedic surgeons.

13.1 Spine

Fractures of the spine constitute 3–6% of skeletal injuries, but carry high morbidity and mortality [1]. Advanced diagnostic imaging is commonly used for the assessment of spinal injury, and has become routine at major trauma centers [2].

Key Point

C2 fractures often involve the odontoid. The "fat" C2 sign is useful on radiographs.

13.1.1 Cervical Spine

The occipital base, C1, and C2, along with several extrinsic and intrinsic ligaments, form the atlantooccipital and atlantoaxial joints. These articulations protect the brainstem, cranial nerves, and blood supply to the brain, while allowing flexibility and movement [3, 4]. C2 fractures account for 17–20% of cervical spine fractures, and approximately 59% of C2 fractures involve the odontoid [5, 6]. The three main C2 fracture types are odontoid fractures, traumatic spondylolysis, and less commonly, vertebral body/lateral mass fractures [4, 5].

Because the most common mechanism of C2 fractures is motor vehicle accident (MVA), mortality of C2 fractures is high—approximately 15% at 30 days and 34% and one year in patients 65 years and older [7]. However, low-energy trauma can result in odontoid fractures in older patients [7]. Figure 13.1 illustrates an 80-year-old man who had a ground-level fall. The fracture in this patient is at the junction of the odontoid process and the C2 vertebral body. According to the Anderson and D'Alonzo classification, this would be considered a Type II fracture [4, 8]. Type II fractures are the most common, constituting up to 63% of C2 fractures; age greater than 50 years, greater than 6 mm of displacement, comminution, and/or con-

M. K. Lowry
University of Colorado, Aurora, CO, USA

C. Y. Chang (✉)
Massachusetts General Hospital, Boston, MA, USA
e-mail: cychang@mgh.harvard.edu

J. Hodler et al. (eds.), *Musculoskeletal Diseases 2026-2029*, IDKD Springer Series,
https://doi.org/10.1007/978-3-032-17040-8_13

comitant ligamentous injury carry a greater risk of nonunion and often require surgical management (Fig. 13.2) [5, 9]. Because the patient in Fig. 13.1 was a low-energy trauma, there can be little or no bone marrow edema on MRI (Fig. 13.1c). Type I fractures are high in the odontoid, are likely due to alar ligament avulsion, and therefore are often considered stable and heal with conservative treatment (immobilization) [5, 6, 8]. Type III (39–42%) fractures are also generally stable, as they are through the cancellous bone of the vertebral body, and they heal with immobilization using a halo [5, 6, 8]. The "fat" C2 sign can be used to detect C2 body fractures on radiographs, and if present, indicates a displaced vertebral fragment, which may be unstable (Fig. 13.3) [10].

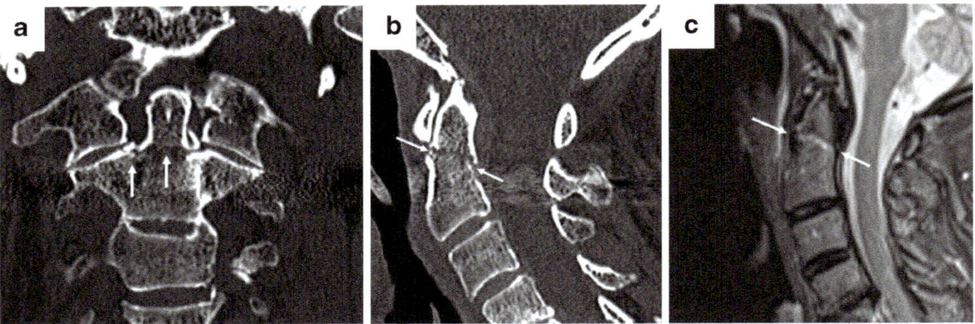

Fig. 13.1 80-year-old man with dementia who had a ground-level fall. (**a**). Coronal noncontrast CT image demonstrates fracture at the base of the odontoid (arrows). This is consistent with a type II fracture. (**b**) Sagittal noncontrast CT image demonstrates approximately 1 mm displacement of the fracture (arrows). Fractures with 6 mm or less displacement can often be managed conservatively. (**c**) Sagittal T2 fat-suppressed image demonstrates the fracture (arrows). There is no substantial prevertebral soft tissue edema or bone marrow edema, probably because this was a low-energy trauma

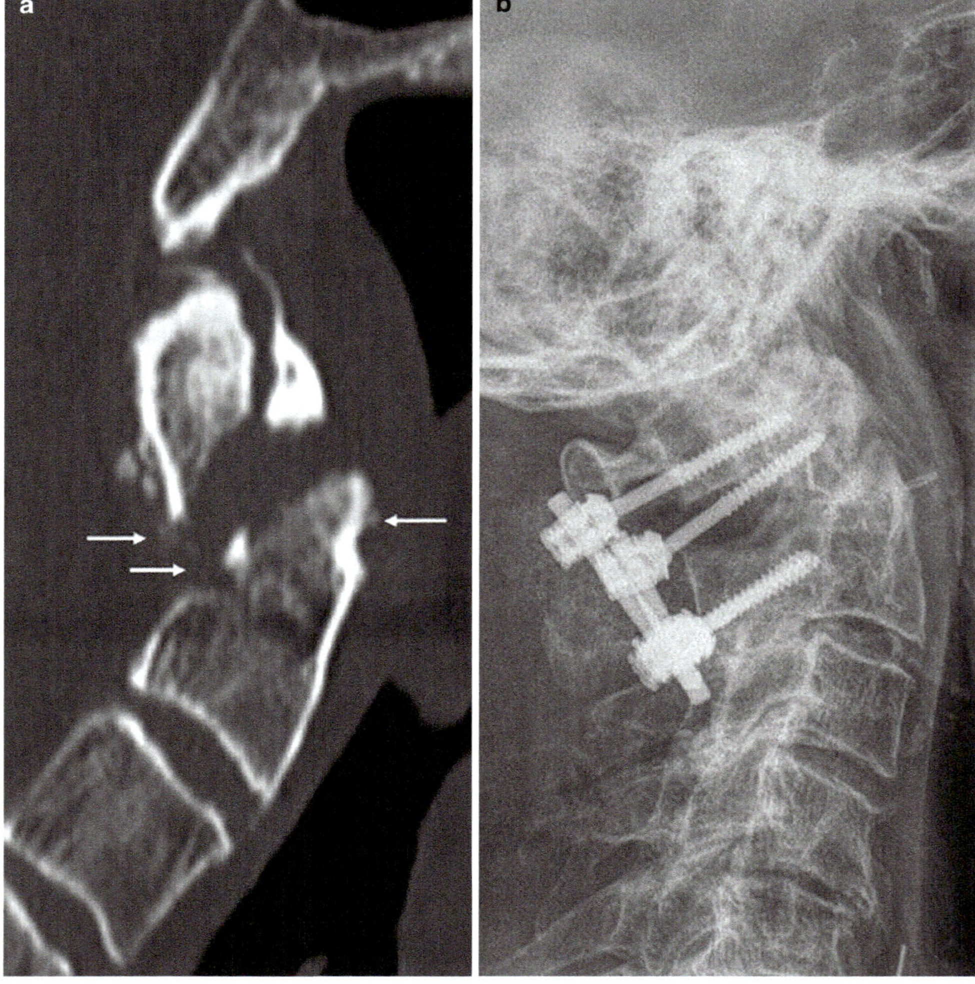

Fig. 13.2 85-year-old man with neck pain after unwitnessed fall. (**a**) Sagittal CT image demonstrates a displaced fracture through the base of the odontoid process, with more than 6 mm of displacement and small chip fragments anteriorly and posteriorly (arrows). This fracture is unstable and requires surgical management. (**b**) Subsequent lateral radiograph demonstrates posterior C1-C2 spinal fusion

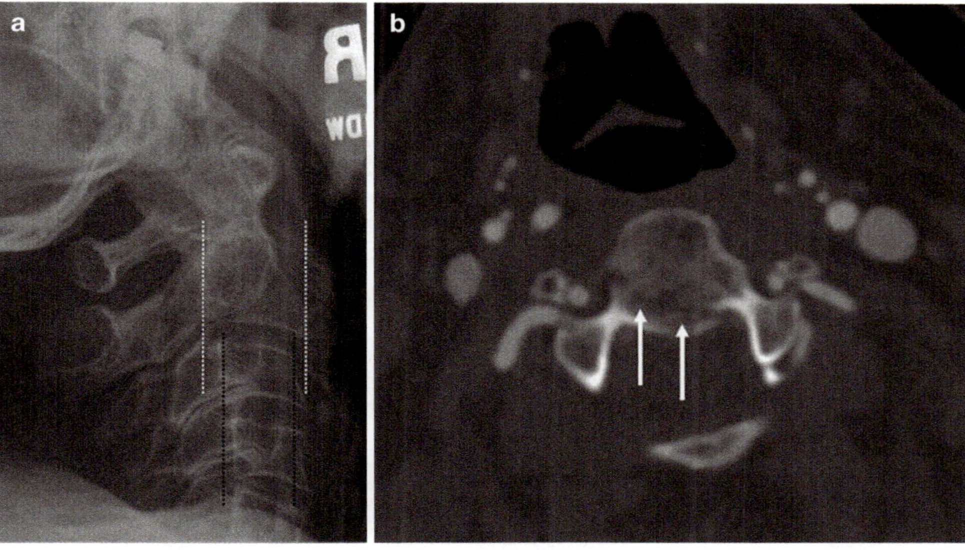

Fig. 13.3 79-year-old woman status post side-impact motor vehicle accident. (**a**) Lateral radiograph of the cervical spine demonstrates wider anterior-posterior (AP) diameter of the C2 vertebral body (white dotted line) compared to the AP diameter of the C3 vertebral body (black dotted line). This is also known as the "fat" vertebral body sign. (**b**) Axial noncontrast CT image through the level of C2 demonstrates a mildly displaced vertebral body fracture (arrows)

The "Hangman fracture", which involves the bilateral pars interarticularis or other posterior elements, is the second most common C2 fracture (~22%) and is most commonly due to MVAs (Fig. 13.4) [3, 11, 12]. Fracture distraction indicates instability, although upright radiographs may be required for diagnosis, as displacement may not be apparent on supine radiographs [3, 13, 14]. Rarely, the C2-C3 facet may also be dislocated [3, 14]. Neurologic injury is less common (26%) and only occurs if there is spinal canal narrowing; most injuries result in spinal canal widening [3]. Hyperflexion injuries that result in vertebral subluxations can lead to vascular injury, and occlusion or distal embolization can lead to cerebrovascular accidents (strokes) [15].

13.1.2 Thoracolumbar Spine

> **Key Point**
> The Thoracolumbar Injury Classification System (TLICS) is clinically relevant and includes an assessment of fracture morphology, posterior ligamentous status, and clinical neurological status.

Spine trauma classification in the thoracic and lumbar regions has undergone numerous revisions over the years, reflecting the ongoing effort to balance accuracy with clinical practicality. Early frameworks, such as the simple two- and three-column theories [16, 17], provided a foundational understanding of spinal stability but lacked nuance for guiding management. These models eventually gave way to the highly detailed and complex Association of Osteosynthesis (AO) classification, finalized in 1994 [18], which included an exhaustive 53 fracture subtypes but proved cumbersome for routine use. In response to the need for morphologic simplification, accountability for neurologic status, and assessment of the posterior ligamentous complex (PLC), the orthopedic community developed and widely adopted the Thoracolumbar Injury Classification and Severity Score (TLICS), a system designed to streamline decision-making while maintaining clinical relevance (Table 13.1) [18].

In the TLICS classification, there are two components that are assessed on imaging: fracture morphology, which can be performed on either CT or MRI, and posterior ligamentous complex (PLC) status, which typically requires MRI but sometimes can be inferred on CT if there is a posterior element fracture or subluxation/dislocation [19]. Fracture morphologies are categorized as compression (Fig. 13.5), compression with burst (Fig. 13.6), translation/rotation (Fig. 13.7), or distraction (Fig. 13.8), which is also the ascending order of severity and are assigned 1, 2, 3, and 4 points in the TLICS scoring, respectively [19]. The PLC status is scored as intact (0 points), indeterminate (2 points), or injured (3 points) [19]. There is also a category for neurological status, which is determined clinically. The combined score places the spine injury in a treatment recommendation category: 0–3 points is nonsurgical, 4 points is either nonsurgical or surgical, and 5 or more points is surgical [18].

While the TLICS classification is arguably the most well-known and uniformly utilized system today, it is important to recognize that additional efforts to improve spine trauma classification have been made in the interim. Notably, in 2013, Vaccaro et al. proposed a hybrid AO/TLICS system aimed at increasing morphologic specificity, enhancing communication between radiologists and surgeons, and simplifying overall applicability [20]. This system organized injuries

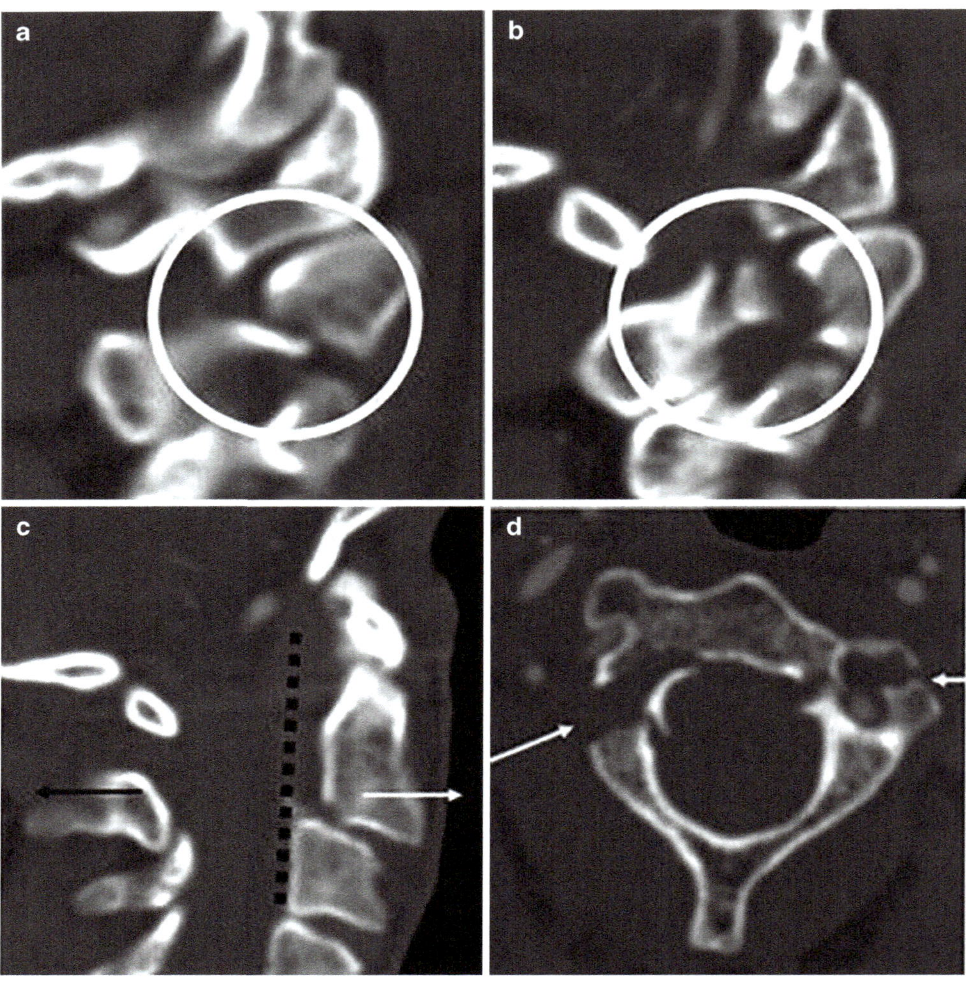

Fig. 13.4 62-year-old woman with multiple sclerosis who fell. (**a**) and (**b**) Sagittal noncontrast CT images of the cervical spine to the right and left of midline, respectively demonstrate bilateral C2 pars interarticularis fractures. (**c**) Sagittal midline noncontrast CT image of the cervical spine demonstrates anterolisthesis (white arrow) and posterior displacement of the C2 posterior elements (black arrow). The posterior margin of C2 should line up with the posterior margin of C3 (dashed black line). Fracture distraction indicates instability. (**d**) Axial noncontrast CT image of the cervical spine demonstrates bilateral comminuted fractures extending into the vertebral foramina. There was no evidence for vertebral artery injury

Table 13.1 Thoracolumbar Injury Classification System (TLICS) [18, 19]

Category	Score
Neurologic status	
Intact	0
Root injury	2
Complete cord injury	2
Incomplete cord injury	3
Cauda equina injury	3
Morphology	
No abnormality	0
Compressed	1
Burst	1
Rotated/translated	3
Distracted	4
Posterior ligamentous complex	
Intact	0
Indeterminate/injury suspected	2
Injury	3

into three broad categories: type A, encompassing compression and burst fractures; type B, representing flexion-distraction injuries with associated posterior ligamentous complex (PLC) involvement; and type C, encompassing translation, rotation, subluxation, dislocation, and other unstable injury patterns. Within type A, subtypes were further defined as A0 (isolated transverse or spinous process fractures), A1 (simple anterior wedge compression), A2 (coronal split) (Fig. 13.9), A3 (burst fracture involving a single endplate), and A4 (burst fracture involving both endplates). Type B was subdivided into B1 (classic Chance fracture), B2 (other flexion-distraction injuries involving any bone-ligament combination), and B3 (hyperextension injuries, such as those associated with ankylosing spondylitis or DISH). Type C included no subtypes, as all such injuries were considered inherently unstable and surgical (Table 13.2). By combining

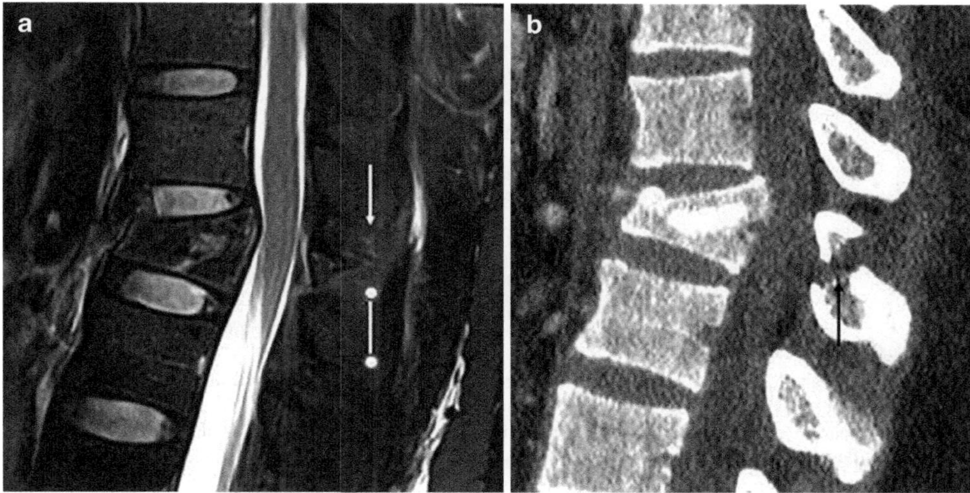

Fig. 13.5 27-year-old who fell from a ladder at a construction site. (**a**) Sagittal T2 fat-suppressed and (**b**) Sagittal noncontrast CT images demonstrate compression fracture of the T12 vertebral body and posterior elements (black arrow). There is also edema of the T11-T12 interspinous ligament (white arrows), consistent with ligamentous injury. (AO/TLICS Type B1)

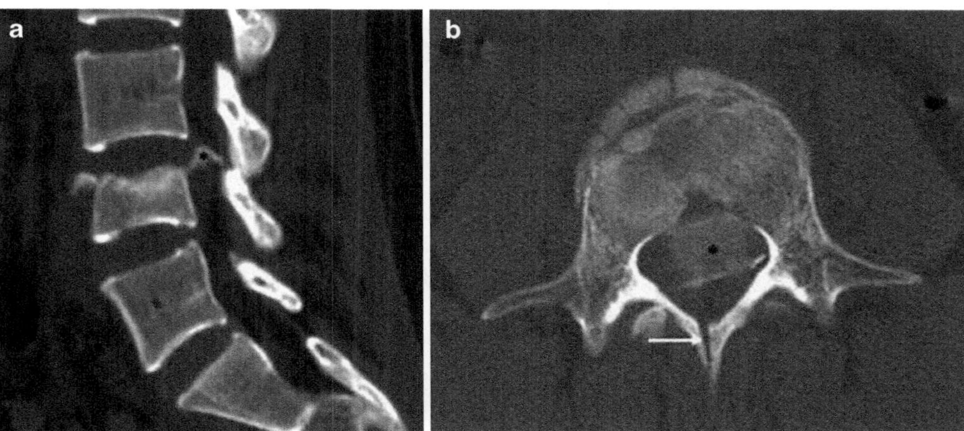

Fig. 13.6 23-year-old man status post fall from a third story window. (**a**) Sagittal and (**b**) Axial noncontrast CT images demonstrate a burst fracture of the L4 vertebral body with retropulsion of a large fragment into the spinal canal (*). The fracture extends into the posterior elements (arrow). This fracture was surgically managed

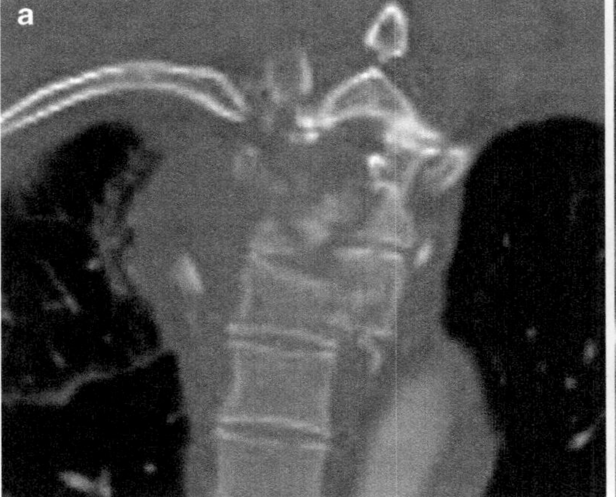

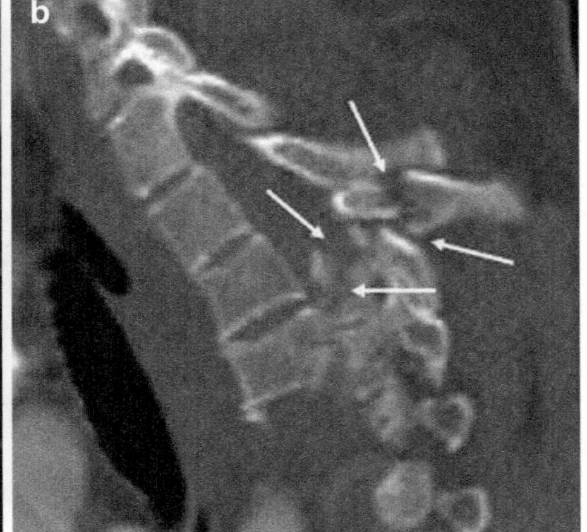

Fig. 13.7 60 -year-old male who collided into a stone wall while trying to avoid other skiers. (**a**) Coronal and (**b**) Sagittal noncontrast CT images of the upper thoracic spine demonstrate a translation/rotation fracture of the upper thoracic spine (AO/TLICS Type C), which also extends into the posterior elements (arrows). The patient was paraplegic at the time of injury

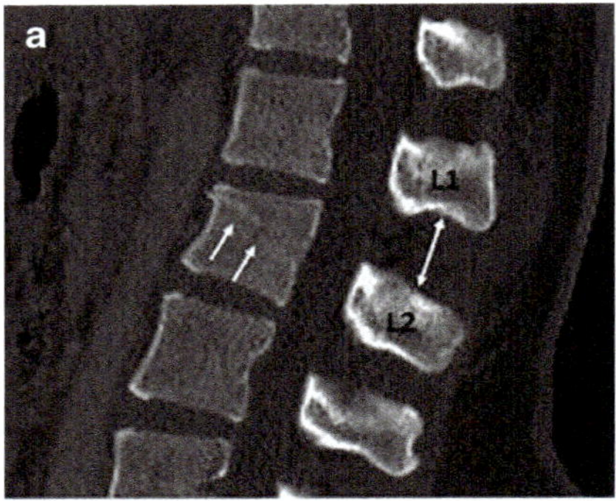

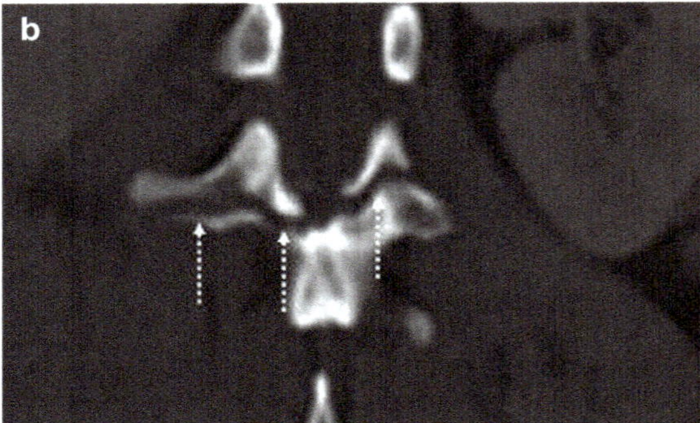

Fig. 13.8 24-year-old woman status post restrained backseat passenger in a high-speed MVA. (**a**) Sagittal and (**b**) Coronal noncontrast CT images demonstrate a fracture through the vertebral body (solid arrows) which extends through the posterior elements (dashed arrows), consistent with a flexion distraction injury. Widening of the L1-L2 interspinous distance is consistent with a ligamentous injury (double-headed arrow). TLICS +3 points, AO/TLICS Type B2. The patient was neurologically intact. Despite the high TLICS score, the patient was successfully treated conservatively using a brace. *TLICS* Thoracolumbar Injury Classification and Severity Score

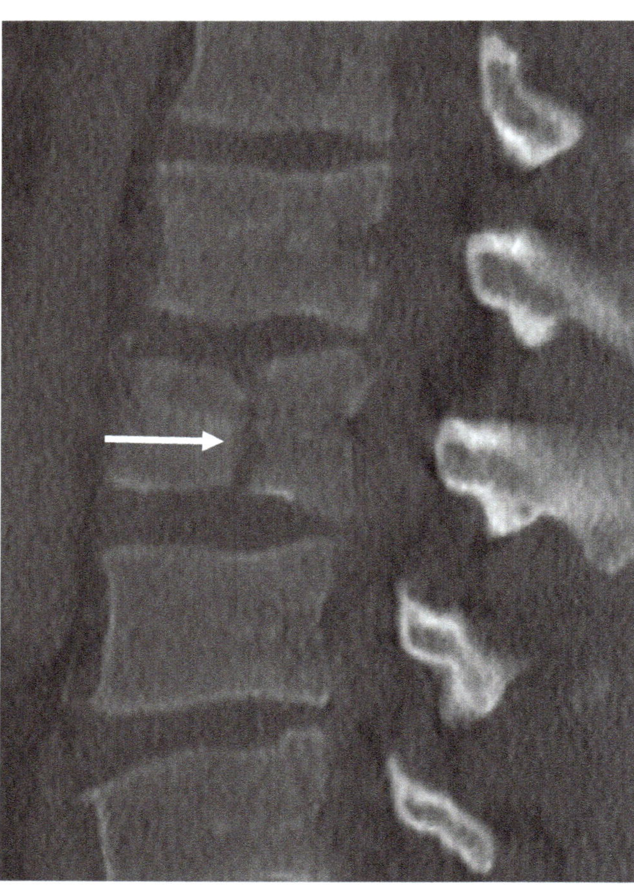

Fig. 13.9 52-year-old male status post horseback riding injury. Sagittal CT image of the lumbar spine demonstrates a coronally oriented split fracture of the L3 vertebral body (white arrow). Coronal split fractures include both the superior and inferior endplates but spare the posterior wall. These are AO/TLICS Type A2

Table 13.2 AO/TLICS classification system [20]

Category
Type A: Compression/burst
A0: Transverse or spinous process only
A1: Simple anterior wedge compression
A2: Coronal split
A3: Burst with one endplate involved
A4: Burst with two endplates involved
Type B: Flexion/distraction injuries
B1: Bony chance fracture
B2: Flexion distraction with PLC injury
B3: Hyperextension injury (as in ankylosing spondylitis, DISH)
Type C: Translation/displacement
No subtypes.

these two classification systems and improving simplicity, this approach sought to better define surgical versus nonsurgical cases and provide a more inclusive framework for imaging interpretation and management.

13.2 Extremities

Key Point

Accurate characterization of fracture patterns, including morphology, displacement, articular involvement, and associated soft-tissue injury, forms the foundation for treatment decisions and is systematically captured by classification systems to standardize communication between radiologists and surgeons.

The treatment plan for extremity fractures depends on multiple factors, including the location of injury, fracture morphology, degree of displacement, articular involvement, and associated soft-tissue damage. Classification systems are designed to capture these critical elements, with the goal of standardizing descriptions, facilitating communication among providers, and guiding appropriate management. Many systems are region-specific and eponymous, such as the Neer classification for proximal humeral fractures, the Garden classification for hip fractures, and the Schatzker classification for tibial plateau fractures, which stratifies fracture types based on patterns of articular depression, split components, and comminution. In contrast, the AO system, developed by Maurice E. Müller and colleagues, sought to create a universal framework applicable across all skeletal trauma, adaptable for both clinical decision-making and electronic data processing. While the AO system is comprehensive and lengthy, and concepts from it will be covered here, the full details of the classification lie beyond the scope of this paper.

Regardless of which system is used, there are fundamental descriptive features of fractures that should always be reported. On plain radiographs, the radiologist should characterize the basic form of the fracture, its complexity, and any associated displacement. Shaft fractures can range from simple two-part injuries, such as transverse, oblique, or spiral patterns, to more complex patterns involving three fragments, including bending wedge or spiral wedge fractures. Multiple fragments may present as segmental, multi-fragmentary, or comminuted fractures.

In addition to the fracture pattern itself, displacement must be assessed in relation to the proximal fragment. This includes lateral displacement, angulation, overriding, rotational malalignment, and impaction, in which fragments are driven into each other. Some displacement patterns carry specific implications: for example, when fracture fragments distract across a gap which may impair healing or in the setting of intra-articular extension associated with joint instability or early degeneration. These may include articular depression fractures, split fractures, or multi-fragmentary/comminuted fractures at the articular surface. Radiologists should report key features such as depression, articular surface distraction, intra-articular fragment position, and any associated soft-tissue signs, including swelling, fat pad displacement, air, or lipohemarthrosis.

Additional special considerations in extremity trauma include apophyseal avulsion fractures, which require attention to the degree and direction of displacement as well as the tendons, muscles, or ligaments involved. Incomplete fractures also form a distinct category, especially in pediatric populations, and include hairline, buckle (torus), and greenstick fractures.

By systematically evaluating these features, radiologists can provide clear, detailed descriptions that not only support accurate classification but also guide clinical decision-making and surgical planning.

13.2.1 Coracoid Fractures

Coracoid fractures are the most commonly missed shoulder girdle fracture, and radiograph sensitivity for coracoid fractures is approximately 40% [21–23]. They are typically associated with other shoulder girdle injuries: acromioclavicular injury (33%), clavicle fracture (17%), lateral scapular spine or acromion (15%), as well as other less common injuries [24–27]. Fractures that extend into the scapular body or glenoid are likely to require surgical intervention [24–27]. Coracoid fractures typically result from high-energy traumas such as MVA, falls, crush injuries, or firearm use [24, 26–28]. The fracture occurs as a combination of upward force from the coracoclavicular ligaments, which insert on the proximal coracoid, the medially directed force from the pectoralis minor, which inserts on the mid-coracoid, and the downward force from the coracobrachialis and short head of the biceps, which insert on the tip of the coracoid [29]. Figure 13.10 is a

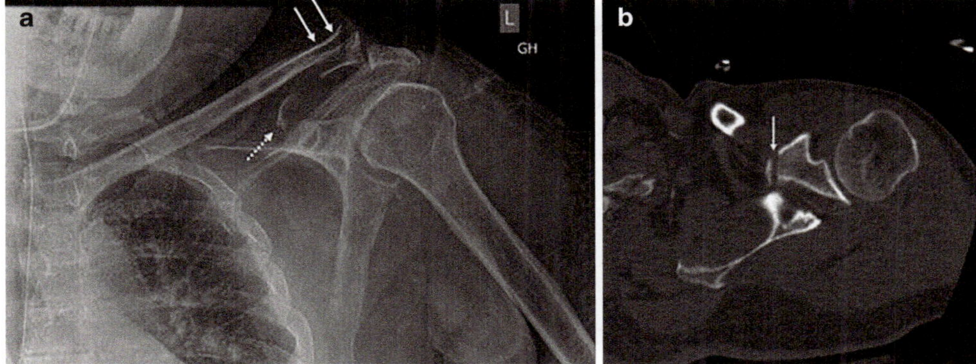

Fig. 13.10 49-year-old man found down, victim of assault, with severe head trauma. (**a**) Frontal radiograph of the left shoulder demonstrates a displaced clavicle distal third fracture (solid white arrows) and a coracoid avulsion fracture (dashed white arrow). (**b**) Axial trauma chest CT image confirms that avulsion fracture is from the proximal coracoid, at the coracoligament attachment (solid white arrow)

case of a 49-year-old man who was likely an assault victim. The avulsed fracture fragment is displaced cranially, suggesting that it is a coracoligament avulsion fracture. Chest trauma CT confirms proximal coracoid location of the fracture, at the coracoid ligament attachment.

13.2.2 Proximal Humeral and Femoral Fractures

Accurate description and classification of fractures involving the proximal humerus and femoral neck are critical, as they directly affect the surgical plan and may influence the development of post-traumatic avascular necrosis (AVN). The Neer classification is widely used for proximal humeral fractures and categorizes fractures based on the number of displaced segments to include either the surgical neck, anatomic neck, lesser tuberosity, or greater tuberosity, and is classified as 1, 2, 3, or 4 part fractures (Fig. 13.11) [30]. This helps determine whether conservative management, percutaneous fixation, or open reduction with internal fixation is appropriate and may help determine risk of AVN seen more commonly in 3 and 4 part fractures [31].

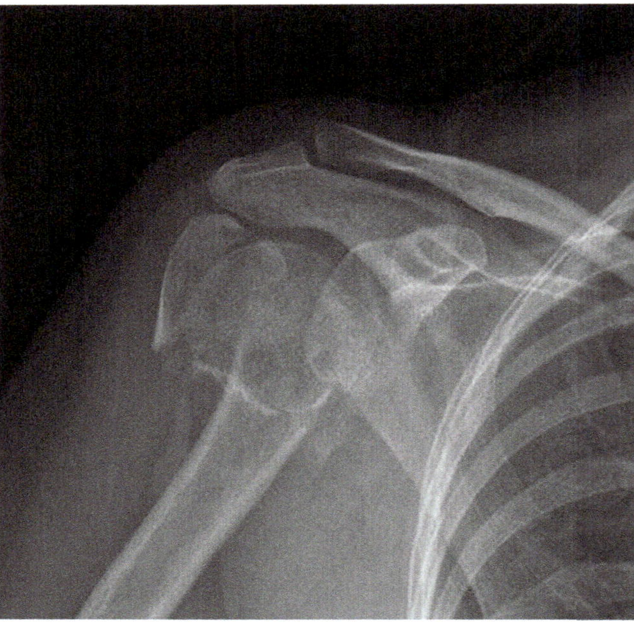

Fig. 13.11 51-year-old woman status post fall. Frontal radiograph of the right shoulder demonstrates a Neer 3-part fracture of the proximal humerus determined by fracture lines involving the surgical neck, greater trochanter, and lesser trochanter (3 parts) of the humerus

Similarly, the Garden classification stratifies femoral neck fractures into four types based on degree of displacement across the epiphyseal and metaphyseal fragments, with higher-grade fractures more likely to require surgical intervention such as internal fixation or arthroplasty due to AVN risk. Accurate assessment of fracture morphology, displacement, and involvement of the articular surface ensures that management strategies optimize functional outcomes while minimizing complications related to disrupted blood supply.

13.2.3 Tibial Plateau Fractures

Tibial plateau fractures encompass 1–2% of all trauma and have association with high-impact trauma [32]. These fractures are problematic in that they involve the articular surface of the proximal tibia and can significantly affect knee stability, alignment, and function. Accurate characterization is critical for guiding treatment, particularly surgical planning. The Schatzker classification is widely used to stratify tibial plateau fractures into six types based on morphology: type I is a lateral split fracture, type II is a lateral split with depression, type III is pure lateral depression, type IV involves the medial plateau, type V is a bicondylar fracture, and type VI includes metaphyseal-diaphyseal dissociation [33, 34]. This classification not only describes fracture morphology but also correlates with fracture severity and the likelihood of soft-tissue compromise, which helps determine the need for open reduction and internal fixation versus conservative management. For example, low-energy lateral plateau fractures (types I–III) are often amenable to minimally invasive or percutaneous techniques, whereas high-energy bicondylar or type VI injuries typically require more complex surgical approaches to restore articular congruity and mechanical alignment (Fig. 13.12). Reporting should emphasize displacement, depression depth, comminution, and associated ligamentous injury, as these factors directly influence surgical planning and postoperative outcomes.

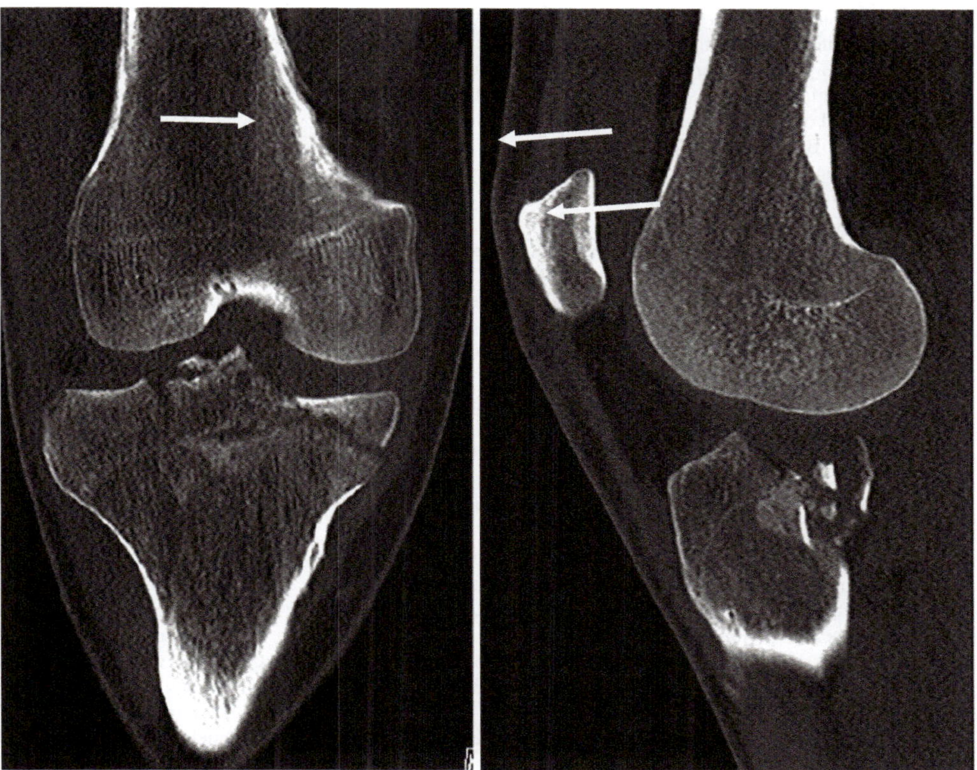

Fig. 13.12 33-year-old male status post paragliding injury. (**a**) Coronal CT image of the knee demonstrates a comminuted fracture of the tibial plateau involving both the medial and lateral articular surfaces (white arrows) classifying as a Schatzker Type VI Bicondylar tibial plateau injury. (**b**) Sagittal CT image in the same patient illustrates the area of severe articular surface depression and comminution at the posterior lateral tibial plateau

13.3 Concluding Remarks

Accurate assessment of musculoskeletal bony trauma relies on systematic imaging and standardized classification systems. In the spine, understanding fracture patterns and stability guides management, while in the extremities, careful evaluation of morphology, displacement, and articular involvement informs treatment. Applying frameworks such as TLICS, Neer, Garden, Schatzker, and AO enhances communication between radiologists and surgeons and supports evidence-based decision-making.

Take Home Messages

1. Cervical spine fractures, particularly C2 injuries, require careful classification (e.g., Anderson and D'Alonzo) to assess stability and guide management.
2. Thoracolumbar fractures should be evaluated using standardized systems such as TLICS and AO/TLICS to inform treatment and communicate stability.
3. Extremity fractures should be appropriately described and classified using frameworks like AO, Neer, Garden, Schatzker, to guide surgical planning and facilitate interdisciplinary communication.

Conflict of Interest I/We declare no competing interests as defined by Springer Nature or other interests that might be perceived to influence results and/or discussion reported in this manuscript.

References

1. Looby S, Flanders A. Spine trauma. Radiol Clin North Am. 2011;49:129–63.
2. Foster G, Russell B, Hibble B, Shaw K, Stella J. Magnetic resonance imaging cervical spine in trauma: a retrospective single-Centre audit of patient outcomes. Emerg Med Australas EMA. 2022;34:65–72.
3. Bransford RJ, Alton TB, Patel AR, Bellabarba C. Upper cervical spine trauma. J Am Acad Orthop Surg. 2014;22:718–29.
4. Dreizin D, Letzing M, Sliker CW, Chokshi FH, Bodanapally U, Mirvis SE, Quencer RM, Munera F. Multidetector CT of blunt cervical spine trauma in adults. Radiographics. 2014;34:1842–65.
5. Greene KA, Dickman CA, Marciano FF, Drabier JB, Hadley MN, Sonntag VK. Acute axis fractures. Analysis of management and outcome in 340 consecutive cases. Spine. 1997;22:1843–52.
6. Pryputniewicz DM, Hadley MN. Axis fractures. Neurosurgery. 2010;66:68–82.
7. Shafafy R, Valsamis EM, Luck J, Dimock R, Rampersad S, Kieffer W, Morassi GL, Elsayed S. Predictors of mortality in the elderly patient with a fracture of the odontoid process. Bone Joint J. 2019;101-B:253–9.
8. Anderson LD, D'Alonzo RT. Fractures of the odontoid process of the axis. J Bone Joint Surg Am. 1974;56:1663–74.
9. Hadley MN, Browner CM, Liu SS, Sonntag VK. New subtype of acute odontoid fractures (type IIA). Neurosurgery. 1988;22:67–71.
10. Pellei DD. The fat C2 sign. Radiology. 2000;217:359–60.

11. James R, Nasmyth-Jones R. The occurrence of cervical fractures in victims of judicial hanging. Forensic Sci Int. 1992;54:81–91.
12. Ferro FP, Borgo GD, Letaif OB, Cristante AF, Marcon RM, Lutaka AS. Traumatic spondylolisthesis of the axis: epidemiology, management and outcome. Acta Ortop Bras. 2012;20:84–7.
13. Riascos R, Bonfante E, Cotes C, Guirguis M, Hakimelahi R, West C. Imaging of Atlanto-occipital and atlantoaxial traumatic injuries: what the radiologist needs to know. Radiographics. 2015;35:2121–34.
14. Levine AM, Edwards CC. The management of traumatic spondylolisthesis of the axis. J Bone Joint Surg Am. 1985;67:217–26.
15. Alexander H, Dowlati E, McGowan JE, Mason RB, Anaizi A. C2-C3 spinal fracture subluxation with ligamentous and vascular injury: a case report and review of management. Spinal Cord Ser Cases. 2019;5:4.
16. Holdsworth F. Fractures, dislocations, and fracture-dislocations of the spine. J Bone Joint Surg Am. 1970;52:1534–51.
17. McAfee PC, Yuan HA, Fredrickson BE, Lubicky JP. The value of computed tomography in thoracolumbar fractures. An analysis of one hundred consecutive cases and a new classification. J Bone Joint Surg Am. 1983;65:461–73.
18. Vaccaro AR, Lehman RA, Hurlbert RJ, et al. A new classification of thoracolumbar injuries: the importance of injury morphology, the integrity of the posterior ligamentous complex, and neurologic status. Spine. 2005;30:2325–33.
19. Khurana B, Sheehan SE, Sodickson A, Bono CM, Harris MB. Traumatic thoracolumbar spine injuries: what the spine surgeon wants to know. Radiographics. 2013;33:2031–46.
20. Vaccaro AR, Oner C, Kepler CK, et al. AOSpine thoracolumbar spine injury classification system: fracture description, neurological status, and key modifiers. Spine. 2013;38:2028–37.
21. Mohammed H, Skalski MR, Patel DB, Tomasian A, Schein AJ, White EA, Hatch GFR, Matcuk GR. Coracoid process: the lighthouse of the shoulder. Radiographics. 2016;36:2084–101.
22. Rabbani GR, Cooper SM, Escobedo EM. An isolated coracoid fracture. Curr Probl Diagn Radiol. 2012;41:120–1.
23. Haapamaki VV, Kiuru MJ, Koskinen SK. Multidetector CT in shoulder fractures. Emerg Radiol. 2004;11:89–94.
24. Ogawa K, Yoshida A, Takahashi M, Ui M. Fractures of the coracoid process. J Bone Joint Surg Br. 1997;79:17–9.
25. Ogawa K, Matsumura N, Yoshida A, Inokuchi W. Fractures of the coracoid process: a systematic review. JSES Rev Rep Tech. 2021;1:171–8.
26. Gil JF, Haydar A. Isolated injury of the coracoid process: case report. J Trauma. 1991;31:1696–7.
27. Ada JR, Miller ME. Scapular fractures. Analysis of 113 cases. Clin Orthop. 1991:174–80.
28. Hill BW, Anavian J, Jacobson AR, Cole PA. Surgical management of isolated acromion fractures: technical tricks and clinical experience. J Orthop Trauma. 2014;28:e107–13.
29. Li CH, Skalski MR, Matcuk GR, Patel DB, Gross JS, Tomasian A, White EA. Coracoid process fractures: anatomy, injury patterns, multimodality imaging, and approach to management. Emerg Radiol. 2019;26:449–58.
30. Kilcoyne RF, et al. The Neer classification of displaced proximal humeral fractures: spectrum of findings on plain radiographs and CT scans. AJR Am J Roentgenol. 1990;154(5):1029–33.
31. Fazzari F, Canton G, Giraldi G, Falcioni N, Clocchiatti S, Rasio N, Murena L. Avascular necrosis of humeral head after proximal humerus fracture: comparison between classification systems in predicting necrosis risk. Acta Biomed. 2023 Jun 23;94(S2):e2023089.
32. Cole P, Levy B, Schatzker J, Watson JT. Tibial plateau fractures. In: Browner B, Levine A, Jupiter J, Trafton P, Krettek C, editors. Skeletal trauma: basic science management and reconstruction. Philadelphia, PA: Saunders Elsevier; 2009. p. 2201–87.
33. Schatzker J. Compression in the surgical treatment of fractures of the tibia. Clin Orthop Relat Res. 1974;105:220–39.
34. Zeltser DW, Leopold SS. Classifications in brief: Schatzker classification of tibial plateau fractures. Clin Orthop Relat Res. 2013 Feb;471(2):371–4.

Degeneration and Inflammation of the Spine

14

Nadja A. Farshad-Amacker and William E. Palmer

Learning Objectives

- To learn the relevant spine anatomy and nomenclature related to degenerative abnormalities.
- To understand that the correlation of clinical symptoms with imaging findings enables the most accurate diagnosis of pain generator.
- To differentiate degenerative disorders from infection and inflammation.

14.1 Introduction

Most individuals experience neck or back pain at least once in their lifetime. Whereas spinal degeneration represents the most common cause of symptoms, inflammatory, infectious, traumatic, metabolic, and neoplastic etiologies must also be considered. In this article, we focus on degenerative and inflammatory disorders, reviewing the imaging findings in patients with spine-related symptoms. Emphasis is placed on magnetic resonance imaging (MRI) as the most important diagnostic imaging modality. We do not address spinal injections for pain management but acknowledge that radiologists can leverage their training in image interpretation to make treatment decisions and perform safe and effective needle placements. Experienced proceduralists develop the skills to correlate symptoms with imaging findings and distinguish incidental abnormalities from actual pain generator [1].

N. A. Farshad-Amacker (✉)
Department of Radiology, Balgrist University Hospital, Zurich, Switzerland
e-mail: Nadja.farshad@balgrist.ch

W. E. Palmer
Department of Radiology, Massachusetts General Hospital, Boston, MA, USA
e-mail: WPALMER@mgh.harvard.edu

14.2 Diagnostic Imaging

Conventional radiography and whole body slot-scanning produce reliable images for screening, diagnosing, and monitoring degenerative changes and alignment abnormalities. They enable measurements of scoliosis, kyphosis, lordosis, and coronal or sagittal balance. To assess dynamic instability, standing radiographs may be compared to supine or prone views, lateral flexion-extension views or lateral sitting views, and anteroposterior side-bending views.

Compared to radiographs, CT provides higher anatomical resolution of complex osseous structures such as posterior elements and higher contrast discrimination of soft tissues. Therefore, CT serves as the modality of choice following spinal trauma. In disc degeneration, it depicts the locations of disc-osteophyte complex, vacuum phenomenon, and endplate sclerosis. In facet degeneration, it characterizes alignment, loss of bone stock, bony proliferation, and crystal deposition. CT can be a valuable alternative in patients with contraindications to MRI. In spinal stenosis, it can distinguish focal disc herniation from diffuse disc bulge and demonstrate ligamentum flavum mineralization. 2D reformats show curvature and alignment abnormalities, while 3D reconstructions help in preoperative planning and hardware positioning.

Spine specialists rely on MRI for diagnosing the cause of symptoms and deciding on treatment. Compared to CT, MRI has the advantage of revealing bone marrow and soft tissue edema or inflammation due to mechanical or inflammatory etiologies. It demonstrates neural structures and signs of mechanical impingement in the setting of central canal, subarticular/recessal zone, and foraminal stenosis. A standard MRI protocol for degenerative change should include a sagittal STIR or T2-weighted fat-suppressed (fluid-sensitive) sequence, a sagittal T1-weighted sequence, a sagittal T2-weighted sequence, and axial T2-weighted sequences through the levels of pathologic changes visualized on sagittal images. Coronal sequences are most valuable in the lum-

J. Hodler et al. (eds.), *Musculoskeletal Diseases 2026-2029*, IDKD Springer Series,
https://doi.org/10.1007/978-3-032-17040-8_14

bar spine to characterize curvature, assess lateral listhesis, and classify lumbosacral transitional vertebra (LSTV). In the cervical spine, oblique sagittal or 3D sequences may compliment axial images and help to evaluate the degree of foraminal stenosis.

A whole-body MRI protocol for inflammatory changes due to spondyloarthropathy is recommended as screening, including sagittal and coronal T2-weighted fat-suppressed or STIR sequences as well as T1-weighted sequences in combination with coronal and axial STIR and coronal T1-weighted sequences along the sacroiliac joints (SIJ).

Key Point

- Although CT is the modality of choice for evaluating bone structures in acute spinal trauma, MRI offers superior soft-tissue resolution, increasing its effectiveness for diagnosing the cause of spinal symptoms and guiding treatment decisions.

14.3 Anatomy and Normal MRI Appearance

The vertebral column serves essential functions. More than a passive scaffolding for muscle attachments, it maintains posture, provides balance, distributes body weight, enables flexibility, absorbs shock, protects neural structures, and allows for a full range of movements and activities. To serve these functions, spinal anatomy is highly complex. The vertebrae, ribs, and sacrum articulate through intervertebral discs, facet joints, costovertebral joints, and SIJ. These articulations, as well as the craniocervical junction, are stabilized by disc material, hyaline cartilage, capsular tissue, ligaments, and muscles.

The intervertebral disc is comprised of the centrally located nucleus pulposus, a soft gelatinous structure consisting mainly of water, proteoglycans, and loosely arranged type II collagen, and the surrounding annulus fibrosus, a firm fibrocartilaginous ring consisting of layered lamellae and tightly arranged type I collagen. Whereas the nucleus pulposus is hyperintense on T2-weighted MR images, the annulus fibrosis is hypointense. The lumbar discs are greater in height compared to cervical and thoracic discs, and the L4-5 disc is often the greatest in height. Nutrients diffuse into the avascular nucleus pulposus across the vertebral endplates, which are normally smooth and covered by a thin layer of cartilage. This cartilage layer is not visible on routine MRI studies.

The articulating processes of the facet joints change in orientation from the cervical to the lumbar spine. Horizontal orientation in the cervical spine shifts to a coronal orientation in the thoracic spine to allow for rotation at the expense of extension. Oblique sagittal orientation in the lumbar spine tends to limit spinal rotation. The tight capsule of the facet joint allows only a small amount of intra-articular fluid.

Numerous ligaments stabilize the spine and SIJ. The longitudinal spinal ligaments course anteriorly and posteriorly to the vertebral bodies. The posterior elements are stabilized by the ligamentum flavum, interspinous, and supraspinous ligaments. Muscles generate motion while providing dynamic stabilization of the spine. Loss of muscle mass results in sarcopenia, chronic weakness, and poor prognosis. The degree of muscle atrophy and fatty replacement is considered important in clinical decision-making [2].

14.4 Degenerative Spinal Diseases and MRI Appearance

Degenerative spinal disease is the most common cause of back pain. Although the etiology is multifactorial, certain factors are known to accelerate the degenerative progress, such as genetics, cumulative mechanical stresses (such as heavy lifting), vascular insufficiency, smoking, advanced age, and lumbar hypolordosis [3, 4].

14.4.1 Degeneration of the Disc

Degeneration and aging of the disc results in a decrease in proteoglycan content and an increase in type I collagen, decreasing the normal high signal intensity on fluid-sensitive MRI sequences and eventually leading to loss of disc space height. The MRI grading system published by Pfirrmann et al. considers the combination of T2-weighted signal intensity, disc space height, and morphology of the annulus fibrosus [5] .

14.4.2 Annulus Fibrosus Tears

Annular tears are characterized by high intensity zones (HIZ) on T2-weighted (fluid-sensitive) MRI sequences. With gadolinium contrast administration, diagnostic sensitivity might increase for those not detected as HIZ on fluid-sensitive images [6]. Also, with discography, annular tears are not accurately characterized as it can produce false-positive and false-negative results and expose patients to unnecessary risks. Therefore, the diagnostic value of annular tears is highly questioned for now, as these changes are often identified in asymptomatic volunteers [7] and remain unchanged over years [8]. There is only innervation of the disc in the annular fibrosis and at the adjacent endplates. The nucleus is avascular and aneural. Therefore, 'discogenic low back pain' is challenging for clinicians and usually a diagnosis of exclusion. The presence of discogenic bone marrow edema can increase diagnostic sensitivity.

14.4.3 Bulging/Protrusion/Extrusion/Sequester of the Disc

Disc herniations are associated with disc degeneration. In the absence of disc degeneration, herniation can result from acute trauma especially in younger individuals. The annular disc bulge commonly occurs in asymptomatic individuals and is related to normal aging. Focal disc herniations can be further categorized as protrusion, extrusion, or sequestration, as summarized in Fig. 14.1 [9, 10].

Why is it important for the radiologist to distinguish between these disc morphologies in MRI reports? The reason is due to the difference in treatment strategy. In the cervical spine, for example, a broad-based disc protrusion (Fig. 14.1a) may require the surgeon to perform ACDF (anterior cervical discectomy and fusion) for stabilization and decompression of neural tissue. In contrast, focal disc extrusion, with or without sequestration, may be adequately addressed by minimally invasive discectomy. Sequestered disc material has the highest likelihood of spontaneous resorption, followed by extruded disc material.

To further guide diagnosis and treatment, the herniated disc should be described according to its location. Although terminology can be confusing and guided by regional customs, common descriptors include central, paramedian/eccentric, subarticular/recessal (lumbar spine) or preforaminal (cervical and thoracic spine), foraminal, and extraforaminal (Fig. 14.1b and c) [10]. The disc fragment can be described in relationship to nerve roots in the setting of mechanical compression (Fig. 14.2). The degree of compromise can be described as mild (touching), moderate (displacement), or severe (mechanical compression) [11]. Whereas the degree of canal stenosis and nerve root compromise are better assessed on axial images, the degree of foraminal stenosis and nerve root compromise are better assessed on sagittal images in the thoracic and lumbar spines (Fig. 14.3).

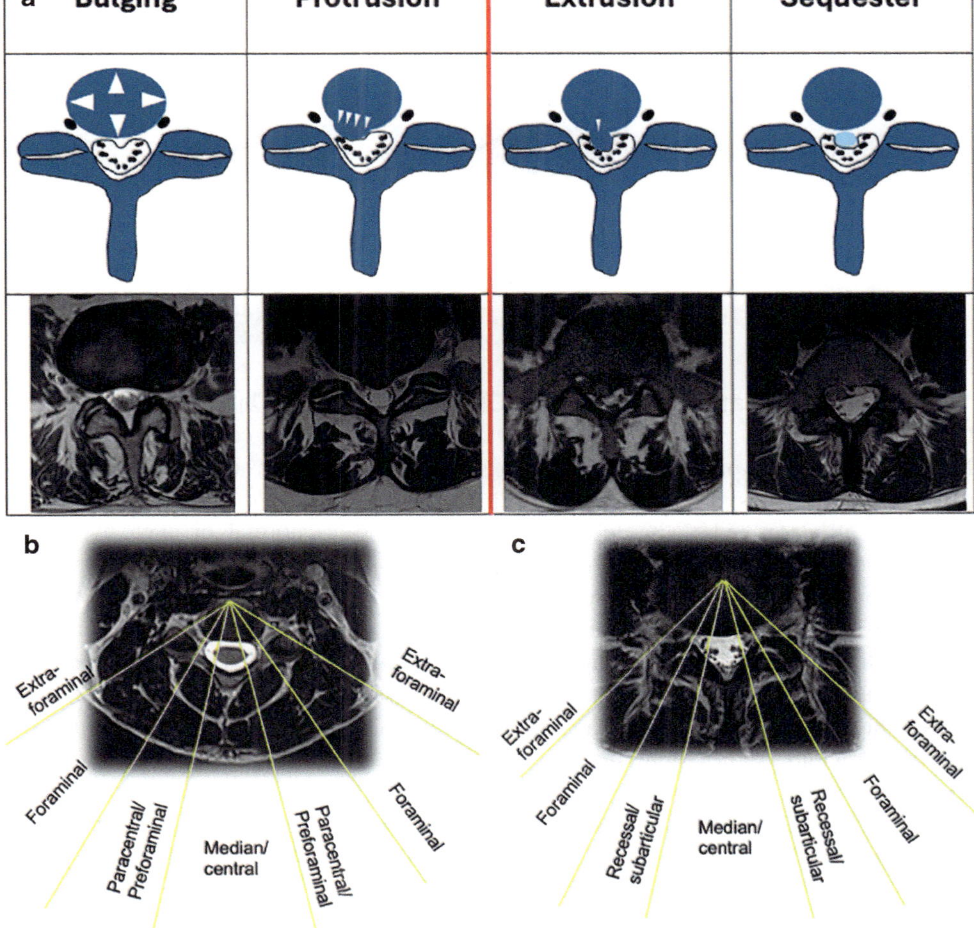

Fig. 14.1 Schematic illustrations (**a**) of the nomenclature of disc pathology with herniations, according to Fardon et al. [9] on axial T2-weighted MR images and (**b** and **c**) schematic illustration to describe the location of the disc hernation (**b**) in the cervical spine and (**c**) lumbar/thoracic spine

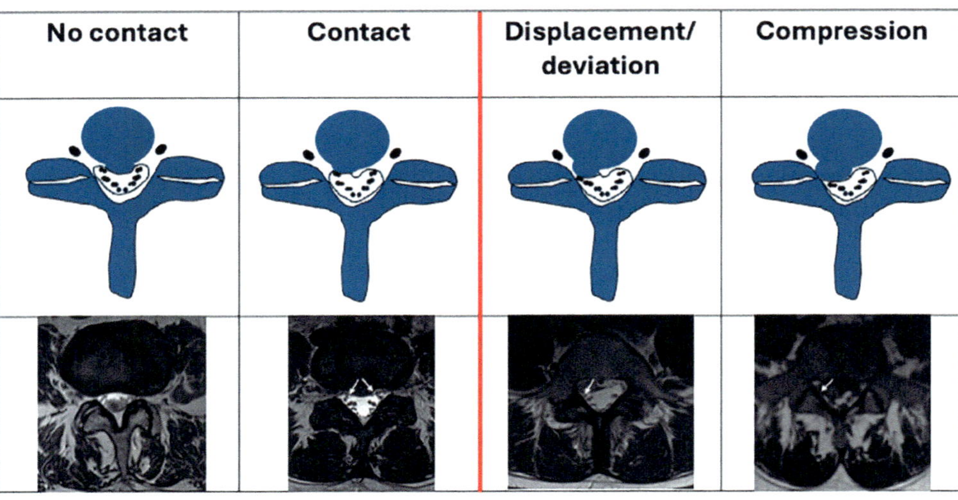

Fig. 14.2 Schematic illustration describing the hernation in relation to the nerve root in the lumbar spine, initally described by Pfirrmann et al. [11]

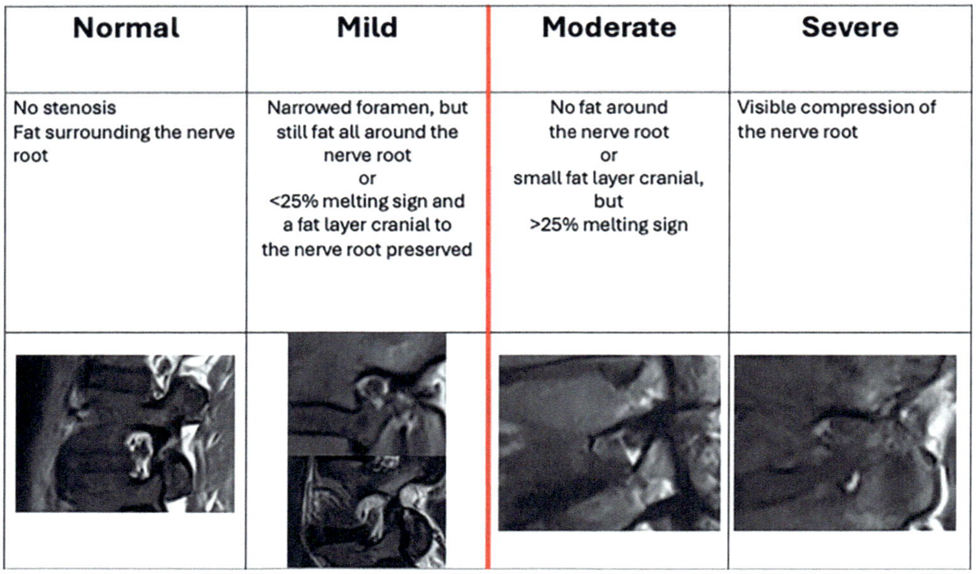

Normal	Mild	Moderate	Severe
No stenosis Fat surrounding the nerve root	Narrowed foramen, but still fat all around the nerve root or <25% melting sign and a fat layer cranial to the nerve root preserved	No fat around the nerve root or small fat layer cranial, but >25% melting sign	Visible compression of the nerve root

Fig. 14.3 Schematic illustration of mild, moderate and severe lumbar foraminal stenosis according to Wildermuth et al. [20] and Farshad et al. [21]

14.4.4 Endplates and Bone Marrow Changes

Disc degeneration is often accompanied by vertebral bone marrow abnormalities (Modic changes) [12]. In the 1980s, Modic et al. described three different types of marrow changes adjacent to the endplates. Whereas Modic type I shows edema-like signal intensity, type II shows fat-like signal intensity. In type 3, normal marrow is replaced by sclerosis-like signal intensity. In longitudinal studies, Modic type 1 usually precedes type 2. Edematous marrow transitions to fatty marrow with loss of the normal erythropoietic marrow. Previous studies suggest that Modic changes are specific (97%) but insensitive (23%) for painful lumbar disc disease [12]. Type 1 and 3 are more likely than type 2 to be associated with low back pain [12]. However, these older studies used spin-echo sequences without fat suppression that could not demonstrate mild bone marrow edema or resolve mixed Modic types.

Unfortunately, some patterns of degenerative bone marrow edema can be confused with spondylodiscitis. In most cases of degeneration, the disc is hypointense, however there could be traumatic bone marrow edema, where the disc stays normal or even hyperintense, as in case of hemorrhage. Vertebral bone marrow edema pattern in degeneration is more bandlike, with sharper margins, and usually not greater than 50% of the vertebral body height. In infection, however, the margins are less distinct and involve more than 50% of the vertebral body height. In difficult cases, intravenous contrast can provide helpful information about adjacent soft tissue inflammation including non-enhancing phlegmon or abscess. Diagnostic criteria are summarized in Table 14.1.

The thin cartilage layer separating the endplates from the disc is not visible on routine MRI sequences. Chondral damage must be assessed indirectly, such as with the endplate damages score [13].

Table 14.1 Differentiation between degenerative intervertebral changes with Modic type 1 changes in contrast to spondylodiscitis

	Degenerative changes with Modic type 1	Spondylodiscitis
CT: Vaccum phenomenon	Yes	No
Disc signal on MRI T2-weighted images	Normal or hypointense	Hyperintense
MRI signal within vertebral endplates	Bandlike, usually not higher than 50% of the vertebral body height	More irregular, often > 50% of vertebral body height
MRI contrast media uptake within vertebral body	Yes	Yes
MRI contrast media uptake of surrounding soft tissue	No	Yes, look for abscesses
Endplate destruction	Nothing/little	Often
Course	Slowly	Rapid

14.4.5 Interaction of Disc Degeneration and Endplate Changes

It has not yet been conclusively established whether disc degeneration begins with the disc or endplate failure resulting in decreased nutrition to the disc. However, it is known that the endplate changes and disc degenerative changes occur together. In other words, greater degrees of disc degeneration are associated with greater degrees of endplate defects and discogenic bone marrow edema [14]. Further, it is known that vascular compromise, as in abdominal aortic aneurysm, accelerates the degenerative process including more severe endplate erosions [3].

14.4.6 Facet Joints and Ligamentum Flavum

Facetogenic pain is a difficult clinical diagnosis. Facet arthropathy and disc degeneration can involve multiple levels of the cervical and lumbar spines, and generate symptoms in identical locations. In patients with facet-related pain, MRI can show cartilage degeneration, synovial inflammation or capsulitis, and bone marrow edema. In osteoarthritis, similar to other diarthrodial joints and can demonstrate chondral defects, joint space narrowing, subchondral bone marrow edema, and marginal osteophyte formation. Bone marrow edema is related to facetogenic pain. When present, it may guide clinicians to consider a facet joint injection for diagnostic information and therapeutic response. Although bone marrow edema is associated with therapeutic response in the small joints of the foot, ongoing research has yet to prove this concept for the facet joints [15].

In advanced osteoarthritis, loss of cartilage and bone stock may lead to degenerative spondylolisthesis. This alignment abnormality, with or without infolding of the ligamentum flavum, may result in spinal stenosis and increase the risk for segmental instability. Therefore, degenerative spondylolisthesis can produce complex pain patterns. In addition to axial pain, radicular pain may result from central canal, subarticular/recessal, or foraminal stenosis. Facet joint synovial cysts are a common cause of nerve root irritation or compression in the subarticular/recessal zone or foraminal zone.

Spine MRI is associated with a high prevalence of structural abnormalities in both symptomatic and asymptomatic individuals. For example, degeneration of the discovertebral unit (nucleus pulposus, annulus fibrosus, cartilaginous plate, endplate, and bone marrow) can lead to the degeneration of posterior structures. Therefore, discogenic change often coexists with other morphological abnormalities that can cause neck or back pain and radicular pain. Because it can be difficult ranking the importance of structural abnormalities during MRI interpretation, radiologists often generate long lists that include all possible pain generators. However, they improve the value of dictated reports and increase diagnostic confidence by correlating clinical information with MRI information [16]. Using symptom knowledge from requisition forms, intake sheets, electronic health records or pre-MRI questionnaires, radiologists are more likely to dismiss incidental findings and agree on the diagnosis of pain generator [17, 18] (Figs. 14.4 and 14.5).

Key Point

- Knowing the anatomy and nomenclature related to degenerative abnormalities is critical in communicating and reporting spine abnormalities.
- Imaging findings should be matched with clinical information to exclude incidental findings.

14.4.7 Spinal Stenosis

14.4.7.1 Foraminal Stenosis

In the cervical spine, foraminal stenosis can be caused by osteoarthrosis of the uncovertebral joints and facet joints. In contrast, uncovertebral joints are absent in the thoracic and lumbar spines. Other common causes of foraminal stenosis include disc-osteophyte complex and disc herniation. Using MRI or CT, grading systems can be used to quantify stenosis based on the degree of effacement of fat surrounding the nerve root, as well as displacement of the nerve root [19, 20]. In the lumbar spine, the so-called melting sign can be further used. If the nerve is in contact with more than 25% with the disc on the sagittal lumbar spine MRI, some nerve irritation is highly possible [21]. So, in the lumbar spine foramina we could describe mild stenosis for contact to the nerve with <25% melting sign and still some fat above the nerve root, moderate if there is >25% melting sign to the nerve root, and severe if there is a compression of the nerve (Figs. 14.3 and 14.4).

14.4.7.2 Canal Stenosis

There are several grading systems for cervical and lumbar spinal canal stenosis, some of which include specific measurements. In the authors' experience, the most effective approach is to quantify the degree of stenosis based on the contact, deviation, or compression of the spinal cord or cauda equina nerve roots. Additionally, special attention should be given to any signal alterations within the spinal cord. Anterior spinal cord ischemia is more common than posterior spinal cord ischemia, primarily due to its reliance on a single artery, resulting in the characteristic 'snake-eye' pattern on imaging. In contrast, the posterior spinal cord is supplied by two arteries and benefits from a broad anastomotic network, making ischemia in this region less frequent. Complete spinal cord ischemia represents the most severe and rare variant.

In the lumbar spine, subarticular/recessal stenosis should be differentiated from central canal stenosis (Fig. 14.5). Central stenosis typically presents with neurogenic claudication causing bilateral buttock and/or lower extremity pain, heaviness or weakness that increases with activity such as walking and decreases with rest. In severe cases, cauda equina syndrome causes bladder and bowel dysfunction. Arterial claudication can produce similar constellation of symptoms. Differentiation is important but can be difficult because of the prevalence of spinal and arterial stenoses in older individuals.

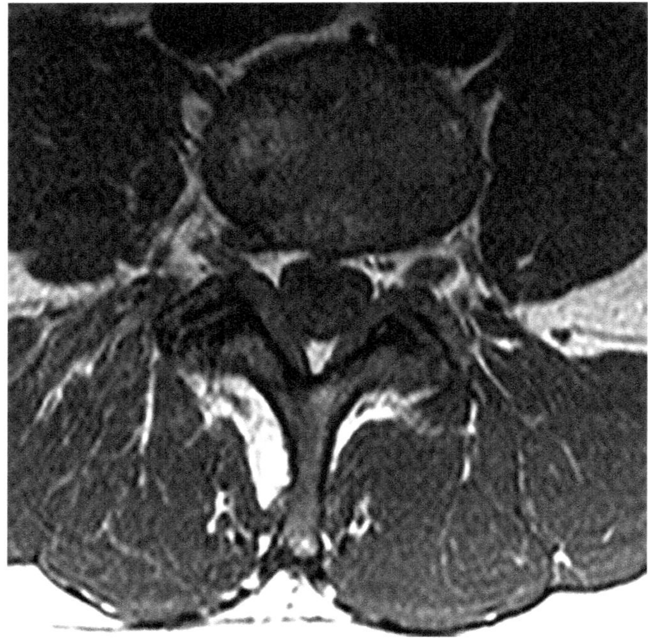

Fig. 14.4 64-year-old male with lumbar spine symptoms. Axial T1-weighted spin-echo MR image at L4-5 shows right-sided, extruded intraforaminal disc fragment causing mechanical nerve impingement. This finding was overlooked and unreported at the time of MRI interpretation. At the time of pain management injection, symptom-MRI correlation enabled the diagnosis and, therefore, selection of the appropriate procedure (right L4-5 transforaminal injection)

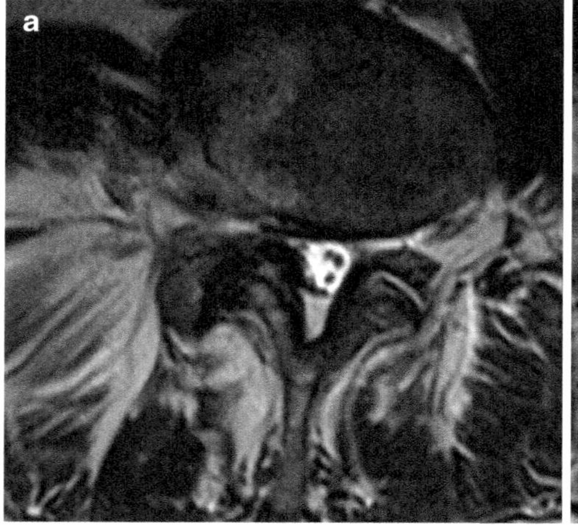

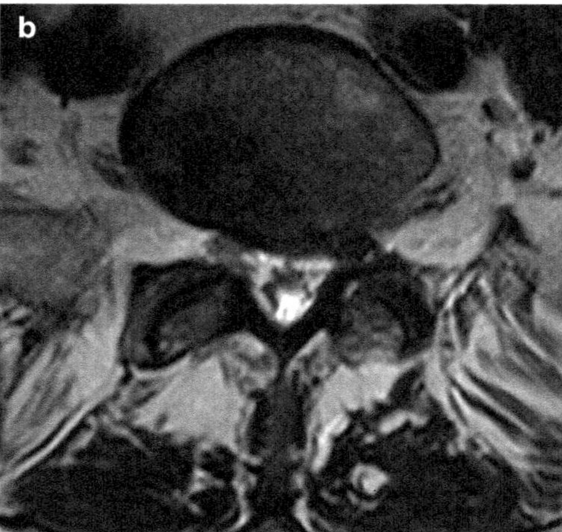

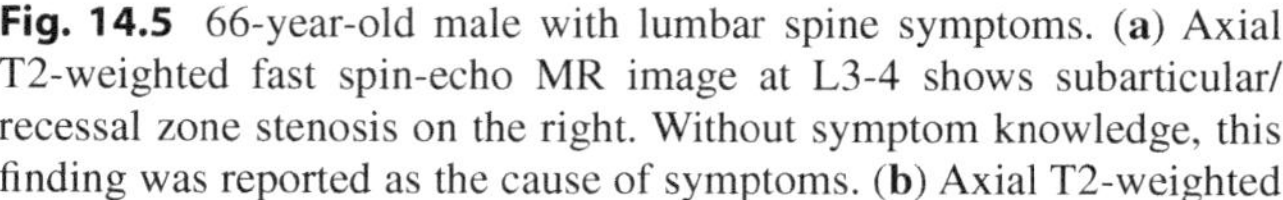

Fig. 14.5 66-year-old male with lumbar spine symptoms. (**a**) Axial T2-weighted fast spin-echo MR image at L3-4 shows subarticular/recessal zone stenosis on the right. Without symptom knowledge, this finding was reported as the cause of symptoms. (**b**) Axial T2-weighted fast spin-echo MR image at L5-S1 shows subarticular/recessal zone stenosis on the left. The patient complained of left-sided leg pain in the S1 distribution. With symptom knowledge, this finding was identified as the cause of symptoms

14.4.8 Most Common Levels of Spinal Degeneration

14.4.8.1 Cervical

Degeneration is most often observed at the levels C4-C7. The loss of T2-weighted signal hyperintensity of a normal intervertebral disc in the cervical spine is in general lower, compared to the lumbar spine. In case of inherited segmentation failure, the so-called Kippel-Feil syndrome, causing the characteristic wasp waist there is an increased risk for accelerated segment degeneration of the adjacent segments, as well as severe neurological damage with already minor trauma, due to the moment arm [22].

14.4.8.2 Thoracic

Segment degeneration in the thoracic spine is less common; due to the rib cage, the thoracic spine is substantially more protected. When observed, it is most often at the lower levels (Th11/12 and Th12/L1) due to free-ending or floating ribs.

14.4.8.3 Lumbar Spine

Degeneration at the lumbar spine is most often observed at the levels L4–5 and L5-S1. Lumbosacral transitional vertebra are present in up to 30% of individuals. The greater the degree of sacralization, the greater the degree of stress on the lowest movable lumbar segment. Similar to the junctional level following spinal fusion, this segment is prone to degeneration. Further, in case of an abdominal aortic aneurysm, the degeneration also shifts to an atypical higher level [23].

14.4.9 Degeneration and Pitfalls After Surgical Decompression or Stabilization

The most common postoperative complications include: recurrent disc herniations, with a frequency of around 10% after decompression surgery, adjacent segment degeneration in case of a fusion, implant failure, pedicle fractures, and pseudoarthrosis.

After foraminotomy or resection of a facet joint, fatty obliteration of the foramen and ghosting of the nerve root should not be misdiagnosed as residual foraminal stenosis [24]. This finding can be expected after surgery. However, in case of persistent radiculopathy of the obliterated nerve root, then contrast administration could help to differentiate granulation tissue which would enhance diffusely, in contrast to a recurrent herniation or sequestered fragment, that would enhance only in the periphery. Further, surgically applied material may be misdiagnosed as hematoma [25].

14.4.10 Inflammatory Spinal Diseases

14.4.10.1 Rheumatoid Arthritis

In rheumatoid arthritis (RA), spinal involvement predominantly affects the cervical spine, particularly the atlantoaxial and craniocervical junctions. Up to 86% of RA patients may show cervical spine involvement [26]. Radiographs remain the first-line imaging tool, but MRI provides superior detail for soft tissue changes, neural compromise, synovitis, erosive changes, and pannus formation.

14.4.10.2 Seronegative Spondyloarthropathies (SpA)

Seronegative SpA have been shown to be genetically predisposed (HLA-B27). Environmental factors, especially prior infections or exposures, may initiate the chronic inflammatory joint disease. It is an immune mediated disease, triggered by a T-cell response to unknown antigens and causes inflammation of peripheral and or axial arthritis and tendinous attachment. Most affected are the SIJ. It often presents in the second to third decades of life with men being much more often involved compared to women and in >90% with presence of the HLA-B27.

There are several types of seronegative spondyloarthropathies, such as

(a) Ankylosing Spondylitis – M. Bechterew
(b) Psoriasis
(c) Reactive SpA (Reiter)
(d) Enteropathic SpA
(e) Undifferentiated SpA
(f) Juvenile SpA

Histologically, there is a chronic synovitis with destruction of articular cartilage and bony ankylosis. Inflammation of tendinous-ligament insertion sites leads to their ossification, producing bony outgrowths, which compound the fibrous and bony ankylosis and results in severe spinal immobility.

In patients with suspected SpA, whole-body MRI is recommended for early diagnosis. We acquire sagittal and coronal T1-weighted and STIR images of the entire spine using a body coil and additional SIJ-aligned sequences generating coronal T1-weighted and STIR images as well as an axial STIR images (Fig. 14.6).

The assessment of SpA in patients with back pain for more than 3 months and age at onset <45 years includes the diagnosis of sacroiliitis with active/acute inflammation on MRI or definite radiographic sacroiliitis according to the modified New York criteria [27] plus ≥ 1 SpA feature, such as inflammatory back pain, arthritis, enthesitis (head), uveitis, dactylitis, psoriasis, Crohn's disease or ulcerative colitis, good response to NSAIDs, family history of SpA, HLA-B27 and elevated CRP (Fig. 14.6). Or alternatively, no radiologic signs, but HLA-B27 plus ≥ 2 Spa feature.

Radiological criteria of SIJ due to the Modified New York criteria [27]:

Grade 0 = normal
Grade 1 = suspicious changes
Grade 2 = minimal abnormalities, like small, localized areas with erosions or sclerosis, without alteration in the joint width
Grade 3 = between Grade 2 and 4
Grade 4 = severe abnormality to total ankylosis

Acute inflammatory MR changes at the SIJ are

- Bone marrow edema signal (osteitis)
- Enthesitis
- Capsulitis with synovitis

Chronic inflammatory MR changes at the SIJ are

- Fatty metaplasia
- Erosions
- Subchondral sclerosis
- Ankylosis

While usually the inflammatory changes involving SIJ are symmetrical, in psoriasis and inflammatory bowel disorders they tend to be asymmetrical.

Acute changes in the spine include:

- Romanus lesion/spondylitis anterior and posterior
- Edema adjacent to facet joints
- Edema around costovertebral joints
- Interspinous edema
- Anderson lesions (discitis)

Chronic changes in the spines include:

- Fatty metaplasia of the bone marrow edema lesions, such as Romanus lesions, around facet joints, around the costovertebral joints
- Syndesmophytes/parasyndesmophytes
- Ankylosis
- Bamboo spine

Other joints involved in SpA include the sternomanubial joints, the sternoclavicular joints, and rarely, the glenohumeral, AC, and hip joints.

Key Point
- Whole-body MRI is the modality of choice assessing inflammatory disease of the spine.

14.4.11 SAPHO

SAPHO is a rare syndrome, as an acronym for synovitis, acne, pustulosis, hyperostosis, and osteitis, with no association to HLA-B27, in contrast to the spondyloarthropathies.

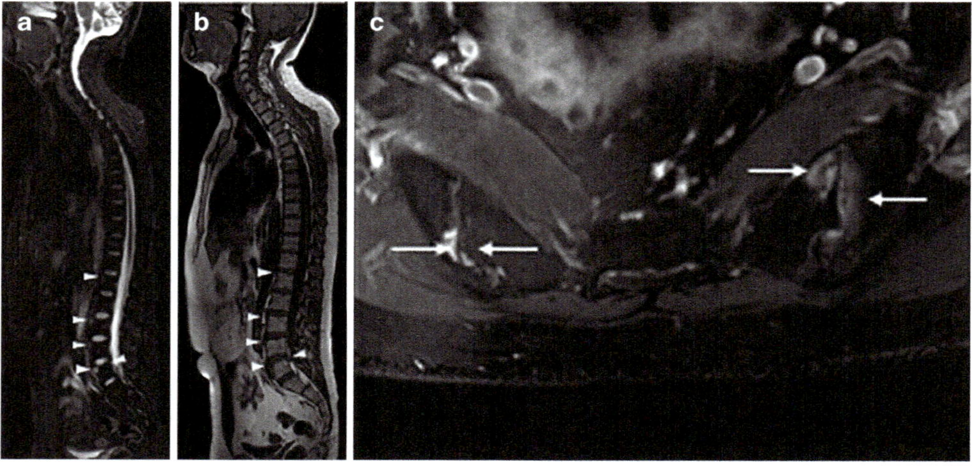

Fig. 14.6 41-year-old male diagnosed with Bechterew disease due to generalized axial pain and HLA-B27 positivity as well as characteristic MRI findings. (**a**) Sagittal STIR and (**b**) T1-weighted MR image demonstrate acute spondylitis anterior and posterior (arrowheads), so called Romanus lesions in the lower spine and (**c**) axial T2-weighted fat suppressed fast-spine echo sequences of the SIJ demonstrated bone marrow edema subchondral along the sacroiliac joint space, giving the diagnosis of active sacroiliac arthritis

The pathogenesis is still not well understood, with potential association to an anti-inflammatory process, potentially triggered by infectious (such as Propionibacterium acnes) or other agents.

In SAPHO the costoclavicular joints followed by the spine and SIJ are most often involved. But also, synchondroses of costochondral joints, symphyses, such as manubriosternal joint and pubic symphyses are often involved. While peripheral arthritis is most often seen in younger adults (<25 years, but not in children) with the knees, hips, and ankles most affected but even the small joints of the hands and feet can be involved [28]. In children and adolescents, long bone metaphyses followed by clavicles are most commonly affected.

14.4.12 CPPD

Calcium pyrophosphate dehydrate crystal deposition around the dens is very common, particularly in older patients, with a prevalence of up to 50% in over 80-year-olds [29]. Usually, they are asymptomatic. The term crowned dens syndrome stands for CPPD deposition together with symptoms such as neck stiffness, and evidence of inflammation such as fever and or elevated C-reactive protein [30].

Key Point

- Calcium pyrophosphate dehydrate crystal deposition around the dens is often an asymptomatic finding.
- The term crowned dens syndrome should only be used when additional symptoms such as neck stiffness and evidence of inflammation (fever and or elevated C-reactive protein) are present.

14.4.13 Calcific Tendinosis of the Longus Colli Muscle

Calcitic tendinosis of the longus colli muscle is a self-limiting disease with neck pain and elevated C-reactive protein. It is diagnosed by typical clinical history and prevertebral edema seen on fluid-sensitive MR images as well as amorphous calcification within the tendon of the longus colli muscles. The calcifications are best seen on radiographs or computed tomography images.

Take Home Messages

- Take a systematic approach to imaging interpretation and reporting.
- Always ask, is there contact, deviation, or compression of a nerve?
- Correlate clinical symptoms with imaging findings to diagnose the actual pain generator.
- When it is not possible to diagnose the exact cause of pain, radiologists create long lists of abnormalities that also include incidental findings.

Conflict of Interest I/We declare no competing interests as defined by Springer Nature or other interests that might be perceived to influence results and/or discussion reported in this manuscript.

Literature

1. Palmer WE. Spinal injections for pain management. Radiology. 2016;281:669–88.
2. Farshad M, Gerber C, Farshad-Amacker NA, Dietrich TJ, Laufer-Molnar V, Min K. Asymmetry of the multifidus muscle in lumbar radicular nerve compression. Skelet Radiol. 2013;43:49–53.
3. Farshad-Amacker NA, Farshad M, Galley J, Sutter R, Götschi T, Pfammatter T, Puippe G, Muehlematter UJ. Atypical patterns of spinal segment degeneration in patients with abdominal aortic aneurysms. Eur Spine J. 2023;32:8–19.
4. Farshad-Amacker NA, Hughes AP, Aichmair A, Herzog RJ, Farshad M. Determinants of evolution of endplate and disc degeneration in the lumbar spine: a multifactorial perspective. Eur Spine J. 2014;23:1863–8.
5. Pfirrmann CW, Metzdorf A, Zanetti M, Hodler J, Boos N. Magnetic resonance classification of lumbar intervertebral disc degeneration. Spine. 2001;26:1873–8.
6. Bartynski WS, Agarwal V, Trang H, Bandos AI, Rothfus WE, Tsay J, Delfyett WT, Nastasi B. Enhancing annular fissures and high-intensity zones: pain, internal derangement, and anesthetic response at provocation lumbar discography. Am J Neuroradiol. 2022;44:95–104.
7. Carragee EJ, Paragioudakis SJ, Khurana S. Lumbar high-intensity zone and discography in subjects without low back problems. Spine. 2000;25:2987–92.
8. Farshad-Amacker NA, Hughes AP, Aichmair A, Herzog RJ, Farshad M. Is an annular tear a predictor for accelerated disc degeneration? Eur Spine J. 2014;23:1825–9.
9. Fardon DF, Milette PC, Neuroradiology CTF of the NASS American Society of Spine Radiology. Nomenclature and classification of lumbar disc pathology. Spine. 2001;26:E93–E113.
10. Farshad-Amacker NA, Farshad M, Winklehner A, Andreisek G. MR imaging of degenerative disc disease. Eur J Radiol. 2015;84:1768–76.
11. Pfirrmann CWA, Dora C, Schmid MR, Zanetti M, Hodler J, Boos N. MR image–based grading of lumbar nerve root compromise

due to disk herniation: reliability study with surgical correlation. Radiology. 2004;230:583–8.
12. Toyone T, Takahashi K, Kitahara H, Yamagata M, Murakami M, Moriya H. Vertebral bone-marrow changes in degenerative lumbar disc disease. An MRI study of 74 patients with low back pain. J bone Jt Surg Br. 1994;76:757–64.
13. Rajasekaran S, Venkatadass K, Babu JN, Ganesh K, Shetty AP. Pharmacological enhancement of disc diffusion and differentiation of healthy, ageing and degenerated discs. Eur Spine J. 2008;17:626–43.
14. Farshad-Amacker NA, Hughes A, Herzog RJ, Seifert B, Farshad M. The intervertebral disc, the endplates and the vertebral bone marrow as a unit in the process of degeneration. Eur Radiol. 2015;27:2507–20.
15. Cieciera M, Sutter R, Wirth SH, Götschi T, Farshad-Amacker NA. Severity of bone marrow edema on MRI predicts the diagnostic potential of foot joint injections. Foot Ankle Int. 2025;46:747–56.
16. Balza R, Palmer WE. Symptom-imaging correlation in lumbar spine pain. Skelet Radiol. 2023;52:1901–9.
17. Balza R, Mercaldo SF, Chang CY, Huang AJ, Husseini JS, Kheterpal AB, Simeone FJ, Palmer WE. Impact of patient-reported symptom information on agreement in the MRI diagnosis of presumptive lumbar spine pain generator. Am J Roentgenol. 2021;217:947–56.
18. Balza R, Mercaldo SF, Huang AJ, Husseini JS, Jarraya M, Simeone FJ, Vicentini JRT, Palmer WE. Impact of patient-reported symptom information on the interpretation of MRI of the lumbar spine. Radiology. 2024;313:e233487.
19. Park H-J, Kim SS, Lee S-Y, Park N-H, Rho M-H, Hong H-P, Kwag H-J, Kook S-H, Choi S-H. Clinical correlation of a new MR imaging method for assessing lumbar foraminal stenosis. AJNR Am J Neuroradiol. 2012;33:818–22.
20. Wildermuth S, Zanetti M, Duewell S, Schmid MR, Romanowski B, Benini A, Böni T, Hodler J. Lumbar spine: quantitative and qualitative assessment of positional (upright flexion and extension) MR imaging and myelography. Radiology. 1998;207:391–8.
21. Farshad M, Sutter R, Hoch A. Severity of foraminal lumbar stenosis and the relation to clinical symptoms and response to periradicular infiltration-introduction of the "melting sign". Spine J. 2017;18:294–9.
22. Samartzis D, Kalluri P, Herman J, Lubicky JP, Shen FH. 2008 Young Investigator Award; The role of congenitally fused cervical segments upon the space available for the cord and associated symptoms in Klippel-Feil patients. Spine. 2008;33:1442–50.
23. Farshad-Amacker NA, Herzog RJ, Hughes AP, Aichmair A, Farshad M. Associations between lumbosacral transitional anatomy types and degeneration at the transitional and adjacent segments. Spine J. 2015;15:1210–6.
24. Farshad-Amacker NA, Sutter R. The great mimickers of spinal pathology. Semin Musculoskelet Radiol. 2022;26:439–52.
25. Altorfer FCS, Sutter R, Farshad M, Spirig JM, Farshad-Amacker NA. MRI appearance of adjunct surgical material used in spine surgery. Spine J. 2022;22:75–83.
26. Shlobin NA, Dahdaleh NS. Cervical spine manifestations of rheumatoid arthritis: a review. Neurosurg Rev. 2021;44:1957–65.
27. Burgos-Vargas R. The assessment of the spondyloarthritis international society concept and criteria for the classification of axial spondyloarthritis and peripheral spondyloarthritis: a critical appraisal for the pediatric rheumatologist. Pediatr Rheumatol. 2012;10:14.
28. Depasquale R, Kumar N, Lalam RK, Tins BJ, Tyrrell PNM, Singh J, Cassar-Pullicino VN. SAPHO: what radiologists should know. Clin Radiol. 2012;67:195–206.
29. Kakitsubata Y, Boutin RD, Theodorou DJ, Kerr RM, Steinbach LS, Chan KK, Pathria MN, Haghighi P, Resnick D. Calcium pyrophosphate dihydrate crystal deposition in and around the atlantoaxial joint: association with type 2 odontoid fractures in nine patients. Radiology. 2000;216:213–9.
30. Matsumura M, Hara S. Crowned dens syndrome. N Engl J Med. 2012;6:367.

Musculoskeletal Infection

15

Aline Serfaty and William B. Morrison

Learning Objectives

1. To recognize appearance of musculoskeletal infection on different modalities
2. To understand basic pathoetiology of musculoskeletal infection (i.e., routes of infection)
3. To be able to generate a differential diagnosis for conditions that can simulate infection

15.1 Introduction

Musculoskeletal infections, encompassing osteomyelitis, septic arthritis, and soft tissue infections, represent a significant source of morbidity worldwide. Their global prevalence is influenced by factors such as population aging, increased prevalence of diabetes and immunosuppressive conditions, and the rising use of orthopedic implants and prosthetic devices. In developing countries, limited access to early diagnostic tools often contributes to delayed diagnoses and worsened outcomes [1].

Key clinical challenges in managing musculoskeletal infections include the nonspecific nature of early symptoms, overlap with noninfectious inflammatory disorders, and the emergence of multidrug-resistant organisms. Delayed or missed diagnosis may lead to irreversible joint damage, chronic osteomyelitis, sepsis, or limb loss. Furthermore, the need for antibiotic stewardship adds complexity, as inappropriate antimicrobial use can exacerbate resistance patterns and hinder treatment efficacy [2, 3].

Early and accurate imaging plays a pivotal role in the diagnostic pathway. Imaging not only helps localize the infection and assess its extent but also guides biopsies, aspirations, and surgical planning. Timely radiological evaluation can significantly improve outcomes by enabling prompt initiation of targeted therapy [4].

This chapter will provide a comprehensive overview of musculoskeletal infections, including their pathophysiology, routes of spread, and characteristic imaging features. We will discuss the role of multiple imaging modalities in diagnosing musculoskeletal infections, including radiography, ultrasound (US), computed tomography (CT), magnetic resonance imaging (MRI), and nuclear medicine, with attention to metal artifact reduction techniques. Common infectious entities such as osteomyelitis, septic arthritis, and soft tissue infections will be addressed, followed by a review of spinal involvement, imaging-guided procedures, and typical vs. atypical infection patterns. Finally, we will outline key imaging mimics, diagnostic pitfalls, and practical pearls to aid clinical interpretation.

15.2 Pathophysiology and Routes of Infection

There are three principal routes by which musculoskeletal infections develop: hematogenous spread, contiguous spread, and direct implantation (inoculation) (Fig. 15.1).

15.2.1 Hematogenous Spread

This is the most common pathway for osteomyelitis in children and immunocompromised adults and frequently affects the spine in all age groups. Pathogens, most commonly *Staphylococcus aureus*, enter the bloodstream and seed highly vascularized regions of the bone, such as the metaphyses of long bones. This results in inflammatory infiltration, marrow edema, and eventual cortical destruction. Hematogenous spread is particularly relevant in systemic

A. Serfaty
Medscanlagos Radiology, Cabo Frio, Rio de Janeiro, Brazil

W. B. Morrison (✉)
Thomas Jefferson University Hospital, Philadelphia, PA, USA
e-mail: William.morrison@jefferson.edu

J. Hodler et al. (eds.), *Musculoskeletal Diseases 2026-2029*, IDKD Springer Series,
https://doi.org/10.1007/978-3-032-17040-8_15

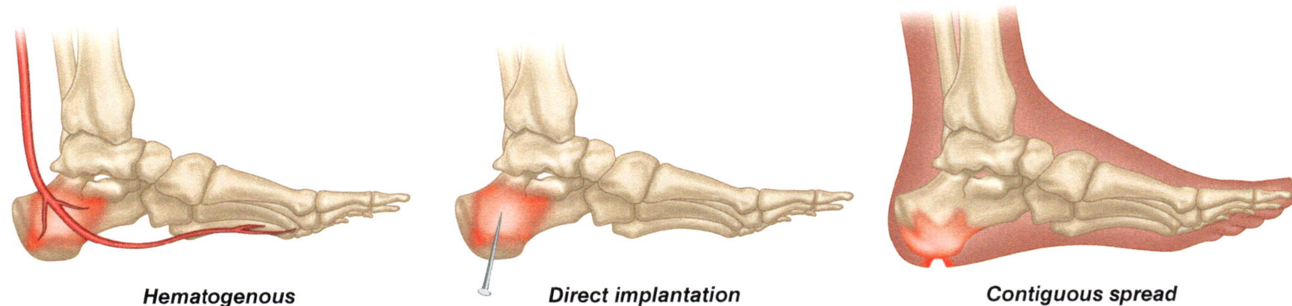

Fig. 15.1 Musculoskeletal infection: modes of spread. Infection can involve the musculoskeletal system though hematogenous spread, direct implantation, or contiguous spread. Hematogenous route is the most common etiology in spinal infection. Direct implantation can result from penetrating injury or surgery. Contiguous spread is the most common route in diabetic patients with pedal ulceration and in paralyzed patients with decubitus ulceration

infections or bacteremia, where there is no obvious local source of infection [5].

15.2.2 Contiguous Spread

Contiguous spread occurs when infection extends from adjacent soft tissues or skin into the musculoskeletal system. It is frequently seen in adults with chronic wounds, such as diabetic foot ulcers or pressure sores in paralyzed patients. These infections often involve polymicrobial organisms and are complicated by poor local vascularity, which hinders both immune response and antibiotic penetration. Common clinical examples include diabetic pedal osteomyelitis and pelvic infections in immobilized individuals [6].

15.2.3 Direct Implantation (Inoculation)

Direct inoculation results from the introduction of pathogens through trauma (e.g., puncture wounds), open fractures, surgical procedures, or percutaneous interventions. This route is relatively common in the hands and feet due to their frequent exposure to penetrating injuries. Iatrogenic infections may also arise following orthopedic surgeries or implantation of prosthetic devices. Diagnosing infection in these cases can be challenging due to overlap with normal postoperative changes on imaging [7].

Key Points

- Three routes for musculoskeletal infection: hematogenous, contiguous spread, and direct inoculation.
- Most common: hematogenous, especially in children and immunocompromised adults; spine often involved.
- Contiguous spread: important in diabetic and paralyzed patients (chronic ulcers, pressure sores), often polymicrobial.
- Direct inoculation: trauma, open fractures, surgery, or procedures; common in hands and feet; consider hardware infection.
- Knowing the route helps anticipate pathogens and select imaging.

15.3 Imaging Modalities

A systematic and multimodal imaging approach is essential for comprehensive assessment. The choice of modality depends on the clinical context, infection location, and presence of metallic implants.

15.3.1 Radiography

Radiography remains the most accessible and cost-effective first-line imaging modality in the evaluation of suspected musculoskeletal infections. Although its sensitivity for early osteomyelitis is relatively low, generally ranging from 43% to 75%, these values are most commonly reported in cases of diabetic foot infections associated with underlying skin ulcers. In such situations, aligning radiographic findings with the precise location of the ulcer can improve diagnostic accuracy by drawing attention to subtle osseous changes [4]. Radiographs also offer a valuable overview of regional anatomy and are instrumental in ruling out alternative diagnoses that may mimic infection, such as fractures, arthritis, or bone tumors. Early radiographic signs of infection include soft tissue swelling and obscuration of fat planes, though these findings are nonspecific and can be seen in various inflammatory or traumatic conditions.

Despite their limitations in detecting early disease, radiographs remain useful for identifying more advanced or chronic changes, including cortical erosion, sequestrum formation, and periosteal reaction. They also aid in the assessment of postoperative complications; in the detection of soft tissue gas, calcifications, or foreign bodies; and in the characterization of arthropathies, including neuropathic osteoarthropathy. While radiographs alone are often insufficient for a definitive diagnosis, they provide important contextual clues and are particularly valuable when interpreted alongside clinical findings. As such, radiography continues to play a crucial role in the initial screening and in guiding decisions regarding further imaging [8].

15.3.2 Ultrasound

Ultrasound remains a valuable imaging modality in the evaluation of musculoskeletal infections, particularly for assessing superficial soft tissue abnormalities and guiding interventions. It is widely accessible, cost-effective, portable, and free of ionizing radiation, making it an ideal bedside tool for critically ill or pediatric patients. US offers high-resolution imaging of superficial structures, making it especially useful for detecting joint effusions, soft tissue abscesses, cellulitis, and tenosynovitis. In pediatric cases, US is often the preferred method for early detection of hip effusions and septic arthritis. When combined with Doppler techniques, it can help demonstrate increased vascularity associated with active inflammation, enhancing diagnostic confidence. One of the most significant advantages of ultrasound is its ability to facilitate real-time image-guided procedures, such as aspiration of joint fluid or drainage of abscesses, directly during the exam [4, 8].

However, ultrasound also has important limitations, particularly in the assessment of deeper or more complex infections. Due to its inability to penetrate cortical bone, US is not suitable for directly evaluating intraosseous involvement, limiting its use to superficial soft tissue and periosteal changes. This becomes especially relevant in suspected osteomyelitis or deeper-seated abscesses, where modalities like MRI or CT offer superior diagnostic value. The effectiveness of ultrasound is also highly dependent on operator expertise and anatomic familiarity, which may reduce diagnostic reliability in less experienced hands. In cases of cellulitis, US may reveal subcutaneous edema, skin thickening, and increased blood flow. A characteristic "cobblestoning" pattern (hypoechoic fluid dissecting between fat lobules) can be seen in inflamed subcutaneous tissues. Abscesses typically appear as hypoechoic or heterogeneously echogenic fluid collections, often with posterior acoustic enhancement and peripheral hyperemia. In cases of necrotizing infections, the presence of gas may be visualized as bright echogenic foci with posterior reverberation artifacts ("dirty shadowing"). While joint effusions can be easily identified with ultrasound, they are nonspecific and may also be seen in noninfectious conditions such as inflammatory arthritis or transient synovitis. In pediatric osteomyelitis, ultrasound can identify periosteal elevation, subperiosteal fluid collections, early cortical breaches, and cloaca formation, often before changes are visible on radiographs [4, 5].

15.3.3 Computed Tomography

Computed tomography plays a critical role in the prompt assessment of musculoskeletal infections, particularly in emergency settings involving acutely ill patients. It is especially helpful when clinical evaluation alone cannot exclude an underlying abscess. CT's high spatial resolution and rapid imaging capability allow for the assessment of large anatomical areas and precise localization of collections that may require intervention. When intravenous contrast is used, CT effectively distinguishes abscesses through their peripheral enhancement, while skin thickening and fat stranding are typical findings in cellulitis. In more severe infections like necrotizing fasciitis, CT can reveal gas in the soft tissues, an important but late and relatively insensitive sign. Although soft tissue gas is present in fewer than half of such cases, its detection is highly specific and aids in assessing the extent of disease spread. CT also serves as a useful tool for guiding percutaneous aspiration or drainage when needed [9].

In the evaluation of osteomyelitis, CT is most valuable in chronic cases and when MRI is contraindicated or limited. While MRI remains the modality of choice for early detection due to its superior soft tissue contrast, CT may demonstrate early cortical bone involvement and medullary changes such as increased attenuation from marrow infiltration. CT is particularly advantageous for evaluating anatomically complex regions like the spine and pelvis or in postoperative settings where metal hardware may cause artifacts on MRI. Furthermore, CT helps assess for hardware complications, including loosening or periimplant lucency. Its ability to detect sequestra (sclerotic, devitalized bone fragments surrounded by radiolucent granulation tissue) is critical, as these require surgical debridement rather than antibiotic therapy alone. CT also visualizes chronic osteomyelitis features such as involucrum (new bone formation encasing a sequestrum) and cloaca (a cortical defect allowing drainage), supporting comprehensive surgical planning and long-term infection control [4, 9].

15.3.4 Magnetic Resonance Imaging

Magnetic resonance imaging (MRI) is a cornerstone in the evaluation of musculoskeletal infections, particularly for detecting and characterizing osteomyelitis and associated soft tissue abnormalities. It is especially useful when initial radiographs are inconclusive or negative, or when soft tissue abscess is suspected [4]. MRI offers exceptional anatomic detail and remains the most accurate imaging modality for diagnosing osteomyelitis, with meta-analyses reporting a sensitivity of 95.6% and specificity of 80.7%. However, its diagnostic accuracy may be limited in patients with prior surgeries, neuropathic arthropathy, or underlying inflammatory diseases such as rheumatoid arthritis [10].

MRI plays a critical role in distinguishing superficial cellulitis from deeper infections and in preoperative planning by defining the extent of disease and surgical margins. T1-weighted sequences reveal low-signal marrow replacement, while T2-weighted and STIR sequences highlight high-signal edema. Postcontrast imaging is essential for delineating necrotic tissue. In diabetic foot infections, which commonly arise from ulceration and contiguous spread, MRI should be tailored to the site of concern. Optimizing the field of view and placing skin markers near superficial ulcers enhance visualization of early infectious changes. Consensus guidelines from the Society of Skeletal Radiology recommend contrast-enhanced MRI in infants for better evaluation of unossified bone and in adults to identify devitalized tissue. MRI is also instrumental in assessing complications such as sinus tracts and abscesses in chronic osteomyelitis. The American College of Radiology supports MRI use through Appropriateness Criteria®, guiding imaging choices in suspected osteomyelitis, septic arthritis, and soft tissue infections [4, 11].

15.3.5 Nuclear Medicine Imaging

Radionuclide imaging is a valuable tool in the assessment of osteomyelitis, particularly in diabetic foot infections where conventional imaging may be inconclusive. Three-phase bone scintigraphy using technetium-99 m-labeled diphosphonates is highly sensitive for detecting osteomyelitis due to its ability to identify early osteoblastic activity. However, its specificity is limited, as increased uptake can also be seen in noninfectious conditions such as recent surgery, trauma, neuropathic osteoarthropathy, and inflammatory arthropathies. Despite these limitations, a normal scan, especially in the absence of severe ischemia, effectively rules out osteomyelitis. A fourth delayed phase (at 24 hours) can sometimes help distinguish osteomyelitis from overlying cellulitis or soft tissue hyperemia in complex cases [12, 13].

Labeled white blood cell (WBC) scintigraphy, typically using 99mTc-labeled leukocytes, offers significantly higher specificity by directly targeting infection-associated leukocyte accumulation. When interpreted in combination with bone scintigraphy, overall diagnostic accuracy improves markedly, with reported specificities reaching 90–100%. Nonetheless, WBC scans can produce false negatives in patients pretreated with antibiotics or with significant ischemia and false positives in settings of sterile inflammation. The addition of SPECT/CT enhances anatomic localization and improves differentiation between soft tissue and bone involvement [14].

FDG-PET/CT offers both high sensitivity and specificity for detecting chronic osteomyelitis and can be particularly useful in patients with equivocal MRI or CT findings or when metallic implants limit image quality. FDG uptake reflects inflammatory and infectious processes rather than bone turnover alone, allowing for better differentiation of infection from postsurgical or degenerative changes. Although more costly and less widely available, FDG-PET/CT is increasingly used in complex or recurrent infections [12].

15.3.6 Metal Artifact Reduction Techniques

Magnetic resonance imaging evaluation in the presence of metallic implants is often limited by significant susceptibility artifacts, which obscure the periprosthetic bone and adjacent soft tissues. Advanced metal artifact–reduction techniques such as Slice Encoding for Metal Artifact Correction (SEMAC) and Multi-Acquisition Variable-Resonance Image Combination Selective (MAVRIC-SL) have been developed to address this issue. These sequences reduce distortion by correcting for in-plane and through-plane artifacts, enabling more accurate visualization of joint effusions, synovial thickening, marrow signal abnormalities, and periimplant collections. Both techniques are effective at 1.5 T and 3 T, significantly improving diagnostic quality in the postoperative setting [15].

These improvements are especially valuable in the evaluation of suspected periprosthetic joint infection (PJI). Studies have shown that MRI with MAVRIC-SL can achieve high diagnostic accuracy, with positive predictive values of up to 81% and negative predictive values approaching 100% in the detection of infection. Imaging features such as lamellated synovitis, pericapsular fluid collections, and bone marrow edema can help differentiate infectious from noninfectious causes of postoperative symptoms. When combined with clinical and laboratory data, advanced MRI techniques play a critical role in the early diagnosis and management of PJI [16].

Key Points

- Radiography is first line. Low early sensitivity. Good for overview, gas, foreign bodies, and chronic change.
- Ultrasound is bedside and accessible. Detects effusions and abscesses. Guides aspiration. Limited for bone.
- CT is fast. Maps collections and gas. Guides drainage. Helpful with hardware and chronic osteomyelitis.
- MRI is most accurate for osteomyelitis and extent. Contrast defines necrosis. Use caution after surgery or in neuropathic joints. Tailor protocols for the diabetic foot.
- Nuclear medicine helps when MRI or CT are equivocal. Bone scan is sensitive but nonspecific. WBC scans are more specific, especially with SPECT/CT. FDG-PET/CT is useful in chronic or implant cases.
- Metal artifact reduction works. SEMAC and MAVRIC-SL improve periprosthetic MRI at 1.5 T and 3 T. They aid early PJI assessment.

15.4 Imaging Appearances of Common Infections

15.4.1 Soft Tissue Infections

15.4.1.1 Cellulitis

Cellulitis is an acute bacterial infection involving the superficial soft tissue (skin, subcutaneous tissues, and superficial fascia), often resulting from minor trauma or skin disruption. It is characterized clinically by erythema, warmth, swelling, and tenderness, with borders that are typically ill-defined. Imaging is not routinely required for diagnosis when clinical presentation is classic, but it plays a vital role when complications such as abscess or necrotizing fasciitis are suspected or in cases with atypical features or poor clinical response to antibiotics. Importantly, cellulitis is confined to the superficial soft tissue layers and does not extend into the deep fascial planes or muscle, whereas necrotizing fasciitis is distinguished by involvement of the deep fascia and underlying musculature, a feature that underscores its severity and the need for prompt recognition [8, 17].

The diagnosis of cellulitis is primarily clinical, with imaging reserved for cases of progression, poor treatment response, or diagnostic uncertainty. Plain radiographs may reveal nonspecific findings such as soft tissue swelling, loss of fat planes, or, less commonly, soft tissue gas, which indicates a more severe infection. Ultrasound typically demonstrates a "cobblestoning" pattern, reflecting fluid tracking between echogenic subcutaneous fat lobules, and is particularly useful when an abscess is suspected; increased vascularity on Doppler may also be present. On CT, cellulitis manifests as skin thickening, fat stranding, and edema of the subcutaneous tissue and superficial fascia, with subtle contrast enhancement helping distinguish it from bland edema. MRI demonstrates similar features, with confluent or reticulated low T1 and high fluid-sensitive signal intensity in the subcutaneous tissues and superficial fascia, often accompanied by skin thickening. Both CT and MRI can delineate abscess formation, detect gas, and evaluate deeper extension. Importantly, cross-sectional imaging helps exclude mimics or associated conditions such as necrotizing soft tissue infection, thrombophlebitis, or osteomyelitis, thereby guiding timely and appropriate management [9, 17].

Key Points

- Acute infection of skin, subcutaneous tissues, and superficial fascia.
- Diagnosis is clinical. Image when atypical, worsening, or to exclude abscess and necrotizing infection.
- Ultrasound shows "cobblestoning" pattern and can detect abscess.
- CT and MRI show skin thickening, fat stranding, and superficial fascial edema.
- Disease is limited to superficial layers. Deep fascia and muscle are not involved.

15.4.1.2 Soft Tissue Abscess

A soft tissue abscess is a localized, encapsulated collection of pus resulting from bacterial invasion, most often *Staphylococcus aureus*, streptococci, or Gram-negative organisms, surrounded by a capsule of inflammatory and granulation tissue. Risk factors include penetrating trauma, ulcers, diabetes, immunosuppression, and bacteremia. Radiographs are nonspecific, typically showing soft tissue swelling, with gas-fluid levels rarely visible but highly suggestive of infection. Ultrasound is highly sensitive, revealing a fluid collection with variable echogenicity, posterior acoustic enhancement, swirling debris on compression, peripheral hyperemia with an avascular core, and occasionally gas as echogenic foci with dirty shadowing. CT depicts a centrally nonenhancing hypodense cavity bounded by a thick, irregular enhancing wall, often with adjacent fat stranding or muscle edema, and is particularly useful for guiding drainage. MRI provides the highest diagnostic accuracy, showing low T1 and high T2/fluid-sensitive signal with a thick enhancing rim and central nonenhancement after contrast; restricted diffusion on DWI further confirms the diagnosis, while the "penumbra sign," a hyperintense T1 rim of granulation tissue, helps distinguish abscess from necrotic tumors. Abscesses are usually subcutaneous, fascial, or intramuscular, often adjacent to skin ulcers or osteomyelitis, and MRI also enables evaluation of associated septic arthritis or bone infection [8, 9, 17].

Key Points

- Localized collection of pus with an inflammatory rim.
- Ultrasound is sensitive and guides aspiration or drainage.
- CT shows a nonenhancing center with a thick-enhancing wall and surrounding stranding.
- MRI shows low T1 and high fluid signal with a thick-enhancing rim and restricted diffusion.
- Consider nearby ulcers, osteomyelitis, and septic arthritis.

15.4.1.3 Necrotizing Fasciitis

Necrotizing fasciitis is a rapidly progressive necrotizing soft tissue infection that primarily targets the deep fascia and adjacent subcutaneous tissues, with potential spread to skin and muscle. Many authors now favor the broader term "necrotizing soft-tissue infection," emphasizing that the process entails tissue death across the skin and superficial soft tissues, both layers of fascia, and even the musculature [17]. It carries substantial morbidity (including amputation) and mortality, especially in the lower limbs, so early recognition and urgent surgical debridement are critical. Risk rises with diabetes, immunosuppression, malignancy, liver disease, alcohol use, obesity, older age, and intravenous drug use. Because presentation can mimic cellulitis or nonnecrotizing fasciitis (pain, swelling, erythema; fever may be absent), a high index of suspicion is essential. The LRINEC score, derived from routine labs, supports risk stratification (≥6 concerning; ≥8 highly suggestive), but definitive diagnosis rests on operative findings of devitalized tissue with easy blunt separation along the deep fascia and "dishwater" fluid [8, 9].

Imaging is adjunctive and should never delay surgery. In the emergency setting, CT is often preferred for speed, availability, and its sensitivity to small volumes of soft tissue gas. Gas tracking along fascial planes is the most specific CT sign, yet it appears in fewer than half of patients; absence of gas does not exclude the disease. Additional CT features include asymmetric deep fascial thickening, subfascial edema, fat stranding, fluid collections, obscured myofascial planes, and the occasional foreign body. Plain radiographs may reveal soft tissue emphysema but are insensitive, and ultrasound can show fascial thickening or fluid while being operator-dependent and less reliable for deep involvement [9].

MRI offers the most detailed soft tissue assessment. Findings that favor necrotizing infection over nonnecrotizing processes include deep fascial thickening (around ≥3 mm), fluid pockets along the deep fascia, heterogeneous or absent fascial enhancement, intrafascial gas, and involvement of multiple fascial compartments (Fig. 15.2). Notably, when MRI shows no deep fascial abnormality, the negative predictive value is high. Integrating MRI features (e.g., deep fascial thickening and multicompartment involvement) with the LRINEC score improves discrimination compared with LRINEC alone. Diffusion-weighted imaging can highlight coexisting abscesses but is not diagnostic by itself. Overall, imaging's role is twofold: confirm deep fascial involvement and map disease extent, while clinical urgency and prompt operative management remain paramount [8].

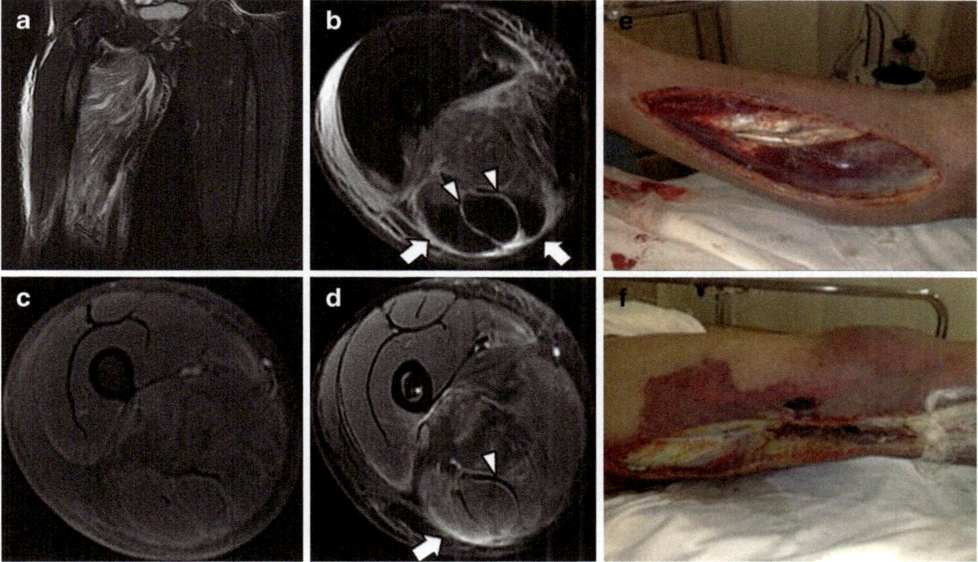

Fig. 15.2 Necrotizing fasciitis of the distal thigh in a 29-year-old man with 1 week of fever and pain. (**a**) Coronal fat-suppressed T2-weighted image shows diffuse high-signal intensity within the muscles of the medial and posterior compartments of the thigh with diffuse high-signal intensity within the subcutaneous tissue. (**b**) Axial fat-suppressed T2-weighted image shows thickening and fluid along the deep peripheral fascia overlying the muscles of the medial and posterior compartments of the thigh (arrows) with extension along the deep intermuscular fascia (arrowheads). (**c** and **d**) Axial pre- and postcontrast T1-weighted image depicts peripheral band-like enhancement (arrow) of involved muscle and thin smooth enhancement of deep fascia (arrowhead), with intervening nonenhancing segments. (**e** and **f**) Intraoperative photographs following urgent fasciotomy/debridement confirm extensive fascial necrosis. Intraoperative cultures grew *Streptococcus pyogenes*. (Case courtesy of Dr. Julio Brandão Guimarães)

Key Points
- Rapidly progressive infection of deep fascia with high morbidity.
- Risk is higher with diabetes, immunosuppression, cancer, liver disease, obesity, older age, alcohol use, and intravenous drug use.
- LRINEC supports risk assessment. Surgical exploration confirms the diagnosis.
- CT detects gas and maps extent. Absence of gas does not exclude disease.
- MRI shows deep fascial thickening, fascial fluid, variable enhancement, gas, and multicompartment spread.
- Imaging must not delay urgent debridement.

15.4.1.4 Pyomyositis

Pyomyositis is a suppurative infection of skeletal muscle that may arise either from hematogenous spread or from extension of infection in adjacent tissues. *Staphylococcus aureus* is the most frequent causative organism. The disease often affects children and young adults, most commonly involving the thigh, calf, or pelvic muscles. Early clinical features may be subtle, such as fever, discomfort, or limping, so imaging plays a central role in diagnosis, guiding interventions (e.g., aspiration or drainage), and monitoring treatment response [9].

On radiographs, findings are nonspecific, usually limited to focal soft tissue swelling. Ultrasound can reveal hypoechoic fluid collections and guide aspiration, but its sensitivity for early or deep abscesses is limited. Contrast-enhanced CT demonstrates muscle enlargement with heterogeneous attenuation, central low-density collections with peripheral rim enhancement, and sometimes gas, though it is less sensitive in early disease. MRI is the most sensitive modality, detecting muscle enlargement and T2 hyperintensity and later showing rim-enhancing intramuscular abscesses. DWI and ADC mapping help distinguish bacterial pyomyositis from necrotic tumors or viral myositis. Thus, MRI not only provides accurate diagnosis and staging but also aids in differentiating pyomyositis from neoplasms and other mimics [9, 18].

Key Points
- Suppurative infection of the skeletal muscle. Often due to *Staphylococcus aureus*.
- Early symptoms can be subtle. Imaging guides diagnosis and intervention.
- Ultrasound can show fluid and helps aspiration.
- CT shows muscle enlargement and rim-enhancing collections.
- MRI is most sensitive for edema and abscess with restricted diffusion.

15.4.1.5 Infectious Tenosynovitis and Bursitis

Infectious tenosynovitis is an infection of the tendon sheath that behaves like a closed-space process: once bacteria seed the sheath, typically after a skin breach such as a laceration, puncture, or bite, the synovial-lined compartment can rapidly fill with inflammatory fluid and organisms, threatening tendon viability and function [17]. It must be distinguished from noninfectious (overuse or inflammatory) tenosynovitis because delay risks rigidity, contractures, and permanent impairment. *Staphylococcus aureus* is the leading pathogen; others include *Pasteurella multocida* (classically cat bites), *Neisseria gonorrhoeae*, *Eikenella corrodens* (human bites), and mycobacteria such as *M. tuberculosis* and *M. marinum* (water exposure). Clinical clues favoring infection over sterile inflammation include overlying cellulitis, a skin defect or foreign body, soft tissue edema, and when present concomitant septic arthritis [9, 19].

Imaging supports but does not replace clinical judgment and microbiologic confirmation. Ultrasound is an excellent first step for superficial tendons: infected sheaths typically show distension with complex fluid/debris, synovial thickening, and hyperemia on Doppler; US also enables targeted aspiration or biopsy. MRI is the most comprehensive modality, demonstrating complex sheath fluid with septations, thick-enhancing synovium, ill-defined perisynovial edema, and possible abscesses or sinus tracts; "rice bodies" (small fibrinous bodies) may appear, particularly with tuberculous or fungal infection (Fig. 15.3). CT depicts tendon thickening, fluid, and abscess, and radiographs are useful to detect retained foreign bodies or osseous involvement. Because imaging appearances overlap with rheumatoid, gouty, and psoriatic tenosynovitis, fluid aspiration for culture remains the diagnostic endpoint when uncertainty persists [8, 19].

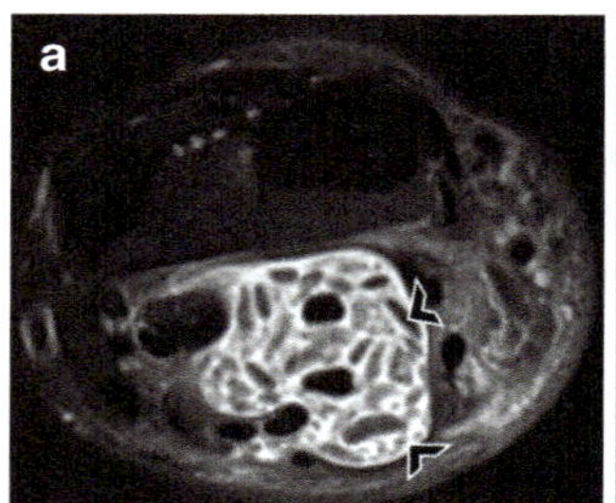

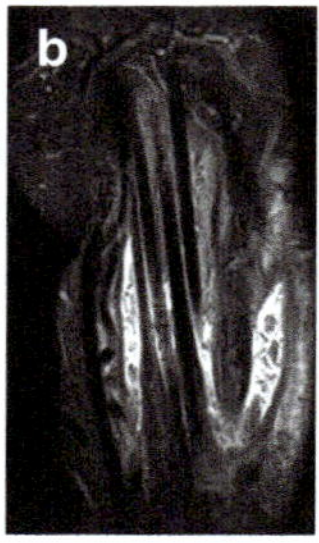

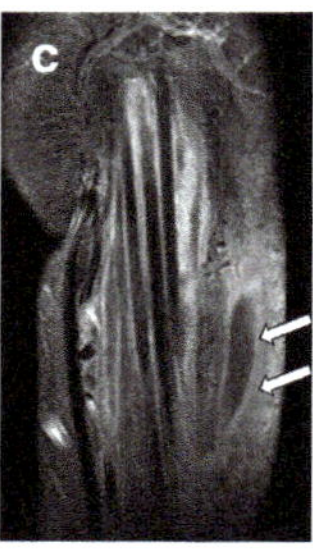

Fig. 15.3 *Mycobacterium kansasii* tenosynovitis in a 22-year-old man with forearm and wrist swelling. Axial fat-suppressed T2-weighted MRI image (**a**) at the distal forearm shows marked distension of the ulnar bursa filled with high-signal fluid containing innumerable low-signal ovoid bodies, consistent with rice bodies (arrowheads). Coronal fat-suppressed T2-weighted image (**b**) demonstrates longitudinal extension of the distended ulnar bursa from the wrist into the proximal forearm with surrounding soft tissue edema. Coronal fat-suppressed postcontrast T1-weighted image (**c**) depicts diffuse tenosynovial thickening with enhancement surrounding the nonenhancing intrabursal rice bodies (arrows). No osseous erosion or marrow edema is identified. (Case courtesy of Dr. Tatiane Cantarelli)

Infectious bursitis mirrors these principles in synovial bursae, presenting as a distended bursa with complex fluid and thick rim enhancement on contrast studies. Across entities, prompt recognition, appropriate imaging to map extent and guide procedures, image-guided aspiration, and timely surgical and antibiotic therapy are the cornerstones of preventing long-term disability [9, 17].

Key Points

- Closed space infection of a tendon sheath or bursa after a skin breach.

Staphylococcus aureus is most common. Animal and human bites and mycobacteria also occur.

- Ultrasound is first line for superficial disease and enables aspiration.
- MRI shows complex fluid, synovial thickening and enhancement, perisynovial edema, and possible abscess or sinus tract.
- Aspiration and culture establish the diagnosis when uncertain.

15.4.1.6 Devitalized Tissue

Devitalized tissue refers to nonviable or critically ischemic soft tissue, most often encountered in the diabetic foot and in peripheral arterial disease. Its recognition matters because mapping the extent of nonviable tissue guides debridement and limb-sparing amputations. On contrast-enhanced MRI, it appears as a geographic region of absent enhancement with a sharp transition to surrounding hyperemic tissue. Subtraction images can make the boundary more conspicuous. Within these nonenhancing zones, superimposed infection, including cellulitis, abscess, or osteomyelitis, will also lack enhancement; therefore diagnosis of infection relies primarily on T1 and fluid-sensitive signal features. Reporting the precise distribution, particularly beneath and beyond ulcer margins, is essential because complete removal of devitalized tissue improves wound healing. Use of the term and its imaging criteria carry some caveats: give intravenous contrast when feasible; recognize that nonenhancement may reflect necrosis, severe ischemia, or venolymphatic congestion; and consider delayed postcontrast images to reduce false interpretations [17].

Key Points

- Most often in the diabetic foot and peripheral arterial disease.
- Contrast-enhanced MRI shows geographic nonenhancement with a sharp transition to hyperemic tissue; subtraction images improve conspicuity.

- Superimposed infection within devitalized areas also does not enhance, so rely on T1 and fluid-sensitive signals to assess cellulitis, abscess, or osteomyelitis.
- Map and report the exact extent, especially beneath and beyond ulcer margins, to guide debridement and limb-sparing surgery.
- Give intravenous contrast when feasible; be aware that nonenhancement may reflect necrosis, severe ischemia, or venolymphatic congestion, and consider delayed images to reduce false readings.

15.4.2 Septic Arthritis

Septic arthritis is an acute infection of the synovial space, most often arising from hematogenous seeding, though direct inoculation from procedures or penetrating injury can also occur. It typically presents as a painful, swollen monoarthritis with elevated inflammatory markers and no antecedent trauma, and it preferentially involves large joints such as the knee and the hip. *Staphylococcus aureus* is the leading pathogen, with Gram-negative organisms, *Neisseria gonorrhoeae* in younger sexually active patients, and regionally prevalent *Borrelia* species as additional considerations. Septic arthritis risk is heightened by immunosuppression (including TNF inhibitors), intravenous drug use, recent intraarticular procedures, and underlying rheumatologic disease [20]. Given that cartilage destruction can progress within days, any rapidly destructive monoarthritis should be managed as septic until proven otherwise, and prompt joint aspiration for Gram stain and culture is essential whenever an effusion is present [9, 17].

Imaging is adjunctive and helps define urgency and extent. Radiographs provide a quick baseline but cannot exclude infection; early changes are often nonspecific, limited to soft tissue swelling or signs of effusion. Ultrasound reliably detects effusions, even in deep joints and in obese patients, and the absence of a joint effusion on ultrasound has a high negative predictive value; it also enables immediate image-guided aspiration. CT and MRI further characterize disease. Septic joints typically show a sizable effusion with synovial thickening and enhancement, and periarticular reaction appears as edema in adjacent soft tissues and in the subchondral bone. On MRI (Fig. 15.4), complex effusion with debris, thick-enhancing synovium, and marrow edema that extends into the medulla raises concern for associated osteomyelitis [9].

In native joints, the absence of a substantial effusion strongly argues against infection. In prosthetic joints, clinical and imaging signs may be subtler despite infection, so a low threshold for aspiration is advised. When ultrasound is equivocal or expertise is limited, proceed to cross-sectional imaging, but imaging should not delay diagnostic aspiration and timely therapy aimed at joint preservation [8, 20].

Key Points

- Acute, usually hematogenous monoarthritis. Large joints are typical. *Staphylococcus aureus* is most common.
- Risk rises with immunosuppression, intravenous drug use, recent procedures, and rheumatic disease.
- Treat any rapidly destructive monoarthritis as septic until proven otherwise.
- Aspirate promptly for Gram stain and culture when an effusion is present.
- Imaging is adjunctive: radiographs for baseline, ultrasound to detect effusion and guide aspiration, and CT/MRI to assess extent. Lack of a substantial effusion in native joints argues against infection.

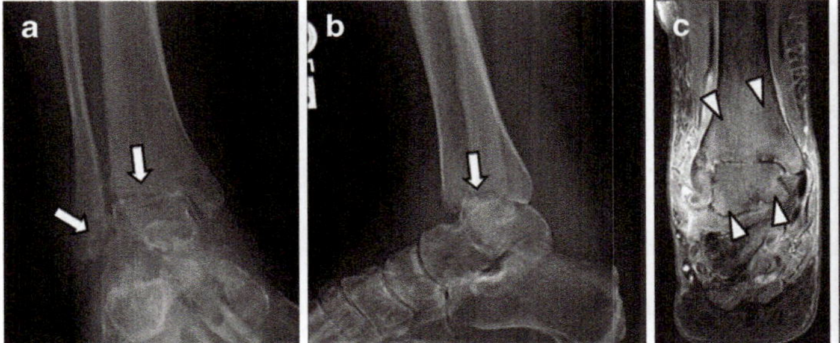

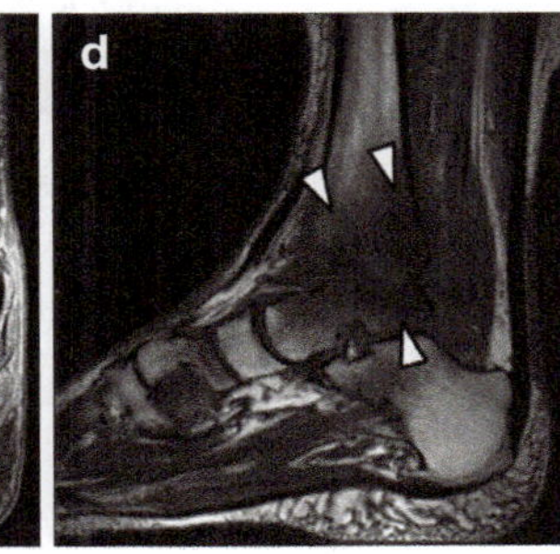

Fig. 15.4 Septic arthritis and osteomyelitis of the ankle in a 34-year-old woman with increasing pain and swelling over a 3-month period. (**a** and **b**) AP and lateral radiographs show diffuse soft tissue swelling at the ankle. Joint space narrowing is present at the ankle joint, with erosions at the articular surface (arrows). Coronal T2-weighted fat-suppressed (**c**) and sagittal T1-weighted (**d**) MRI images show marked bone marrow edema and marrow replacement (arrowheads) around the ankle joint with erosions and surrounding soft tissue edema consistent with septic arthritis and secondary osteomyelitis

15.4.3 Osteomyelitis

Osteomyelitis is an infection of bone centered in the medullary cavity. It reaches bone by three main routes: direct inoculation from trauma or surgery, spread from adjacent infected soft tissues, and hematogenous seeding. Contiguous spread dominates in the foot, especially in diabetes with ulcers or postoperative wounds; an ulcer that probes to bone or is large increases the likelihood of underlying infection. Hematogenous disease is more frequent in children and immunocompromised adults, with a tendency for metaphyseal regions and the spine. *Staphylococcus aureus* is the leading pathogen, although Gram-negative organisms are important in adults and intravenous drug users, and *Kingella* and streptococci feature in children [5, 17, 21].

Diagnosis integrates clinical context, laboratory markers, and targeted sampling. Elevated ESR and CRP support suspicion, but organism confirmation comes from culture. Yields are imperfect, so biopsy is reserved for cases in which results will change management, ideally after withholding antibiotics. Acute disease evolves over days to weeks, whereas chronic infection persists for longer and often presents more subtly [9, 21].

Imaging is staged: radiographs first for overview and complications, followed by MRI when questions remain or to map extent. The most specific MRI indicator of osteomyelitis is confluent T1 marrow replacement in a medullary distribution with matching high signal on fluid-sensitive sequences, often with enhancement; isolated subcortical or patchy T1 changes are less specific and prompt a search for supportive signs such as an adjacent ulcer or sinus tract. CT is helpful when MRI is limited, for detecting gas, foreign bodies, or cortical detail and for chronic features such as sequestra. Dual-energy CT can depict marrow edema with virtual noncalcium techniques and may assist when MRI is contraindicated. Interpretation must account for vascular status: poor perfusion can blunt expected T1 changes or enhancement and lead to false-negative studies [9, 17].

Chronic osteomyelitis (Fig. 15.5) is characterized by necrotic bone (sequestrum), reactive new bone (involucrum), and cortical drainage tracts (cloaca), with possible Brodie abscess. Additional chronic manifestations include reactive bone sclerosis, sinus tracts to the skin, and abscesses within bone or adjacent soft tissues. These findings carry therapeutic implications: antibiotics penetrate poorly into nonviable bone, making surgery central to definitive control, whereas uncomplicated acute hematogenous infection may respond to antimicrobial therapy alone. In children, a classic subacute form is the Brodie abscess, usually metaphyseal. MRI shows an ovoid fluid cavity, and radiographs depict a lucent focus with a sclerotic rim that may extend toward the physis. Special scenarios require caution. In children, infection may spread subperiosteally and lead to pathologic fractures, and neuropathic osteoarthropathy may mimic infection. Correlation with clinical data and, when indicated, interval follow-up imaging is essential [5, 17, 21].

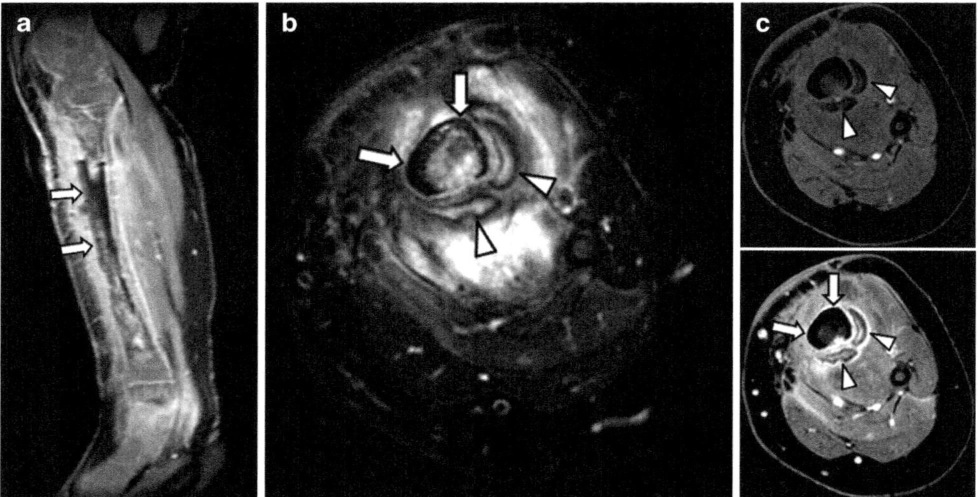

Fig. 15.5 Chronic osteomyelitis of the tibia in a five-year-old boy. Sagittal T1-weighted postcontrast MRI image (**a**), axial T2-weighted fat-suppressed MRI image (**b**), and axial pre- and postcontrast T1-weighted fat-suppressed images (**c**) of the lower leg show diffuse soft tissue edema and enhancement representing cellulitis. There is marrow edema within the tibia but lack of enhancement of a segment (arrows) representing devitalization (sequestrum). Note edematous, enhancing new bone formation (arrowheads) surrounding the sequestrum representing an involucrum

Key Points

- Infection of bone marrow space. Routes: direct inoculation, contiguous spread, and hematogenous seeding.
- Contiguous spread dominates in the diabetic foot. Hematogenous disease is common in children and the immunocompromised. *Staphylococcus aureus* is primary.
- Diagnose with clinical context, ESR/CRP, and culture when feasible. Reserve biopsy for cases that change management.
- Imaging pathway: radiographs first; MRI best for detection and mapping. Confluent T1 marrow replacement with matching fluid-sensitive hyperintensity is most specific. CT helps with gas, foreign bodies, cortex, and sequestra.
- Chronic disease shows sequestrum, involucrum, and cloaca; surgery is often required. Beware mimics such as neuropathic arthropathy and consider follow-up imaging when uncertainty remains.

15.4.4 Mimickers of Infection

15.4.4.1 Neuropathic Osteoarthropathy

Differentiation of osteomyelitis and neuropathic osteoarthropathy can be difficult, because both can demonstrate marrow abnormality, joint effusion, and surrounding soft tissue edema. Some rules may be used to help differentiate these entities on MRI images. First, the vast majority of cases of osteomyelitis of the foot and ankle are due to contiguous spread. Therefore, a bone marrow abnormality without adjacent skin ulceration, sinus tract, or soft tissue inflammation is less likely to represent infection. This concept is particularly useful when there are extensive bone marrow signal abnormalities and lack of subcutaneous tissue involvement. Second, neuropathic osteoarthropathy is predominantly an articular process manifesting as instability, often with multiple regional joints involved (e.g., the Lisfranc, Chopart, or multiple adjacent metatarsophalangeal joints). This and other articular manifestations of neuropathic disease (subluxation, cysts, necrotic debris) are not as common in infection. Associated neuropathic marrow changes can be extensive (especially at the midfoot) but tend to be centered equally about a joint and at the subarticular bone. Osteomyelitis shows more diffuse marrow involvement, and unless there is a primary septic arthritis, the marrow changes are generally greater on one side of the joint. Finally, location of disease is important. Neuropathic osteoarthropathy by far is most common at the Lisfranc and Chopart joints. Osteomyelitis occurs predominantly at the metatarsal heads, toes, calcaneus, and malleoli, a distribution that mirrors that of friction, callus, and ulceration. However, contiguous spread of infection can occur at atypical sites if there is a foot deformity (e.g., the cuboid in cases of rocker-bottom deformity).

15.4.4.2 Renal Failure

Chronic renal failure can lead to resorption of bone at the joints and enthesial attachments, as well as the intervertebral discs, leading to an appearance on imaging similar to that of infection. This is also referred to "dialysis-associated spondyloarthropathy" or "spondylosis of renal failure" due to high incidence in the spine. However, other joints with high stress and bone turnover can be involved, including the sacroiliac joints. The appearance is related to bone resorption, hyperemia, and instability due to secondary hyperparathyroidism. Radiographs show bone resorption that can simulate erosion. Edema and joint effusion is observed. A background of altered bone density typical of secondary hyperparathyroidism can be sought (i.e., "rugger jersey spine"). There may also be amyloid deposition within or around the joints or discs; amyloid is low signal on T1- and T2-weighted images. If there is history of renal failure, this diagnosis can be entertained in the setting of imaging features concerning for infection. However, if the clinical picture is compatible with infection (increased WBCs, fever, positive blood culture), biopsy may be needed. The pathologist should be prompted to look for amyloid and perform a Congo Red stain.

15.4.4.3 Crystalline Disorders

Crystalline diseases can simulate infection on various modalities. Gout (monosodium urate crystal deposition) can present in various ways including tophaceous versus nontophaceous and intraarticular versus extraarticular. Extraarticular involvement can include infiltration of tendons and bursae. Cases with more severe involvement can present with bone destruction and even a "mutilans" pattern of joint erosion. Intraarticular crystal deposition can simulate infection, with joint effusion and erosions. The inflammatory nature of the arthritis also results in subchondral bone marrow edema as well as periarticular edema which can be very difficult to differentiate from osteomyelitis. Demonstration of tophi, which are mass-like foci in or around the joint, can suggest the true diagnosis; tophi demonstrate low signal on T1- and T2-weighted images, unlike infection-related abscess or phlegmon. Additionally, since gout is a systemic disease, involvement of other joints should be sought in the patient's imaging file. Recently dual-energy CT has proven useful for diagnosis and determination of extent of involvement.

CPPD (calcium pyrophosphate deposition) and HADD (hydroxyapatite deposition disease) are calcium-based crystal disorders involving joint cartilage (CPPD) and tendons/bursae (HADD). In the case of CPPD, inflammatory involvement can lead to joint effusion and periarticular edema that can simulate gout or infection; the clinical manifestation is often referred to as "pseudogout" due to paroxysmal pain and swelling. Radiographs can be helpful in this circumstance with demonstration of chondrocalcinosis (calcium deposition in fibrocartilage and/or articular cartilage); this appearance is nonspecific and is often incidental in older patients. However, association with soft tissue swelling/joint effusion with the typical clinical presentation can reveal the diagnosis. HADD is also characteristic on radiographs, with focal calcification at a tendon attachment or bursa. This most commonly occurs at the rotator cuff; but if the location is atypical (i.e., hand tendon or gluteal attachment), the clinical presentation can mimic infection.

15.4.4.4 Inflammatory Arthropathies

Rheumatoid arthritis, reactive arthritis, and psoriatic arthritis (as well as less common arthropathies resulting in synovial proliferation) can simulate septic arthritis and osteomyelitis on imaging exams, with joint effusion, joint space narrowing, erosions, and subchondral bone marrow edema. One useful differentiating feature is periarticular edema. Inflammatory arthropathies are generally chronic processes with slow distention of the joint capsule, whereas (at least bacterial infection) it results in marked hyperemia and rapid joint distention resulting in aggressive appearing pericapsular edema ("angry effusion"). This effect is accentuated in smaller, lower capacity joints (i.e., the sacroiliac joint). Additionally, chronic inflammatory arthropathies (especially rheumatoid arthritis) may exhibit synovial proliferation with a mass-like quality, whereas bacterial arthritis progresses rapidly without proliferative synovial hyperplasia, except in later stages or in poorly treated cases. Finally, septic arthritis, except in rare circumstances of disseminated infection, is a monoarticular process. Chronic inflammatory arthropathies listed above are associated with systemic disease and can exhibit similar findings in other joints and locations such as tendon sheaths and enthesial attachments.

15.4.4.5 Neoplasm

Certain neoplasms can have characteristics similar to infection on imaging exams. Imaging findings that can be seen in both infection and tumor include bone destruction, periosteal reaction, fluid collections and necrosis, and soft tissue mass effect. Tumor is generally easily differentiated from septic arthritis or discitis because neoplasms rarely cross joints. Involvement of both sides of a joint therefore indicates an arthritic process, inflammatory or degenerative. However, tumors involving the shaft of a bone can result in destruction and periosteal reaction similar to osteomyelitis. Tumors at the epiphysis can cause a joint effusion (i.e., osteoid osteoma). Small round cell tumors result in a permeative pattern similar to infection. Classic lesions simulating osteomyelitis include Ewing sarcoma, leukemia and lymphoma, and Langerhans cell histiocytosis. Conversely, atypical infections such as tuberculosis and fungal and parasitic infections can cause focal bone destruction simulating tumor. When biopsy is performed, one should always consider sending samples for both histologic and microbiologic analyses.

Key Points

- There are various noninfectious inflammatory and noninflammatory conditions that can simulate musculoskeletal infection on imaging modalities.
- Differential diagnosis to be considered includes neuropathic osteoarthropathy (Charcot arthropathy), renal failure (especially in the spine), crystal deposition diseases, various inflammatory arthropathies including rheumatoid arthritis, and neoplasm.
- History, clinical signs, and imaging findings can be used to help differentiate infection from other conditions.

15.5 Conclusion

In the acute setting, musculoskeletal infection requires urgent attention and demands prompt and accurate assessment by the radiologist. Rapid diagnosis and treatment can prevent significant morbidity and even mortality. Radiologists should have a high suspicion for infection when imaging features outlined in this chapter are demonstrated. Subsequent communication with the referring physician is essential, with discussion of additional imaging or biopsy that may need facilitation.

Take-Home Points

- Musculoskeletal infection can arise from hematogenous spread, contiguous spread, or direct implantation.
- Infection is an urgent condition and must be diagnosed rapidly with effective communication of findings.
- Differential diagnosis should be considered, with clinical and laboratory data taken into consideration.

Conflict of Interest Statement I/We declare no competing interests as defined by Springer Nature or other interests that might be perceived to influence results and/or discussion reported in this manuscript.

References

1. Poultsides LA, Liaropoulos LL, Malizos KN. The socioeconomic impact of musculoskeletal infections. J Bone Joint Surg Am. 2010;92(11):e13. https://doi.org/10.2106/JBJS.I.01131.
2. Shihabul Hassan M, Stevenson J, Gandikota G, Veeratterapillay A, Bhamidipaty KDP, Botchu R. Current updates in MSK infection imaging: a narrative review. J Clin Orthop Trauma. 2024;51(102396):102396. https://doi.org/10.1016/j.jcot.2024.102396.
3. Klontzas ME, Vassalou EE, Spanakis K, Alpantaki K, Karantanas AH. Musculoskeletal infection: the great mimickers on imaging. J Clin Med. 2024;13(18):5424. https://doi.org/10.3390/jcm13185424.
4. Jardon M, Alaia EF. Approach to imaging modalities in the setting of suspected infection. Skeletal Radiol. 2024;53(10):1957–68. https://doi.org/10.1007/s00256-023-04478-2.
5. Restrepo R, Park HJ, Karakas SP, Cervantes LF, Rodriguez-Ruiz FG, Zahrah AM, Inarejos-Clemente EJ, Laufer M, Shreiber VM. Bacterial osteomyelitis in pediatric patients: a comprehensive review. Skeletal Radiol. 2024;53(10):2195–210. https://doi.org/10.1007/s00256-024-04639-x.
6. Matcuk GR Jr, Katal S, Gholamrezanezhad A, Spinnato P, Waldman LE, Fields BKK, Patel DB, Skalski MR. Imaging of lower extremity infections: predisposing conditions, atypical infections, mimics, and differentiating features. Skeletal Radiol. 2024;53(10):2099–120. https://doi.org/10.1007/s00256-024-04589-4.
7. Sabir N, Akkaya Z. Musculoskeletal infections through direct inoculation. Skeletal Radiol. 2024;53(10):2161–79. https://doi.org/10.1007/s00256-024-04591-w.
8. Kompel A, Guermazi A. Imaging of MSK infections in the ER. Skeletal Radiol. 2024;53(10):2039–50. https://doi.org/10.1007/s00256-023-04554-7.
9. Matcuk GR Jr, Skalski MR, Patel DB, Fields BKK, Waldman LE, Spinnato P, Gholamrezanezhad A, Katal S. Lower extremity infections: essential anatomy and multimodality imaging findings. Skeletal Radiol. 2024;53(10):2121–41. https://doi.org/10.1007/s00256-024-04567-w.
10. Llewellyn A, Jones-Diette J, Kraft J, Holton C, Harden M, Simmonds M. Imaging tests for the detection of osteomyelitis: a systematic review. Health Technol Assess (Winchester, England). 2019;23(61):1–128. https://doi.org/10.3310/hta23610.
11. Expert Panel on Musculoskeletal Imaging, Pierce JL, Perry MT, Wessell DE, Lenchik L, Ahlawat S, Baker JC, Banks J, Caracciolo JT, DeGeorge KC, Demertzis JL, Garner HW, Scott JA, Sharma A, Beaman FD. ACR appropriateness criteria® suspected osteomyelitis, septic arthritis, or soft tissue infection (excluding spine and diabetic foot): 2022 update. J Am Coll Radiol: JACR. 2022;19(11S):S473–87. https://doi.org/10.1016/j.jacr.2022.09.013.
12. Palestro CJ. Radionuclide imaging of osteomyelitis. Semin Nucl Med. 2015;45(1):32–46. https://doi.org/10.1053/j.semnuclmed.2014.07.005.
13. Love C, Palestro CJ. Radionuclide imaging of infection. J Nucl Med Technol. 2004;32(2):47–57.; quiz 58–9. PMID: 15175400
14. Glaudemans AWJM, de Vries EFJ, Vermeulen LEM, Slart RHJA, Dierckx RAJO, Signore A. A large retrospective single-Centre study to define the best image acquisition protocols and interpretation criteria for white blood cell scintigraphy with 99mTc-HMPAO-labelled leucocytes in musculoskeletal infections. Eur J Nucl Med Mol Imaging. 2013;40(11):1760–9. https://doi.org/10.1007/s00259-013-2481-0.
15. Feuerriegel GC, Sutter R. Managing hardware-related metal artifacts in MRI: current and evolving techniques. Skeletal Radiol. 2024;53(9):1737–50. https://doi.org/10.1007/s00256-024-04624-4.
16. Inaoka T, Kitamura N, Sugeta M, Nakatsuka T, Ishikawa R, Kasuya S, Sugiura Y, Nakajima A, Nakagawa K, Terada H. Diagnostic value of advanced metal artifact reduction magnetic resonance imaging for periprosthetic joint infection. J Comput Assist Tomogr. 2022;46(3):455–63. https://doi.org/10.1097/RCT.0000000000001297.
17. Alaia EF, Chhabra A, Simpfendorfer CS, Cohen M, Mintz DN, Vossen JA, Zoga AC, Fritz J, Spritzer CE, Armstrong DG, Morrison WB. MRI nomenclature for musculoskeletal infection. Skeletal Radiol. 2021;50(12):2319–47. https://doi.org/10.1007/s00256-021-03807-7.
18. Soler R. Magnetic resonance imaging of pyomyositis in 43 cases. Eur J Radiol. 2000;35(1):59–64. https://doi.org/10.1016/s0720-048x(99)00108-4.
19. Patel DB, Emmanuel NB, Stevanovic MV, Matcuk GR Jr, Gottsegen CJ, Forrester DM, White EA. Hand infections: anatomy, types and spread of infection, imaging findings, and treatment options. Radiogr: Rev Publ Radiol Soc North Am. 2014;34(7):1968–86. https://doi.org/10.1148/rg.347130101.
20. Chan BY, Crawford AM, Kobes PH, Allen H, Leake RL, Hanrahan CJ, Mills MK. Septic arthritis: an evidence-based review of diagnosis and image-guided aspiration. AJR Am J Roentgenol. 2020;215(3):568–81. https://doi.org/10.2214/AJR.20.22773.
21. Desimpel J, Posadzy M, Vanhoenacker F. The many faces of osteomyelitis: a pictorial review. J Belg Soc Radiol. 2017;101(1):24. https://doi.org/10.5334/jbr-btr.1300.

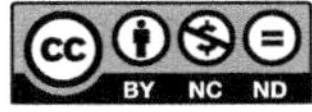

Muscle Imaging

16

James Teh and David Rubin

Learning Objectives

- To understand the imaging modalities used for muscle assessment and their respective strengths and limitations
- To recognize the characteristic imaging features of traumatic, inflammatory, infectious, and metabolic muscle disorders, as well as denervation and ischemic myopathies
- To appreciate the imaging hallmarks of various types of muscle injury and learn how MRI contributes to injury grading and prognosis
- To differentiate idiopathic inflammatory myopathy subtypes based on MRI and ultrasound patterns
- To apply imaging findings to guide diagnosis, biopsy planning, and treatment monitoring for muscle disorders

A broad variety of disorders affect skeletal muscle including traumatic, inflammatory, infectious, congenital, metabolic, vascular, neoplastic, and denervation-related conditions. Clinical features such as pain, swelling, and weakness are nonspecific, so imaging plays a key role in identifying the relevant abnormalities, narrowing the differential diagnosis, grading disease, guiding biopsy, and monitoring treatment.

J. Teh
Department of Radiology, Nuffield Orthopaedic Centre, Oxford, UK
e-mail: james.teh@ouh.nhs.uk

D. Rubin (✉)
Department of Radiology, NYU Grossman School of Medicine, New York, NY, USA
e-mail: drubin@radsource.us

16.1 Imaging Techniques

16.1.1 Ultrasound

Ultrasound offers unique advantages for evaluating muscle disorders: Doppler vascular evaluation, easy contralateral comparison, and improved visualization through extended field-of-view imaging [1, 2]. Dynamic assessment, carried out both at rest and during contraction, can highlight abnormalities such as muscle herniation or rupture. Broadband high-frequency linear array probes (5–10 MHz) are generally preferred for evaluating muscle, as they provide excellent resolution and detail. In larger patients, or when deeper muscles need to be assessed, a lower-frequency curvilinear probe (2–4 MHz) can provide greater penetration. To reduce anisotropy—which leads to signal drop off and can mimic disease—the transducer should be positioned as close to perpendicular as possible to the muscle's long axis [1]. Evaluation should be performed in both short axis and long axis.

On longitudinal ultrasound, the perimysium surrounding the muscle fascicles (which are organized bundles of muscle fibers) appears as fine, linear hyperechoic lines [1, 3]. In short axis, the muscle fibers appear as fine lines and small echogenic dots. Occasionally, thicker reflective septa can be seen within the muscle belly, creating a characteristic reticular pattern. The epimysium, which envelops the entire muscle belly, is also highly reflective. These connective tissue layers are continuous throughout the muscle and contribute to the formation of tendons at sites of attachment.

Sonography can detect changes in muscle size, echogenicity, architecture, and perfusion for both diagnosing and monitoring neuromuscular disease, myopathies, and myositis [4]. Muscle atrophy, fatty infiltration, fibrosis, and increased echogenicity are common ultrasound findings in late-stage disease due to multiple causes. After injury, in addition to identifying muscle tears, lacerations, and contu-

J. Hodler et al. (eds.), *Musculoskeletal Diseases 2026-2029*, IDKD Springer Series,
https://doi.org/10.1007/978-3-032-17040-8_16

sions, ultrasound is particularly useful for characterizing hematomas and detecting complications such as myositis ossificans [5].

16.1.2 MRI

MRI provides a comprehensive evaluation of muscle. A standard MRI protocol should include axial imaging and at least one orthogonal plane and whenever possible comparison with the contralateral limb. Both T1-weighted and fluid-sensitive (e.g., fat-suppressed intermediate/T2-weighted or STIR) sequences should be obtained routinely [6, 7]. For certain clinical indications, quantitative sequences (Dixon fat fraction mapping to quantify fatty infiltration, T2 relaxometry for edema, diffusion imaging for fiber architecture, and MR spectroscopy for metabolic assessment) may be useful [8]. Intravenous contrast is not typically needed for muscle assessment, unless there is clinical suspicion of necrotic tissue.

On MRI, normal skeletal muscle is intermediate-signal intensity on both T1- and T2-weighted images, typically with visible striations and interspersed fat [6, 9]. Increased signal on T1-weighted images can indicate fatty infiltration, methemoglobin, or proteinaceous material. Edema appears bright on fluid-sensitive images. Fibrosis and calcification are typically low-signal intensity on all sequences.

16.1.3 Radiographs and Computed Tomography (CT)

Radiographs and CT may not be able to detect early muscle injury or disorders, but they remain indispensable for characterizing mineralization and ossification and detecting gas [10]. CT can also show alterations in muscle size (atrophy or hypertrophy) and fatty infiltration [11].

16.1.4 Positron Emission Tomography-Computed Tomography (PET-CT)

PET-CT in muscle imaging is primarily a research tool, with particular utility in systemic muscle disorders [6]. Its main clinical value lies in detecting early metabolic and inflammatory changes in muscle, often before structural abnormalities are apparent on other imaging modalities. In patients with idiopathic inflammatory myopathy (IIM), PET-CT can identify active muscle inflammation, guide biopsy of metabolically active regions, and screen for associated malignancy [9]. PET-CT may also provide quantitative assessment of muscle metabolism and perfusion, which can help monitor disease activity and therapeutic response. Pitfalls include physiologic FDG uptake in muscle commonly due to recent exercise, insulin administration, or even shivering [12].

Key Point

- While MRI is the gold standard for muscle imaging, offering excellent sensitivity for edema, fatty infiltration, necrosis, and architectural change, ultrasound allows for dynamic imaging and assessment of vascularity using Doppler and is particularly useful for trauma, superficial lesions, and biopsy guidance.

16.2 Muscle Strains and Tendon Avulsions

The most common myotendinous injuries in sports are due to eccentric activities, those that occur while a muscle is being lengthened or stretched at the same time as the muscle belly is contracting [13]. Rapid acceleration, deceleration, and cutting (sudden changes in direction) are the typical causes. This mechanism can produce damage anywhere along the muscle-tendon-bone chain. Injuries within the tendon proper typically only affect tendons that are already degenerated; common examples include rotator cuff, patellar, and Achilles' tendon tears. Fractures due to eccentric activity are mainly seen in skeletally immature individuals and occur at the apophyseal growth plates, such as those in the pelvis. But in skeletally mature athletes, injuries predominate at the interfaces between different tissue types (Fig. 16.1). The most common tear locations are at the junctions between the muscle and main tendon (the main myotendinous junction), between the muscle and its surrounding fascia (the myofascial junction), and within the muscle belly surrounding the intramuscular tendon and aponeurotic fibers (the central myotendinous junction). These injuries comprise the common "muscle strain" or "pulled muscle." While most muscle strains are treated nonsurgically, imaging plays a key role in staging and prognosis, as well as evaluation of healing and later complications. A tendon can also avulse from its bone insertion. Identification of tendon avulsions is critical because treatment is often surgical repair.

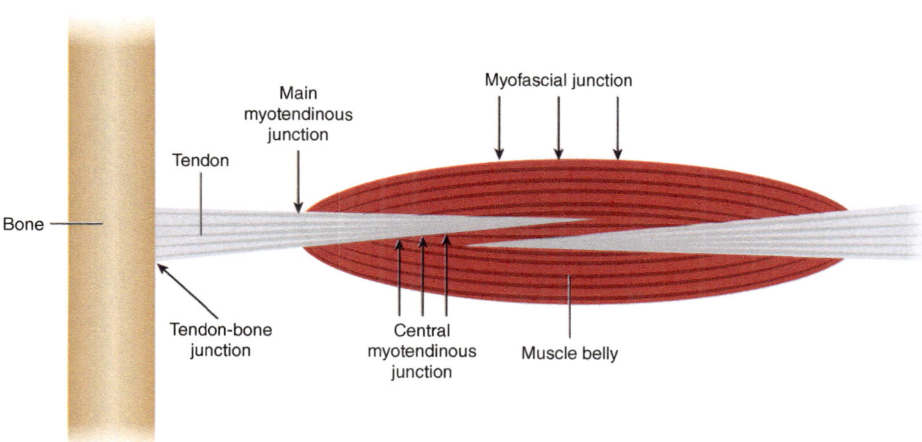

Fig. 16.1 Drawing showing the common locations of injuries along the muscle-tendon-bone axis. Injuries occurring at the various tissue junctions will have unique imaging findings, as well as different implications for management and recovery

16.2.1 Imaging Findings

Acute tendon avulsions from bone are relatively easy to recognize. On ultrasound the echogenic tendon will no longer attach to the bone and may be retracted; comparison with the contralateral side is often useful. MRI demonstrates partial or complete separation of the usually low-signal intensity tendon from its insertion site with adjacent soft tissue edema on water-sensitive sequences. Marrow edema within the underlying bone, if present, is typically less severe compared to a bone contusion. Edema and/or hemorrhage will be present in the gap in acute injuries. With complete tears, the tendon will be retracted a variable amount from the bone. The amount of edema within the muscle depends on the amount of retraction and is typically located close to the main myotendinous junction. A small cortical bone fragment accompanying the torn tendon may be easier to identify on radiographs. In children, fractures through the apophyseal growth plates are more common than tendon avulsions.

Muscle strains characteristically appear as ill-defined muscle edema extending along the muscle fibers, often with a "feathery" morphology on MRI [14, 15]. The location of the muscle edema is an important clue to the anatomic interface involved (Fig. 16.2), which in turn affects prognosis. Edema primarily in the muscle periphery indicates a myofascial injury. Edema centered at the main myotendinous junction predicts injury to that structure. An edema pattern centrally within the muscle belly or paralleling a tendon or aponeurosis within the muscle represents injury to the central myotendinous junction. Gaps between the edematous muscle fibers or focal disruptions of the intramuscular tendon elements are critical to recognize for grading and prognostication [14]. "Loss of tension" manifest as laxity or waviness of any portion of the intramuscular tendon is a clue to fiber disruption. Similarly, a hematoma within the muscle indicates macroscopic fiber disruption. On ultrasound, increased echogenicity is seen at the site of muscle injury, with a focal hypoechoic or anechoic focus indicating macroscopic fiber disruption [2, 15].

Key Point

- Muscle strains occur at tissue interfaces, most commonly involving the peripheral myofascial junction, the main myotendinous junction, or the central myotendinous junction.

16.2.2 Injury Grading

There are two main goals for grading an injury: guiding management and informing prognosis, including return-to-play time and risk of recurrent injury. Acute tendon avulsions and some complete muscle tears (especially those involving the main myotendinous junction) are often treated with surgical repair because these injuries take longer to heal compared to others. Most muscle strains will be managed conservatively with initial rest, physiotherapy, and gradual rehabilitation. Some clinicians utilize injections with substances like platelet-rich plasma, although strong scientific evidence for a positive effect of intramuscular injections is lacking [16]. In cases where a large hematoma has formed, aspiration (typically using ultrasound guidance) may be performed once the hematoma has liquified [17].

Predicting return to play after a conservatively managed muscle strain is influenced by many factors in addition to imaging severity of the injury. Athletes in individual sports like sprinting must essentially be back to 100% health to effectively complete, while players on a team sport may be able to contribute even before complete recovery. Different

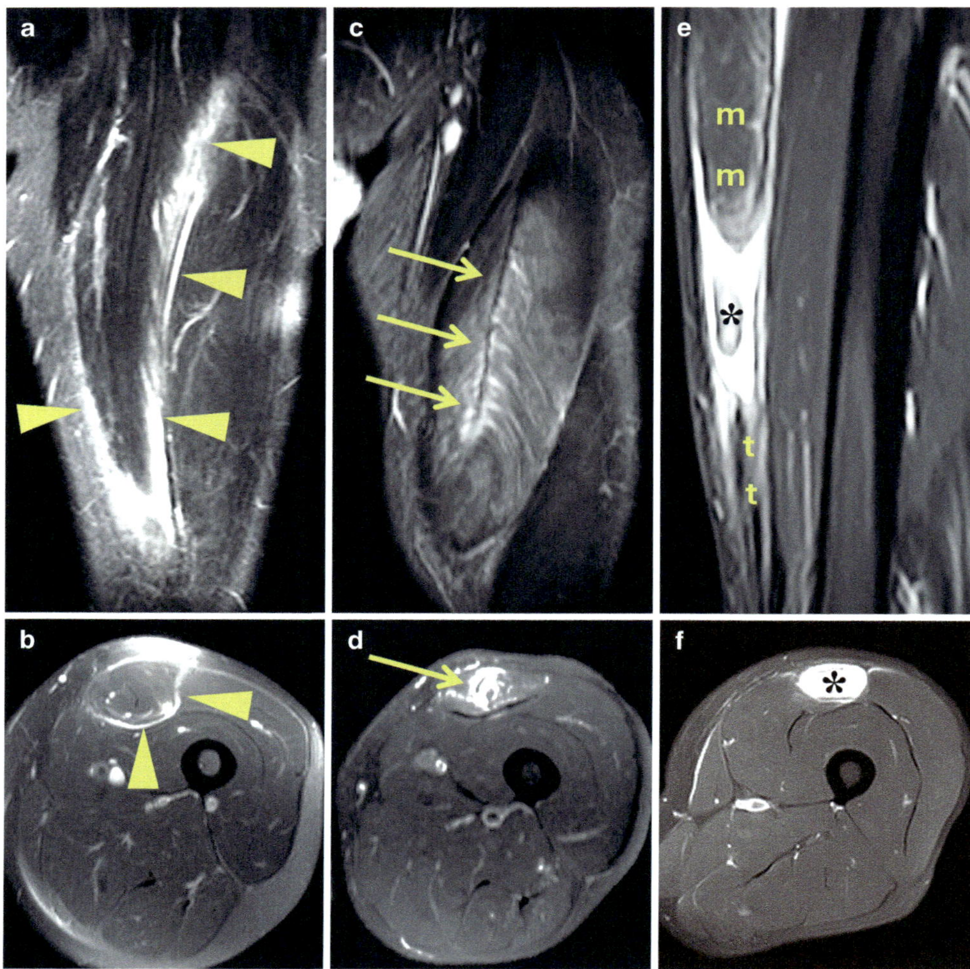

Fig. 16.2 (**a**–**f**) Rectus femoris muscle strains in three anatomic locations on fat-suppressed, fluid-sensitive pulse sequences. (**a**) Coronal and (**b**) axial images of a myofascial injury with edema in the muscle periphery (arrowheads). Peripheral injuries have a better prognosis compared with central injuries. (**c**) Coronal and (**d**) axial images of an injury involving the central myotendinous junction with muscle edema surrounding the intramuscular portion of the tendon (arrows). (**e**) Sagittal and (**f**) axial images of an injury at the main myotendinous junction, with a complete tear of the muscle fibers (m) from the distal tendon (t), separated by a fluid collection and hematoma (asterisks). Complete tears have a worse prognosis compared to partial tears

positions in many team sports require varying amounts of running and cutting, which can affect return-to-play decisions. The timing of the injury with respect to the athletic calendar (e.g., in preseason compared to playoffs compared to just before a trading deadline) often influences roster decisions. The athlete's age, coexistent injuries, and pressure from coaches, agents, and sporting organizations are also important. The decision to clear an athlete to participate in sports is currently made based on clinical assessment, without input from imaging studies; indeed at the time of return to play most injured muscles will show persistent signal abnormalities on MRI [18].

A few general observations seem to hold true for many muscle injuries [19]: (1) The initial clinical severity and physical exam findings are poor predictors of recovery time. (2) Complete tears—whether tendon avulsions or at the main myotendinous junction—take longer to heal compared to partial tears. (3) Peripheral (myofascial) injuries heal faster than central injuries (at least for rectus femoris injuries). (4) Muscle contusions (due to blunt force trauma) heal faster than muscle strains (due to eccentric stretching). (5) Disruption of intramuscular tendon or aponeurotic fibers negatively affects recovery time. (6) The total extent of muscle edema has some influence on healing rates.

Several imaging-based grading systems attempt to capture the major factors that influence return to play. None of these provides a perfect predictor of recovery times and most demonstrate only moderate interobserver agreement [20]. One of the most widely used and studied is the British Athletics Muscle Injury Classification (BAMIC) (Table 16.1) [21]. A recent systematic review found consistent evidence that BAMIC grading offers useful prognostic information concerning return to play [22]. While the system was designed to evaluate hamstring injuries, many radiologists and sports physicians now apply it to other sites. A BAMIC grade 0 injury describes an athlete with a clinical muscle injury but either a normal MRI or only patchy muscle edema. Grade 0 injuries have the best prognosis with the fastest recovery times. Grades 1–3 describe increasingly severe injuries based on how much of the muscle belly's cross section is edematous, the maximum longitudinal extent of the muscle edema, and the length of macroscopic fiber disrup-

Table 16.1 Summary of the British Athletics Muscle Injury Classification (BAMIC)

	Anatomic modifier	a	b		c
Grade		Myofascial (peripheral)	Main myotendinous junction		Intramuscular tendon (central)
1 (small)	Maximum muscle cross-sectional area edema	<10%	<10%		
	Longitudinal length of edema	<5 cm	<5 cm		
	Length of fiber disruption	None	<1 cm		
2 (moderate)	Maximum muscle cross-sectional area edema	10–50%	10–50%	Cross section of tendon involvement	<50%
	Longitudinal length of edema	5–15 cm	5–15 cm		
	Length of fiber disruption	<5 cm	<5 cm	Longitudinal length of intratendinous signal abnormality	<5 cm
3 (extensive)	Maximum muscle cross-sectional area edema	>50%	>50%	Cross section of tendon involvement	>50% or loss of tension
	Longitudinal length of edema	>15 cm	>15 cm		
	Length of fiber disruption	>5 cm	>5 cm	Longitudinal length of intratendinous signal abnormality	>5 cm
4 (full thickness)			Complete discontinuity of muscle with retraction		Complete tendon discontinuity with retraction

tion. Grade 4 injuries are full-thickness muscle or tendon tears. In addition to the numerical grade, a letter is affixed indicating the anatomic location of the injury: (a) for myofascial (peripheral), (b) for main myotendinous, and (c) for intramuscular tendinous (central) injuries [21]. Whether or not a radiologist uses the actual BAMIC classifications in a report or simply describes the different injury elements is a stylistic choice.

Key Point

- The anatomic location of muscle injuries, the amount of associated edema, and the extent of fiber disruption influence injury grading and help predict return to play.

16.2.3 Injury Healing

As an injured muscle recovers, the high-signal intensity edema decreases on fluid-sensitive MRI sequences [23]. Healing involves a combination of muscle regeneration, fibrosis, and fatty replacement [24]. On MRI and ultrasound, regenerated muscle appears identical to normal muscle. Fibrosis is typically linear and low-signal intensity on all pulse sequences, usually oriented along injured intramuscular tendon and aponeurosis fibers, making them appear focally thickened [25]. Fibrotic scarring does not seem to increase the risk of recurrent injury to the same muscle [26]. Fatty infiltration shows high-signal intensity on T1-weighted images and increased echogenicity on ultrasound. Macroscopic hematomas usually completely resorb but occasionally may result in fluid collections (seromas), fibrosis, or myositis ossificans (see below) [2].

16.2.4 Injuries in Specific Muscles

While strains can involve any skeletal muscle in the body, certain muscles are at higher risk. Injuries are most common in the lower extremities and in muscles that are eccentrically activated during sports. Muscles that cross two joints and have a high percentage of type II fast twitch fibers are particularly susceptible [15].

16.2.4.1 Hamstring Injuries

Hamstring injuries show extensive variability on imaging studies (Fig. 16.3). Proximal tendon avulsions—of the semimembranosus and/or conjoint tendon origins from the ischial tuberosities—are most common in activities with like water skiing, gymnastics, and track and field [27]. These injuries often require surgical repair [28]. In sprinters

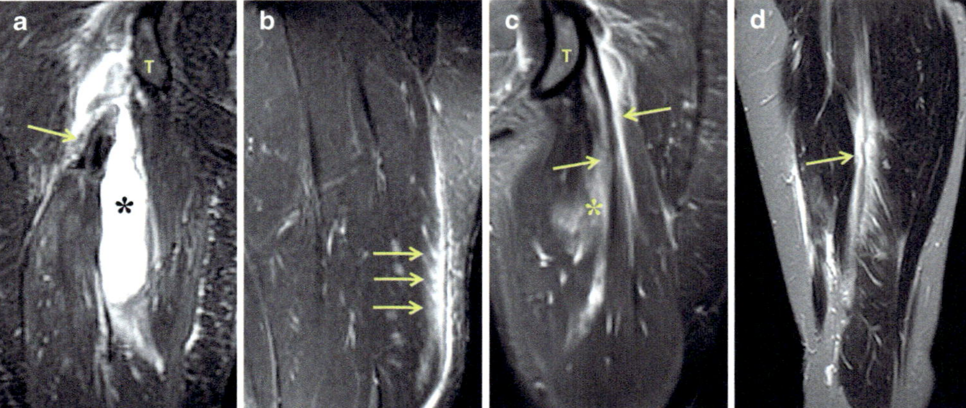

Fig. 16.3 (**a-d**) Examples of hamstring injuries on coronal fat-suppressed, fluid-sensitive sequences. (**a**) Complete proximal tendon avulsion in a water skier (BAMIC 4c). The entire proximal tendon complex (arrow) is torn and retracted from the ischial tuberosity (T) with surrounding hemorrhage (asterisk). (**b**) Low-grade myofascial injury involving the proximal long head biceps femoris in an American football player (BAMIC 1a). Note the edema confined to the muscle periphery (arrows), which measured less than 5 cm in length. (**c**) Moderate atypical hamstring injury in a yoga instructor (BAMIC 2b). Edema is located at the proximal semimembranosus myotendinous junction (asterisk), but injury extends into and surrounding the proximal tendon (arrows); T, ischial tuberosity. (**d**) Extensive injury involving the central myotendinous junction in the distal biceps femoris in a soccer player (BAMIC 3c). Edema surrounds the intramuscular portion of the tendon, which has a wavy appearance (arrow) indicating loss of tension

and other speed athletes, the long head biceps femoris muscle is most frequently injured, with tears occurring at either the proximal or distal main myotendinous junction or at the myofascial or central myotendinous junctions [27, 29]. Injuries to the distal muscle can extend into the aponeurosis between the long and short heads; these tears have a particularly high recurrence rate [30]. An atypical type of strain occurs with extreme stretching, as may occur in professional dancers and sports that emphasize high kicking or front splits [27]. These atypical injuries involve the proximal myotendinous junction of the semimembranosus and extend to involve the proximal tendon; while they may be relatively mild initially, recovery is especially prolonged and may take more than one year [31].

16.2.4.2 Quadriceps Injuries

Athletes who participate in sports that include repetitive kicking and high-speed running are susceptible to quadriceps muscle injuries, with the rectus femoris most frequently affected. Like the hamstrings, both proximal tendon avulsions (of the direct or indirect heads) [32] and injuries to any of the three main tissue interfaces occur (Fig. 16.2). Complete ruptures and tears involving the intramuscular tendon have prolonged recovery times, especially compared to myofascial injuries [33]. A unique "degloving" pattern of injury has been reported in the rectus femoris where a central core of the muscle (representing the indirect head and its central tendon) becomes separated from the surrounding muscle belly by a cone of fluid, which allows the inner muscle belly to retract proximally [34]. These delaminating injuries do not fit neatly into classification systems.

16.2.4.3 Calf Muscle Injuries

Athletic injuries in the calf primarily involve the posterior musculature, most commonly the medial gastrocnemius or soleus muscles [35]. Tears occur in many sports and over a wide age range, but one characteristic circumstance is an acute injury during racket sports, known as "tennis leg." The soleus and gastrocnemius muscles have multiple aponeuroses within the muscle bellies as well as between the muscles, and injuries that disrupt these structures take longer to heal [36]. Strains affecting more than one muscle also have more prolonged recovery times [37]. Most injuries are managed nonoperatively, unless a compartment syndrome develops from a large hematoma.

16.2.4.4 Pectoralis Major Injuries

The pectoralis muscle is the most frequently injured chest wall muscle. Injuries are highly associated with weightlifting, especially bench press exercises. Tears occur predominantly as either tendon avulsions from the humerus or at the main myotendinous junction (Fig. 16.4). Distinguishing these injuries is important because the former are treated with surgical repair while the latter are usually managed conservatively [38]. In both types of injury, hemorrhage and edema occur around the myotendinous junction, so they may be difficult to separate based on imaging findings. The most useful signs suggesting a tendon avulsion on MRI are high-signal edema along the anterior margin of the humeral shaft and lack of a visible tendon insertion on the bone [39].

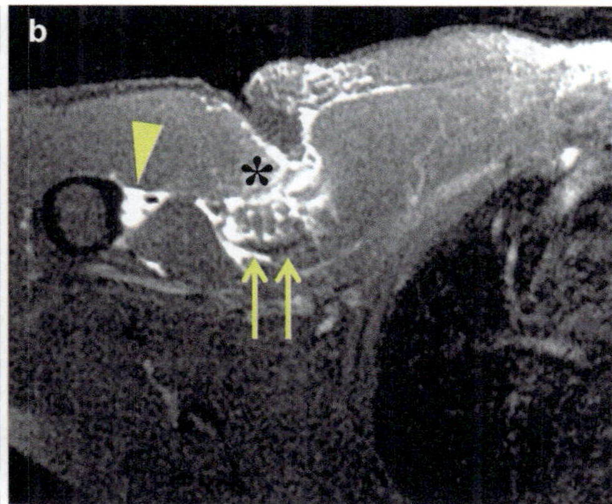

Fig. 16.4 (**a–b**) Axial fat-suppressed, fluid-sensitive images of pectoralis major muscle injuries that occurred during bench pressing in two different athletes. (**a**) Myotendinous injury. Edema (asterisk) is located at the myotendinous junction, and an intact tendon (arrows) is visible inserting on the humerus. (**b**) Tendon avulsion. Edema is again present at the myotendinous junction (asterisk) but a high-signal intensity fluid collection (arrowhead) along the anteromedial humerus is visible instead of an intact tendon. The retracted tendon (arrows) is located more medially

16.3 Myopathy

Myopathy refers to dysfunction of skeletal muscle and represents a broad spectrum of diseases, including hereditary, endocrine, drug-induced, and idiopathic conditions [40]. Clinical features typically include myalgia, tenderness, and weakness. The principal subtypes of idiopathic inflammatory myopathies (IMM) include dermatomyositis (DM), antisynthetase syndrome (ASS), immune-mediated necrotizing myopathy (IMNM), inclusion body myositis (IBM), overlap myositis, and antimitochondrial antibody (AMA)-associated myositis [41]. Almost all patients who would previously have been labelled as having "polymyositis" are now understood to have one of these other conditions. The diagnosis of IMM is often delayed because early symptoms overlap with aging, occasionally leading to inappropriate treatment.

Imaging can identify characteristic distribution patterns (Fig. 16.5), determine disease activity, and assist in guiding biopsy and therapy decisions. Radiographs and CT play a limited role but can identify calcinosis, especially in dermatomyositis. Ultrasound can evaluate vascularity but lacks sensitivity for diffuse edema. MRI is the gold standard, with sensitivity exceeding manual muscle testing or electromyography and excellent tissue contrast [41]. T1-weighted sequences demonstrate chronic changes such as fatty degeneration and atrophy while fluid-sensitive sequences show acute inflammation indicating active disease, correlating with serum creatine kinase levels. MRI also has an invaluable role in guiding biopsy, monitoring treatment, and differentiating between disease subtypes. Whole-body MRI demonstrates the global disease burden, and quantitative fat-fraction mapping provides reproducible metrics now required in clinical trials. Integrating the imaging findings with the clinical features and serology (e.g., myositis-specific antibodies) is the most accurate strategy for classification and management [42, 43].

16.3.1 Dermatomyositis (DM)

DM is classically bimodal in onset (5–15 years and 40–50 years), with a female predominance (F:M ratio ~ 2:1) [9, 41, 44]. Classic features include a heliotrope rash (a violaceous eye lid rash), Gottron's papules, and photosensitive skin changes, combined with progressive proximal thigh weakness. Approximately 80% of patients demonstrate DM-specific autoantibodies, including Mi-2, MDA5, NXP2, TIF1-γ, and SAE [45]. Symmetrical proximal muscle involvement commonly affects the quadriceps and gluteal muscles [6, 41]. On MRI, muscle edema is often patchy with preferential involvement of perimysial and epimysial regions (Fig. 16.5a). Fasciitis and subcutaneous edema may precede intramuscular changes. Chronic disease is characterized by mild muscle atrophy and fatty infiltration. In children, dense sheet-like calcifications can occur, easier to appreciate on radiographs or CT than on MRI. DM is associated with an increased risk of malignancy, especially with anti-TIF1γ antibodies, particularly within the first few years of Diagnosis [45].

16.3.2 Antisynthetase Syndrome (ASS)

ASS typically presents in the fourth to seventh decade, with extramuscular manifestations such as interstitial lung

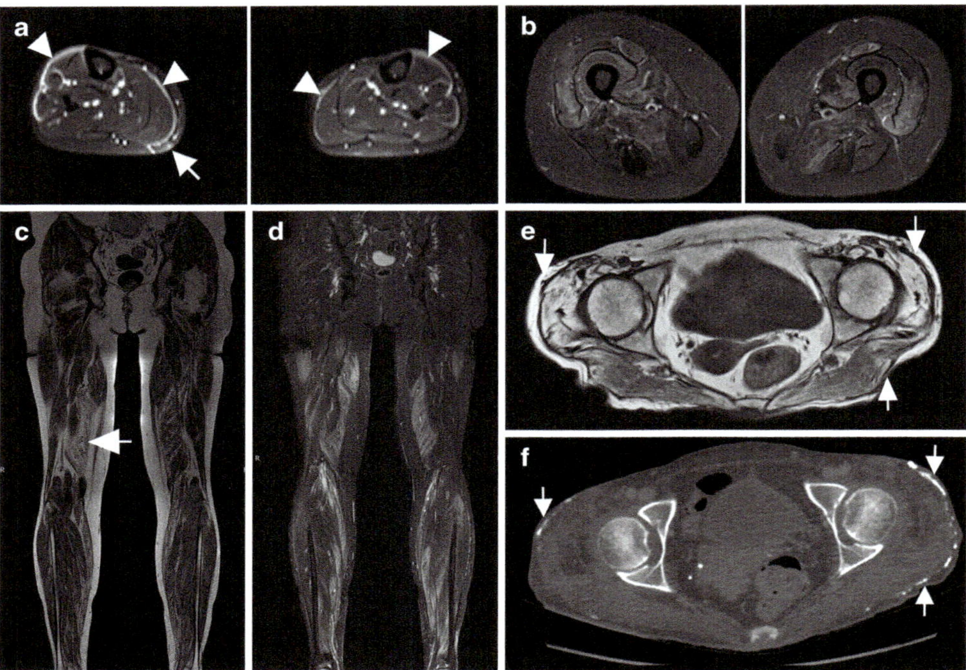

Fig. 16.5 (**a**–**f**) Comparison of idiopathic inflammatory myopathy subtypes. (**a**) Dermatomyositis with epimysial distribution. Axial fat-suppressed proton density-weighted image of the calves demonstrates bilateral epimysial and perimysial inflammatory changes (arrowheads). There is also a region of subcutaneous edema (arrow). (**b**) Immune-mediated necrotizing myositis. Axial fat-suppressed proton density-weighted image demonstrates bilateral asymmetric myositis in the thighs. (**c**–**d**) Inclusion body myositis. (**c**) Coronal T1-weighted image shows patchy profound fatty infiltration of the lower extremity muscles particularly affecting the right semimembranosus (arrow). (**d**) Coronal STIR image showing patchy, multifocal muscle edema. (**e**–**f**) Overlap myositis in a patient with systemic sclerosis and myositis. (**e**) T1-weighted axial image demonstrates low-signal thickening of the deep fascia (arrows) in addition to patchy muscle atrophy. (**f**) CT demonstrates calcinosis in the deep fascia (arrows) not appreciated on the MRI

disease, arthritis, Raynaud's phenomenon, and "mechanic's hands" [41]. Anti-Jo-1 is the most frequent antibody. On MRI, muscle edema is bilateral but patchy, and fasciitis is present in up to 90% of cases. Fatty infiltration is present in up to 69% of cases and subcutaneous edema in up to 61% of cases. ASS characteristically spares the adductor muscles with a predilection for involvement of the tensor fascia lata, producing a pattern that may be useful for differentiation from other IMM [46].

16.3.3 Immune-Mediated Necrotizing Myopathy (IMNM)

IMNM presents in the fourth to sixth decade, with a female predominance [41]. It is often severe, rapidly progressive, and refractory to steroids. IMNM may be associated with statins, malignancy, or specific antibodies—SRP and HMGCR [45]. On MRI there is diffuse, often asymmetric muscle edema (Fig. 16.5b), especially in the gluteal and thigh compartments, with intense edema at times predicting a favorable treatment response [41, 46]. Fascial involvement is typically minimal, which may allow differentiation from DM or ASS. Severe proximal atrophy can develop early in the disease process, especially in SRP-positive cases.

16.3.4 Inclusion Body Myositis (IBM)

IBM usually affects individuals over 50 years, with a male-to-female ratio of 2:1 [47]. It progresses slowly, often with diagnostic delays exceeding five years. Dysphagia and distal muscle weakness (notably involving the finger flexors) are common. Tau and amyloid protein can accumulate in muscle, similar to their buildup in Alzheimer's disease within the brain. Anti-cN1A antibodies are present in a subset of patients [45]. On MRI, there is often profound fatty infiltration and atrophy (>90%) at presentation (Fig. 16.5c–d) [41]. Residual muscle edema may be present in up to one-third of patients. The distribution is usually bilateral but asymmetric, with a predilection for the quadriceps, sartorius, medial gastrocnemius, and forearm flexors [6, 41]. Fascial edema is absent, allowing differentiation of IBM from DM and ASS [48].

16.3.5 Overlap Myositis

Overlap myositis occurs when IIM features coexist with a systemic autoimmune disease such as systemic lupus erythematosus, systemic sclerosis, or Sjögren's syndrome [49]. There is a female predominance, with most patients presenting in the fourth to sixth decades. The MRI features vary, but bilateral gluteal and thigh involvements are considered typical [6, 49]. The distribution often reflects the underlying connective tissue disease. Soft tissue mineralization may be appreciated on CT (Fig. 16.5e–f).

16.3.6 Antimitochondrial Antibody (AMA)-Associated Myositis

This is a rare form of IIM which usually presents in middle age (40–65 years), predominantly in women, and often with cardiac involvement and primary biliary cholangitis [50]. On MRI, there is symmetric proximal muscle involvement, with the pelvis and thighs more often affected than the lower legs. Fasciitis is frequently seen [51]. Fatty degeneration is less pronounced than in IMNM [41].

Key Point

- Inflammatory myopathies show distinctive patterns of muscle and fascial involvement (Table 16.2); integrating imaging findings with clinical and laboratory data (myositis-specific antibodies) is critical for accurate diagnosis.

Table 16.2 Distinguishing features of idiopathic inflammatory myopathies subtypes

Subtype	Symmetry	Fasciitis	Fatty change	Distinctive features
DM	Symmetric	Prominent	Mild	Cutaneous signs, perimysial edema
ASS	Symmetric, patchy	Most	Majority	Extramuscular manifestations
IMNM	Often asymmetric	Minimal	Severe, early	Rapid progression
IBM	Asymmetric	Absent	90–100%	Hand flexors, sartorius, vastus lateralis
AMA	Symmetric	Frequent	Mild	Cardiac involvement and primary biliary cholangitis

- *DM* dermatomyositis, *ASS* antisynthetase syndrome, *IMNM* immune-mediated necrotizing myopathy, *IBM* inclusion body myositis, *AMA* antimitochondrial antibody-associated myositis

16.4 Denervation Syndromes

Denervation can result from various causes such as spinal cord injury, peripheral nerve injury or compression (especially entrapments in the upper extremity), and inflammatory neuritis. The muscle imaging findings depend on the stage of denervation. After losing nerve supply, predictable muscle changes occur although timescales may differ between individuals [52]. In the acute and subacute phases, MRI demonstrates increased signal intensity on fluid-sensitive sequences, reflecting muscle edema, while T1-weighted images typically remain normal [53, 54]. Chronic denervation is characterized by muscle atrophy and fatty infiltration, which appear as increased signal intensity on T1-weighted images and reduced muscle volume (Fig. 16.6). Importantly, the muscle findings should occur in the distribution of the affected nerve(s). Quantitative MRI techniques show elevated T2 relaxation times and decreased apparent fiber diameter in denervated muscle, correlating with severity on electromyography [8]. On ultrasound, denervated muscle initially appears swollen and hypoechoic, later becoming echogenic due to fatty infiltration with loss of the normal muscle architecture [4, 55].

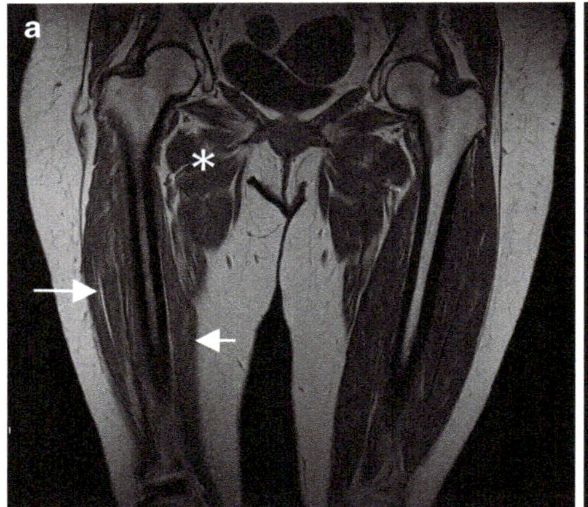

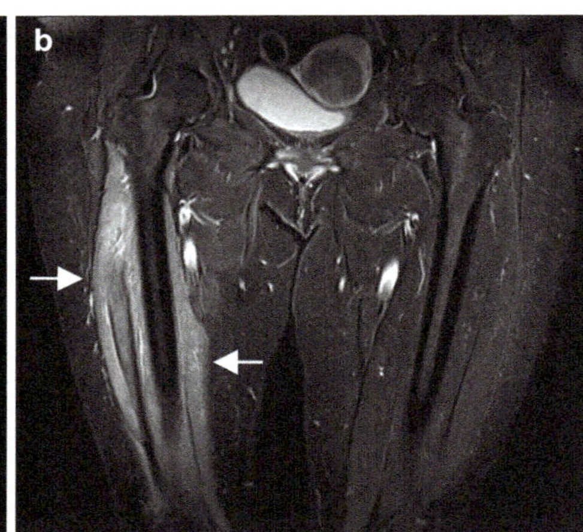

Fig. 16.6 (**a**–**b**) Subacute muscle denervation in the femoral nerve distribution. (**a**) Coronal T1-weighted image shows decreased muscle bulk and slight fatty infiltration of the left quadriceps (arrows). Note sparing of the adductor muscles (asterisk), which are supplied by the obturator nerve. (**b**) Coronal STIR image shows diffuse muscle edema of the quadriceps (arrows)

Key Point

- Muscle imaging findings of denervation should conform to a peripheral nerve distribution, with muscle edema predominating in subacute disease, and fatty atrophy indicating chronic disease.

16.5 Diabetic Myonecrosis

Diabetic myonecrosis, also known as diabetic muscle infarction, is a rare but increasingly recognized microvascular complication of long-standing, poorly controlled diabetes mellitus [56, 57]. A systematic review of 126 cases found the mean age at presentation to be in the fifth decade [58]. There is a slight female preponderance. Almost all patients exhibit other microvascular complications—most frequently nephropathy and retinopathy. The presentation overlaps with more common causes of acute limb pain such as deep venous thrombosis, cellulitis, or soft tissue infection. Diabetic myonecrosis carries important prognostic significance, as it often heralds advanced systemic microangiopathy and is associated with a poor long-term outcome for the patient.

Clinically, patients report abrupt onset of focal pain and swelling without preceding trauma or infection. The quadriceps muscles of the thigh are involved in approximately 60% of cases, followed by hip adductors (15%) and hamstrings (10%) [58]. Approximately 90% of cases are unilateral. MRI typically demonstrates diffuse enlargement of the affected muscle with high-signal intensity on fluid-sensitive sequences (Fig. 16.7) [44]. T1-weighted images usually show isointense or hypointense signal relative to normal muscle, though focal hyperintensity may appear in necrotic regions. The findings are similar to pyomyositis, so clinical history is key. When characteristic clinical findings are present, biopsy is not necessary [56]. Management consists of rest, analgesia, and optimization of glycemic control, with spontaneous recovery usually in 5–13 weeks [58].

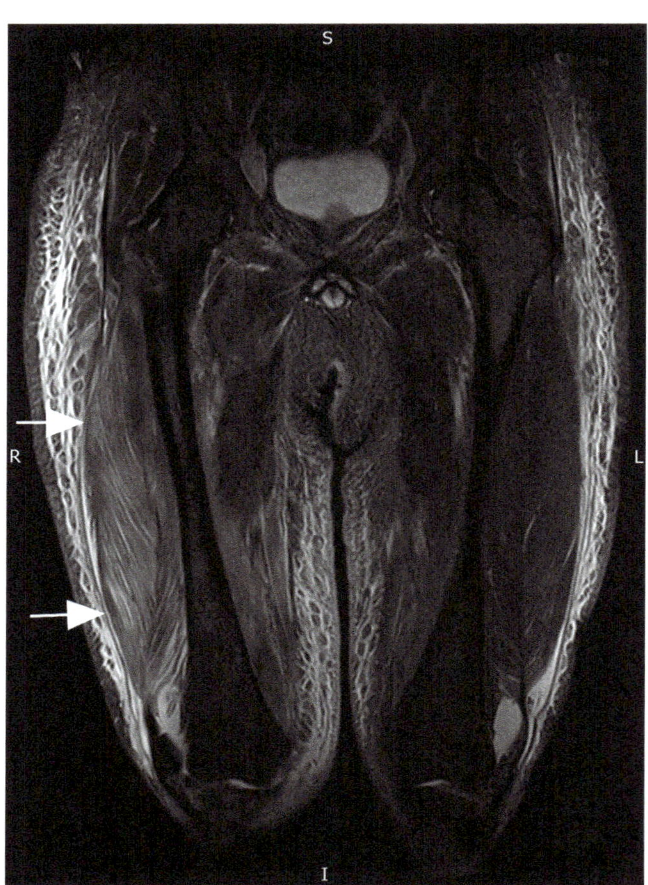

Fig. 16.7 Diabetic myonecrosis. Coronal STIR image demonstrates extensive muscle edema and swelling in the quadriceps compartment (arrows) in a poorly controlled type 1 diabetic with acute-onset pain. There is extensive subcutaneous edema and perifascial edema

Key Point

- The imaging findings of diabetic myonecrosis overlap with other conditions like pyomyositis, but the typical clinical scenario of a poorly controlled diabetic patient with acute onset pain should suggest the diagnosis.

16.6 Infectious Myopathies

16.6.1 Necrotizing Fasciitis

Necrotizing fasciitis is a life-threatening condition due to infection with bacteria that release toxins leading to vascular thrombosis, ischemia, and widespread necrosis of the deep fascia and subcutaneous tissues [59]; the muscles may be spared in the early stages [60]. It most commonly affects the middle-aged and elderly males. Risk factors include diabetes, obesity, immunosuppression, peripheral vascular disease, and intravenous drug use. Clinically, there is swelling, erythema, and severe pain out of proportion to the clinical examination. Rapid progression with systemic toxicity leads to death in 11–20% of patients, and emergent surgical debridement should not be delayed by imaging when there is a high clinical suspicion [61].

Radiographic evidence of soft tissue gas is highly specific (94%) but not sensitive (49%), with gas present in less than 25% of cases [62]. When imaging confirmation is needed, CT is usually faster and safer than MRI for critically ill patients [10] and is more sensitive than radiographs for gas as well as for fascial enhancement, fat stranding, and edema [63]. MRI may show thickening and hyperintensity of deep fascia, fascial fluid, and peripheral band-like hyperintense signal in the muscles on fluid-sensitive sequences. Variable contrast enhancement often with nonenhancing deep fascia may be present [64, 65]. Ultrasound can be performed at the bedside and may demonstrate fluid along the fascial planes and subcutaneous gas but may be limited by poor visualization due to subcutaneous gas and edema [66].

16.6.2 Pyomyositis

Pyomyositis is a primary bacterial infection of skeletal muscle, most commonly caused by gram-negative organisms, with abscess formation within the muscle [61]. It is often preceded by local trauma or penetrating injury, or vigorous muscle use, and typically presents with localized muscle pain, swelling, tenderness, and fever. Pyomyositis is most common in the pelvis and lower extremities. Risk factors include intravenous drug use, immunosuppression, and diabetes. Endemic forms occur in tropical regions. MRI is the preferred imaging modality and demonstrates diffuse muscle hyperintensity on fluid-sensitive images, diffuse muscle enhancement, and intramuscular abscesses (Fig. 16.8). Fascial involvement is typically irregular or limited, and gas is rare [61, 62]. Less common causes of muscle infection include viruses (influenza, HIV), parasites (trichinosis, cysticercosis), and fungi (typically in immunocompromised individuals).

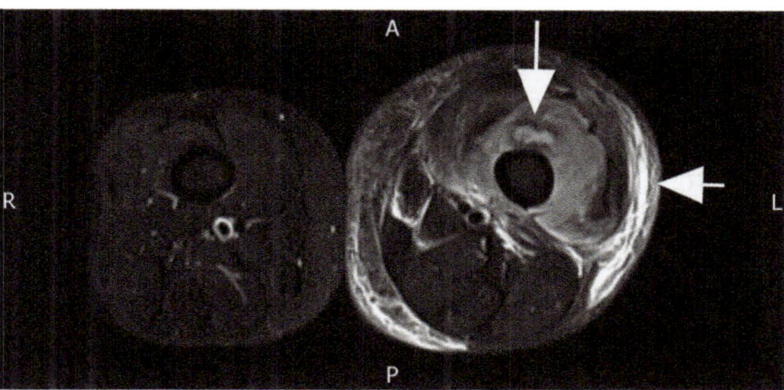

Fig. 16.8 Pyomyositis. Axial fat-suppressed proton density-weighted image demonstrates edema throughout the left quadriceps muscles with an intramuscular abscess in the vastus intermedius (long arrow). There is associated cellulitis (short arrow)

Key Point

- Necrotizing fasciitis and pyomyositis are distinct entities in terms of pathogenesis, clinical presentation, and imaging findings.

16.7 Congenital and Metabolic Myopathies and Muscular Dystrophy

Congenital myopathies due to genetic defects are a heterogeneous group of early-onset muscle disorders defined by specific histopathological features [67]. These conditions typically present in neonates or children with hypotonia and proximal muscle weakness, but severity and age of onset can vary. Progressive respiratory involvement is common, and cardiac and extraocular muscle involvement may occur in specific subtypes.

Metabolic myopathies are caused by inherited defects in muscle energy metabolism, most commonly involving glycogen storage or fatty acid oxidation pathways [68]. They present with exercise intolerance, episodic rhabdomyolysis, and variable weakness, often in childhood or adolescence. Symptoms may be triggered by exertion, fasting, or illness. The clinical spectrum ranges from mild, isolated muscle involvement to severe, multisystem disease.

Duchenne muscular dystrophy (DMD) is an X-linked genetic disorder with near-complete loss of functional dystrophin, resulting in progressive muscle weakness, degeneration, and replacement of muscle with fat and fibrous tissue (Fig. 16.9) [69]. The typically presentation is with delayed milestones, proximal weakness, and scoliosis; patients become wheelchair bound by early adolescence. Complications include cardiomyopathy, respiratory failure, and occasional cognitive impairment. In Becker dystrophy, there is partially functional dystrophin, with a later onset of less severe muscle disease.

In these disorders, whole-body MRI is increasingly used to map disease distribution and severity and may help direct biopsy [70]. Central core disease shows selective involvement of gluteus maximus and adductor magnus, while nemaline myopathy demonstrates diffuse anterior thigh and axial muscle involvement [71]. Increased T1 signal indicates fatty replacement, and T2/STIR hyperintensity reflects edema or inflammation [72]. Dixon fat fraction mapping is becoming the standard outcome measure in therapeutic trials. In metabolic myopathies, MRI may show transient muscle edema during acute episodes and patchy or diffuse fatty infiltration in chronic disease [73]. Between attacks imaging may appear normal.

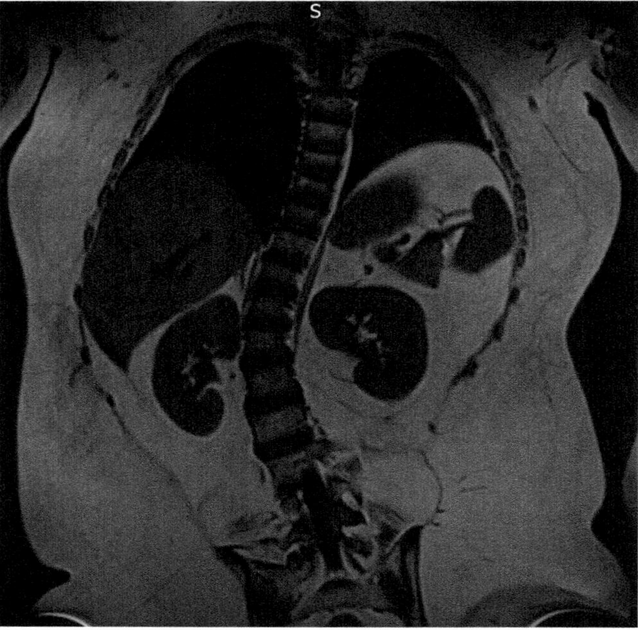

Fig. 16.9 Duchenne muscular dystrophy. A coronal T1-weighted image demonstrates extensive fatty replacement of the trunk skeletal muscles and scoliosis

16.8 Myositis Ossificans

Myositis ossificans is a benign, heterotopic ossification occurring in muscle that can mimic soft tissue tumors both clinically and on imaging studies. It typically presents as a painful, rapidly growing inflammatory mass, with a history of trauma in approximately half of the cases [74]. Males under 30 years are most affected, usually in the lower limb, especially the quadriceps muscles. The lesion evolves through three phases—acute, subacute, and maturation—producing the characteristic "zone phenomenon" (peripheral ossification with a central myxoid or fibroblastic core) [75–77]. This pattern helps distinguish myositis ossificans from extraskeletal osteosarcoma, where ossification occurs centrally.

In mature lesions, radiographs show peripheral zonal ossification with a lucent center, typically 2–6 weeks after the onset of symptoms. CT and ultrasound can detect early mineralization before radiographs [77, 78]. MRI is most useful in the early phase, before ossification is radiographically apparent. The characteristic findings include an intramuscular mass with preserved muscle fascicles, with isointense signal on T1-weighted images, heterogeneous hyperintensity on fluid-sensitive images, and a distinctive "striate" and "checkerboard-like" pattern paralleling the muscle fibers (Fig. 16.10) [75, 79]. Extensive perilesional muscle edema, with an edema:lesion ratio >2, is considered highly specific

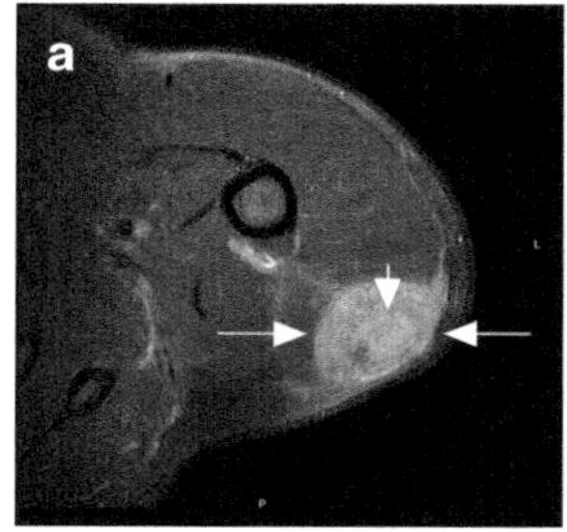

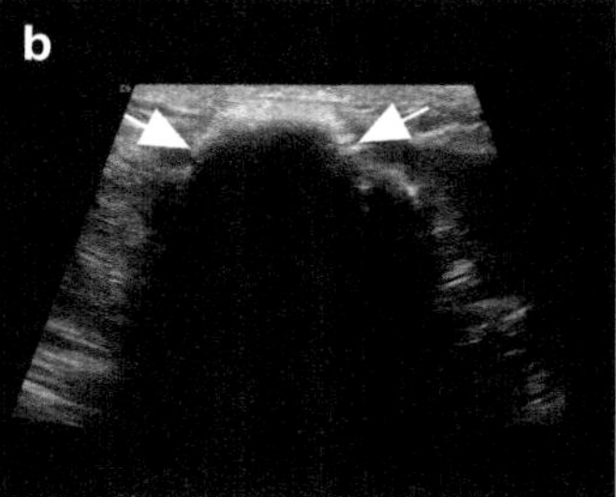

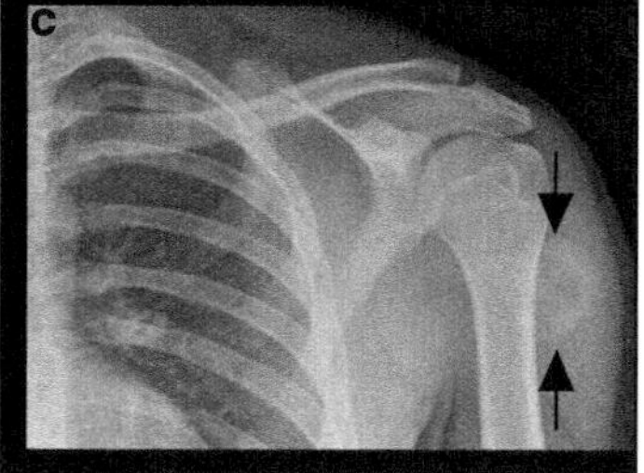

Fig. 16.10 (**a**–**c**) Myositis ossificans in the deltoid muscle. (**a**) Axial fat-suppressed proton density-weighted image demonstrates a heterogeneous high-signal intensity inflammatory mass (long arrows) with a central rounded low signal rim (short arrow) indicating mineralization in the acute phase. (**b**) Ultrasound demonstrates rim mineralization (arrows) with posterior acoustic shadowing in the maturation phase. (**c**) An AP radiograph shows well-circumscribed peripheral mineralization (arrows) surrounding a lucent center in the maturation phase

in the early/intermediate stage and helps differentiate myositis ossificans from malignant soft tissue tumors [80]. Histopathological features may be confused with osteosarcoma, and biopsy should be avoided when there are typical imaging findings. The presence of COL1A1::USP6 fusion may be considered diagnostic for myositis ossificans in the appropriate clinical context [81].

Key Point

- In the initial stages, myositis ossificans can mimic a tumor on imaging studies, but extensive surrounding edema is a characteristic finding; if suspected, a search for peripheral mineralization with ultrasound, CT, or short-term follow-up radiographs should be performed in lieu of immediate biopsy.

16.9 Concluding Remarks

MRI is the gold standard for muscle imaging, providing high sensitivity for detecting edema, inflammation, fatty infiltration, and atrophy. It allows pattern recognition for diagnosis and disease monitoring in traumatic, congenital, metabolic, ischemic, and inflammatory myopathies. Ultrasound offers real-time, bedside evaluation but it has lower sensitivity for deep or early lesions. Computed tomography is less commonly used but remains valuable for quantifying muscle mass and detecting gas, calcification, or ossification. The integration of imaging findings with clinical and laboratory data is essential for accurate diagnosis, guiding biopsy, and informing management decisions in muscle disorders.

Conflict of Interest Statement I/We declare no competing interests as defined by Springer Nature or other interests that might be perceived to influence results and/or discussion reported in this manuscript.

References

1. Vlychou M, Teh J. Ultrasound of muscle. Curr Probl Diagn Radiol. 2008;37:219–30.
2. Peetrons P. Ultrasound of muscles. Eur Radiol. 2002;12:35–43.
3. Campbell RSD, Wood J. Ultrasound of muscle. Imaging. 2014;14:229–40.
4. Gunreben G, Bogdahn U. Real-time sonography of acute and chronic muscle denervation. Muscle Nerve. 1991;14:654–64.
5. Campbell SE, Adler R, Sofka CM. Ultrasound of muscle abnormalities. Ultrasound Q. 2005;21:87–94.
6. Albayda J, Demonceau G, Carlier PG. Muscle imaging in myositis: MRI, US, and PET. Best Pract Res Clin Rheumatol. 2022;36:101765.
7. Kalia V, Advanced MRI. Techniques for muscle imaging. Semin Musculoskelet Radiol. 2017;21:459–69.
8. Tan ET, Serrano KC, Bhatti P, Pishgar F, Vanderbeek AM, Milani CJ, et al. Quantitative MRI differentiates electromyography severity grades of Denervated muscle in neuropathy of the brachial plexus. J Magn Reson Imaging. 2022;56:1104–15.
9. Tan AL, Matteo AD, Wakefield RJ, Biglands J. Update on muscle imaging in myositis. Curr Opin Rheumatol. 2023;35:395–403.
10. Curry CA, Corl FM, Fishman EK. CT diagnosis of necrotizing fasciitis: spectrum of CT findings. Emerg Radiol. 2000;7:369–75.
11. West ATH, Marshall TJ, Bearcroft PW. CT of the musculoskeletal system: what is left is the days of MRI? Eur Radiol. 2008;19:152–64.
12. Parida GK, Roy SG, Kumar R. FDG-PET/CT in skeletal muscle: pitfalls and pathologies. Semin Nucl Med. 2017;47:362–72.
13. Kirkendall DT, Garrett WE Jr. Clinical perspectives regarding eccentric muscle injury. Clin Orthop Relat Res. 2002;403:S81–9.
14. Mueller-Wohlfahrt HW, Haensel L, Mithoefer K, Ekstrand J, English B, McNally S, et al. Terminology and classification of muscle injuries in sport: the Munich consensus statement. Br J Sports Med. 2013;47:342–50.
15. Guermazi A, Roemer FW, Robinson P, Tol JL, Regatte RR, Crema MD. Imaging of muscle injuries in sports medicine: sports imaging series. Radiology. 2017;282:646–63.
16. Hotfiel T, Seil R, Bily W, Bloch W, Gokeler A, Krifter RM, et al. Nonoperative treatment of muscle injuries - recommendations from the GOTS expert meeting. J Exp Orthop. 2018;5:24.
17. Dave RB, Stevens KJ, Shivaram GM, McAdams TR, Dillingham MF, Beaulieu CF. Ultrasound-guided musculoskeletal interventions in American football: 18 years of experience. AJR Am J Roentgenol. 2014;203:W674–83.
18. Zein MI, Reurink G, Suskens JJM, Monte JRC, Smithuis FF, Buckens S, et al. 3.0-tesla MRI observation at return to play after hamstring injuries. Clin J Sport Med. 2025;35:119–26.
19. Reurink G, Brilman EG, de Vos RJ, Maas M, Moen MH, Weir A, et al. Magnetic resonance imaging in acute hamstring injury: can we provide a return to play prognosis? Sports Med. 2015;45:133–46.
20. Binkert OA, Pfirrmann CWA, Fierstra S, Higashigaito K, Rosskopf AB. Classification systems for assessing acute muscle injuries: a retrospective comparison of inter-reader agreements. Skeletal Radiol. 2025;55:191–203.
21. Pollock N, James SL, Lee JC, Chakraverty R. British athletics muscle injury classification: a new grading system. Br J Sports Med. 2014;48:1347–51.
22. Hollabaugh WL, Sin A, Walden RL, Weaver JS, Porras LP, LeClere LE, et al. Outcomes of activity-related lower extremity muscle tears after application of the British athletics muscle injury classification: a systematic review. Sports Health. 2024;16:783–96.
23. Connell DA, Schneider-Kolsky ME, Hoving JL, Malara F, Buchbinder R, Koulouris G, et al. Longitudinal study comparing sonographic and MRI assessments of acute and healing hamstring injuries. AJR Am J Roentgenol. 2004;183:975–84.
24. Flores DV, Mejia Gomez C, Estrada-Castrillon M, Smitaman E, Pathria MN. MR imaging of muscle trauma: anatomy, biomechanics, pathophysiology, and imaging appearance. Radiographics. 2018;38:124–48.
25. Blankenbaker DG, Tuite MJ. Temporal changes of muscle injury. Semin Musculoskelet Radiol. 2010;14:176–93.
26. Reurink G, Almusa E, Goudswaard GJ, Tol JL, Hamilton B, Moen MH, et al. No association between fibrosis on magnetic resonance imaging at return to play and hamstring reinjury risk. Am J Sports Med. 2015;43:1228–34.
27. Rubin DA. Imaging diagnosis and prognostication of hamstring injuries. AJR Am J Roentgenol. 2012;199:525–33.
28. Chang JS, Kayani B, Plastow R, Singh S, Magan A, Haddad FS. Management of hamstring injuries: current concepts review. Bone Joint J. 2020;102-B:1281–8.

29. Malliaropoulos N, Papacostas E, Kiritsi O, Papalada A, Gougoulias N, Maffulli N. Posterior thigh muscle injuries in elite track and field athletes. Am J Sports Med. 2010;38:1813–9.
30. Entwisle T, Ling Y, Splatt A, Brukner P, Connell D. Distal Musculotendinous T junction injuries of the biceps Femoris: an MRI case review. Orthop J Sports Med. 2017;5:2325967117714998.
31. Askling CM, Tengvar M, Saartok T, Thorstensson A. Proximal hamstring strains of stretching type in different sports: injury situations, clinical and magnetic resonance imaging characteristics, and return to sport. Am J Sports Med. 2008;36:1799–804.
32. Begum FA, Kayani B, Chang JS, Tansey RJ, Haddad FS. The management of proximal rectus femoris avulsion injuries. EFORT Open Rev. 2020;5:828–34.
33. McAleer S, Macdonald B, Lee J, Zhu W, Giakoumis M, Maric T, et al. Time to return to full training and recurrence of rectus femoris injuries in elite track and field athletes 2010-2019; a 9-year study using the British athletics muscle injury classification. Scand J Med Sci Sports. 2022;32:1109–18.
34. Kassarjian A, Rodrigo RM, Santisteban JM. Intramuscular degloving injuries to the rectus femoris: findings at MRI. AJR Am J Roentgenol. 2014;202:W475–80.
35. Delgado GJ, Chung CB, Lektrakul N, Azocar P, Botte MJ, Coria D, et al. Tennis leg: clinical US study of 141 patients and anatomic investigation of four cadavers with MR imaging and US. Radiology. 2002;224:112–9.
36. Prakash A, Entwisle T, Schneider M, Brukner P, Connell D. Connective tissue injury in calf muscle tears and return to play: MRI correlation. Br J Sports Med. 2018;52:929–33.
37. Waterworth G, Wein S, Gorelik A, Rotstein AH. MRI assessment of calf injuries in Australian football league players: findings that influence return to play. Skeletal Radiol. 2017;46:343–50.
38. Chadwick N, Weaver JS, Shultz C, Morag Y, Patel A, Taljanovic MS. High-resolution ultrasound and MRI in the evaluation of pectoralis major injuries. J Ultrason. 2023;23:e202–e13.
39. Baker JC, Pacheco RA, Bansal D, Shah VA, Rubin DA. The diagnostic performance of MRI signs to distinguish pectoralis major tendon avulsions from myotendinous injuries. Skeletal Radiol. 2021;50:2395–404.
40. Ziemian M, Szmydtka J, Snoch W, Milner S, Wojciechowski S, Dłuszczakowska A, et al. Integrative approaches to myopathies and muscular dystrophies: molecular mechanisms, diagnostics, and future therapies. Int J Mol Sci. 2025;26:7972.
41. Hamano T, Kamisawa T, Sanada S, Hayashi K. Muscle magnetic resonance imaging findings in patients with idiopathic inflammatory myopathies. Clin Exp Neuroimmunol. 2025;16:72–83.
42. Vlekkert JVD, Maas M, Hoogendijk JE, Visser MD, Schaik INV. Combining MRI and muscle biopsy improves diagnostic accuracy in subacute-onset idiopathic inflammatory myopathy. Muscle Nerve. 2015;51:253–8.
43. Filli L, Maurer B, Manoliu A, Andreisek G, Guggenberger R. Whole-body MRI in adult inflammatory myopathies: do we need imaging of the trunk? Eur Radiol. 2015;25:3499–507.
44. Rilland EDZ, Yao L, Stevens KJ, Chung LS, Fiorentino DF, Boutin RD. Myositis and its mimics: guideline updates, MRI characteristics, and new horizons. Am J Roentgenol. 2024;223:e2431359.
45. Halilu F, Christopher-Stine L. Myositis-specific antibodies: overview and clinical utilization. Rheumatol Immunol Res. 2022;3:1–10.
46. Zhang W, Zheng Y, Wang Y, Xiong H, Que C, Zhang X, et al. Thigh MRI in antisynthetase syndrome, and comparisons with dermatomyositis and immune-mediated necrotizing myopathy. Rheumatology. 2022;62:310–20.
47. Naddaf E. Inclusion body myositis: update on the diagnostic and therapeutic landscape. Front Neurol. 2022;13:1020113.
48. Dion E, Cherin P, Payan C, Fournet J-C, Papo T, Maisonobe T, et al. Magnetic resonance imaging criteria for distinguishing between inclusion body myositis and polymyositis. J Rheumatol. 2002;29:1897–906.
49. Nuño-Nuño L, Joven BE, Carreira PE, Maldonado-Romero V, Larena-Grijalba C, Cubas IL, et al. Overlap myositis, a distinct entity beyond primary inflammatory myositis: a retrospective analysis of a large cohort from the REMICAM registry. Int J Rheum Dis. 2019;22:1393–401.
50. Nagai A, Nagai T, Yaguchi H, Fujii S, Uwatoko H, Shirai S, et al. Clinical features of anti-mitochondrial M2 antibody-positive myositis: case series of 17 patients. J Neurol Sci. 2022;442:120391.
51. Nomiya H, Hamano T, Takaku N, Sasaki H, Usui K, Sanada S, et al. Magnetic resonance imaging findings of the lower limb muscles in anti-mitochondrial M2 antibody-positive myositis. Neuromuscul Disord. 2023;33:74–80.
52. Fleckenstein JL, Watumull D, Conner KE, Ezaki M, Greenlee RG, Bryan WW, et al. Denervated human skeletal muscle: MR imaging evaluation. Radiology. 1993;187:213–8.
53. Kamath S, Venkatanarasimha N, Walsh MA, Hughes PM. MRI appearance of muscle denervation. Skeletal Radiol. 2008;37:397–404.
54. Kim S-J, Hong SH, Jun WS, Choi J-Y, Myung JS, Jacobson JA, et al. MR imaging mapping of skeletal muscle denervation in entrapment and compressive neuropathies. Radiographics. 2011;31:319–32.
55. Klauser A, Buzzegoli T, Taljanovic M, Strobl S, Rauch S, Teh J, et al. Nerve entrapment syndromes at the wrist and elbow by sonography. Semin Musculoskelet Radiol. 2018;22:344–53.
56. Kempegowda P, Melson E, Langman G, Khattar F, Karamat M, Altaf Q-A. Diabetic myonecrosis: an uncommon diabetic complication. Endocrinol Diabetes Metab Case Rep. 2019;2019:19–0067.
57. Rahman I, Narasimhan K, Bair C, Phillips JW. Diabetic myonecrosis. Endocrinologist. 2009;19:169–70.
58. Horton WB, Taylor JS, Ragland TJ, Subauste AR. Diabetic muscle infarction: a systematic review. BMJ Open Diabetes Res Care. 2015;3:e000082.
59. Allaw F, Wehbe S, Kanj SS. Necrotizing fasciitis: an update on epidemiology, diagnostic methods, and treatment. Curr Opin Infect Dis. 2024;37:105–11.
60. McDermott J, Kao LS, Keeley JA, Grigorian A, Neville A, Virgilio C. Necrotizing soft tissue infections: a review. JAMA Surg. 2024;159:1308–15.
61. Stevens DL, Bisno AL, Chambers HF, Dellinger EP, Goldstein EJC, Gorbach SL, et al. Practice guidelines for the diagnosis and management of skin and soft tissue infections: 2014 update by the Infectious Diseases Society of America. Clin Infect Dis. 2014;59:e10–52.
62. Goh T, Goh LG, Ang CH, Wong CH. Early diagnosis of necrotizing fasciitis. Br J Surg. 2014;101:e119–e25.
63. Bruls RJM, Kwee RM. CT in necrotizing soft tissue infection: diagnostic criteria and comparison with LRINEC score. Eur Radiol. 2021;31:8536–41.
64. Seok JH, Jee W-H, Chun K-A, Kim J-Y, Jung C-K, Kim YR, et al. Necrotizing fasciitis versus pyomyositis: discrimination with using MR imaging. Korean J Radiol. 2009;10:121–8.
65. Ali SZ, Srinivasan S, Peh WCG. MRI in necrotizing fasciitis of the extremities. Br J Radiol. 2013;87:20130560.
66. Malghem J, Lecouvet FE, Omoumi P, Maldague BE, Berg BCV. Necrotizing fasciitis: contribution and limitations of diagnostic imaging. Joint Bone Spine. 2013;80:146–54.
67. Claeys KG. Congenital myopathies: an update. Dev Med Child Neurol. 2020;62:297–302.
68. Canda E, Köse M, Diniz G. Clues for differential diagnosis of neuromuscular disorders. Cham: Springer; 2023. p. 249–73.
69. Polavarapu K, Manjunath M, Preethish-Kumar V, Sekar D, Vengalil S, Thomas P, et al. Muscle MRI in Duchenne muscular dystrophy: evidence of a distinctive pattern. Neuromuscul Disord. 2016;26:768–74.

70. Tomas X, Milisenda JC, Garcia-Diez AI, Prieto-Gonzalez S, Faruch M, Pomes J, et al. Whole-body MRI and pathological findings in adult patients with myopathies. Skeletal Radiol. 2019;48:653–76.
71. Leung DG. Magnetic resonance imaging patterns of muscle involvement in genetic muscle diseases: a systematic review. J Neurol. 2017;264:1320–33.
72. Aivazoglou LU, Guimarães JB, Link TM, Costa MAF, Cardoso FN, Badia BML, et al. MR imaging of inherited myopathies: a review and proposal of imaging algorithms. Eur Radiol. 2021;31:8498–512.
73. Bhai SF, Vissing J. Diagnosis and management of metabolic myopathies. Muscle Nerve. 2023;68:250–6.
74. Saad A, Azzopardi C, Patel A, Davies AM, Botchu R. Myositis ossificans revisited—the largest reported case series. J Clin Orthop Trauma. 2021;17:123–7.
75. De Smet AA, Norris MA, Fisher DR. Magnetic resonance imaging of myositis ossificans: analysis of seven cases. Skeletal Radiol. 1992;21:503–7.
76. Kransdorf MJ, Meis JM, Jelinek JS. Myositis ossificans: MR appearance with radiologic-pathologic correlation. AJR Am J Roentgenol. 1991;157:1243–8.
77. Parikh J, Hyare H, Saifuddin A. The imaging features of post-traumatic myositis ossificans, with emphasis on MRI. Clin Radiol. 2002;57:1058–66.
78. Tyler P, Saifuddin A. The imaging of myositis ossificans. Semin Musculoskelet Radiol. 2010;14:201–16.
79. Wang H, Nie P, Li Y, Hou F, Dong C, Huang Y, et al. MRI findings of early myositis ossificans without calcification or ossification. Biomed Res Int. 2018;2018:4186324.
80. Zubler V, Mühlemann M, Sutter R, Götschi T, Müller DA, Dietrich TJ, et al. Diagnostic utility of perilesional muscle edema in myositis ossificans. Skeletal Radiol. 2020;49:929–36.
81. Ledinek Ž, Stefanović M, Mavčič B, Mazić MČ, Gazikalović A, Šekoranja D, et al. Diagnosis of pediatric myositis ossificans based on cytomorphology and molecular analysis from FNAB sample: a case report. Diagn Cytopathol. 2025;53:E138–E43.

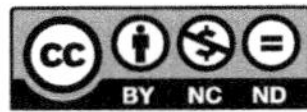

Common Mistakes in MSK Imaging

17

Robert D. Boutin and Marcelo Bordalo-Rodrigues

Learning Objectives

- Discuss perceptual (detection) errors and cognitive errors that occur every day in radiology, emphasizing musculoskeletal (MSK) MRI.
- Promote a healthy work culture with a growth mindset that acknowledges errors (learning from our mistakes) and celebrates diagnostic excellence.
- Use "simulation-based learning" to challenge ourselves with specific cases and discuss strategies for minimizing common mistakes when interpreting MSK MRI.

We must become connoisseurs of our own ignorance.... We need to seek out and explore what we do not know [1].

Socrates famously declared that he was the wisest man in all of Athens precisely because he recognized that he did not know everything [1]. Now, just like in the fifth century BCE, our quest for knowledge often is motivated when we acknowledge our nescience (ignorance).

Inappropriate overconfidence can contribute to harmful diagnostic errors. Interestingly, as radiologists gain expertise, we are actually more likely to acknowledge our limitations with increasing humility. By promoting this mature, healthy attitude toward uncertainty and our mistakes, we can improve our diagnostic accuracy—and actually heighten happiness for ourselves [2].

Despite our best efforts, errors are common. In daily radiology practice, the general interpretation error rate is ~4%, but reportedly increases to ~30% when imaging exams are abnormal [3–6].

Misdiagnosis can be attributed to numerous factors. The root causes contributing to misdiagnosis are sometimes beyond our control, but we can often optimize elements of our work environment. Well-known factors contributing to misdiagnosis (and frustration!) among radiologists can include:

- Healthcare system factors (e.g., incomplete patient history, limitations in access to prior imaging).
- Human factors (e.g., interruptions, distractions, high volume, fatigue).
- Technical factors (e.g., metal artifacts, imaging equipment limitations).

What can we do TODAY to minimize errors? Within our daily direct control, we can learn from our mistakes, including with "simulation-based learning", to mitigate two crucial categories of errors: ***perceptual (detection) errors*** (~70%) and ***cognitive errors*** (~30%) [3–6].

After a brief overview of these errors and general opportunities for self-improvement, we examine mistakes that matter in musculoskeletal radiology. While many excellent publications review errors made with musculoskeletal radiography [7], our objectives here are to focus on common mistakes we see with musculoskeletal MRI and strategies to minimize those misses.

17.1 Tip 1: To Err Is Human [8]

Mistakes can be mitigated by acknowledging errors and celebrating excellence. This acknowledgement helps propel focused, continuous quality improvement. Indeed, collecting and sharing feedback from all stakeholders enhances early correction of errors [9].

R. D. Boutin (✉)
Department of Radiology, Stanford University, Stanford, CA, USA
e-mail: boutin@stanford.edu

M. Bordalo-Rodrigues
Department of Radiology, Aspetar Orthopaedic and Sports Medicine Hospital, Doha, Qatar

J. Hodler et al. (eds.), *Musculoskeletal Diseases 2026-2029*, IDKD Springer Series,
https://doi.org/10.1007/978-3-032-17040-8_17

Although errors are inevitable, failure to learn from our mistakes can be inexcusable. It is our professional duty to mitigate mistakes that might cause harm to our patients (*primum non nocere*). Importantly, we are best equipped to improve patient care when we acknowledge our own mistakes — both perceptual and cognitive.

17.1.1 Perceptual Errors

Perceptual (detection) errors occur when an abnormality is missed at the time of primary interpretation but is "visible in retrospect". As recognized by Weber [7], 70% of fractures missed during the initial interpretation can be identified during a second review.

Failure to recognize an abnormality is more likely with *poor lesion conspicuity* (e.g., small lesion, non-displaced fracture).

Strategies to minimize such errors include being aware of blind spots, reading images systematically, and making time for careful analysis of images.

- Reviewing serial exams can be helpful. For example, with postop imaging looking for subsidence of hardware (e.g., arthroplasty, spinal instrumentation), reviewing the *original postop baseline* exam may help avoid mistakes that can occur when only reviewing the most recent comparison exam.
- Reviewing cross-sectional imaging in all planes can be important. For example, with knee MRI, diagnostic improvements can occur when viewing axial images for a radial meniscus tear and coronal images for a cruciate ligament injury.

17.1.2 Cognitive Errors

Cognitive errors are failures in reasoning that cause misinterpretation. With imaging, this generally means we may observe an abnormal finding, but we assign the wrong meaning to what we see. Misdiagnosis here may be related to a lack of knowledge (e.g., radiologist expertise, poor clinical history) or propagating an error from a previous imaging report.

Radiologists should be aware of three common types of faulty reasoning ("cognitive biases") threatening diagnosis accuracy: (1) **anchoring bias** (e.g., fixating on an early impression of "just osteoarthritis" while ignoring findings that may point to a different type of arthritis), (2) **confirmation bias** (e.g., overcalling degenerative meniscal signal as a tear owing to a history of a positive McMurray test, even though MRI diagnostic criteria for a tear are not satisfied), and (3) **framing bias** (e.g., assuming bone marrow edema in an athlete with is due to trauma or repetitive microtrauma) (Fig. 17.1).

Strategies to minimize such errors include continuing medical education, seeking second opinions, keeping an open mind when formulating a working diagnosis, and reviewing the examination before being biased by previous reports or contemporaneous AI results. In some settings, you may want to consider at least one alternative diagnosis before finalizing your report.

Key Point

- Perceptual errors predominate, especially with poor conspicuity of a finding, so use structured search, check all planes, and perform a targeted secondary search. Cognitive errors resulting in misinterpretation are often driven by biases; counter them by staying open-minded, strengthening domain knowledge, and deferring exposure to previous reports (and AI results) until after your own read.

17.2 Tip 2: Anatomy Is Foundational

Anatomy is the foundation for all that we do — the entire edifice of radiology. You cannot be a good musculoskeletal radiologist unless you are a good musculoskeletal anatomist.

Knowledge of normal anatomy underpins recognizing abnormal findings and enables us to report imaging findings using a universal language. Most anatomic knowledge remains remarkably consistent from your first day in medical school until the day you retire, but the best musculoskeletal radiologists constantly push themselves to refine this knowledge as treatment strategies evolve.

- For example, with knee MRI, anatomic knowledge of the meniscus root attachments is now particularly important owing to innovations in arthroscopic treatments. This awareness helps us avoid *missing* posterior root tears (false-negative interpretation) and *overcalling* anterior root tears (false-positive interpretation) [10].

17.2.1 Entheses and Apophyses

Entheses (tendon or ligament attachments to bone) may have seemed arcane during medical school, but mastering the location of these anatomic footprints is essential for interpreting musculoskeletal MRI.

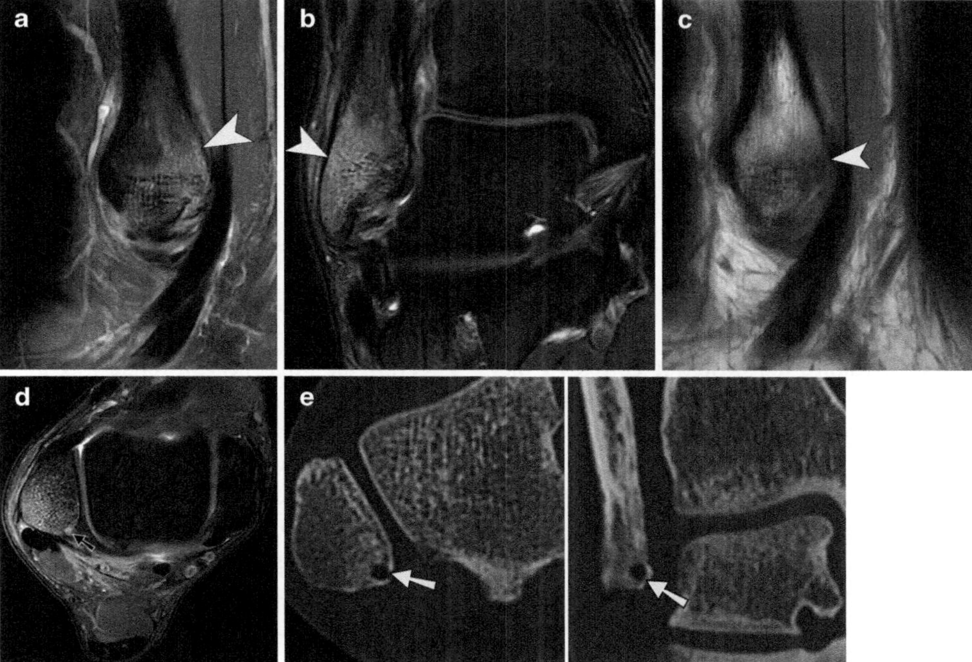

Fig. 17.1 Osteoid osteoma. (**a**) Sagittal, (**b**) coronal T2-weighted fat-suppressed, and (**c**) sagittal T1-weighted MR images of the ankle in a soccer player presenting with lateral ankle pain following trauma during a match. The initial MRI revealed diffuse bone marrow edema in the distal fibula, with intermediate signal on T1-weighted imaging (arrowheads) and no visible fracture line. The findings were interpreted as post-traumatic bone edema. Due to persistent symptoms after 1 month, a second MRI was performed. On the axial T2-weighted fat-suppressed image (**d**), the edema remained, but a small, round lesion was identified in the posterior aspect of the distal fibula (black arrow). Retrospective review confirmed that the lesion was already present on the initial scan. A subsequent CT scan of the ankle (E, axial and coronal reformatted images) revealed a small lytic lesion (white arrows), suggestive of osteoid osteoma. The diagnosis was confirmed by histopathology performed before radiofrequency ablation

- For example, if an MRI shows fluid-equivalent signal on an osseous anatomic attachment site for a tendon or ligament, the radiologist should suspect that tendon or ligament is torn. Focal fluid covering an enthesis means that normal soft tissue is not attached there. In other words, if fluid can go there, a surgeon's probe can go there, too.

Apophyses are normal developmental bony prominences arising from secondary ossification centers at a tendon or ligament attachment. By definition, apophyses do not contribute to the length of long bones, do not form part of the joint surface, and typically fuse at skeletal maturity.

During adolescence, apophyses are subject to traction forces that may result in avulsion fractures or apophysitis. Because the "weak link" in the "kinetic chain" is commonly the apophyseal physis in adolescent patients, awareness of apophyseal anatomy is crucial for avoiding misdiagnosis.

In the subacute or chronic setting, an avulsion injury potentially may resemble a neoplastic process, especially when no history of trauma is available or the radiologist is not familiar with apophyseal anatomy.

- Characteristic locations for avulsion fractures include the pelvis (e.g., ischial tuberosity, anterior inferior iliac spine, anterior superior iliac spine), knee (e.g., tibial tubercle, inferior pole of the patella), foot (e.g., fifth metatarsal base), and elbow (e.g., medial humeral epicondyle).

17.2.2 Ossicles

Knowledge of normal ossicles is crucial every day in musculoskeletal imaging. This understanding helps us accurately distinguish incidental ossicles from avulsion fractures and other clinically relevant derangements.

- In the knee, our understanding of meniscal ossicles has evolved. Once considered a vestigial (congenital) remnant, we now know that meniscal ossicles can develop in adults over time and are highly associated with adjacent posterior root injuries, meniscus extrusion, and progressive osteoarthritis [10].

17.2.3 Anatomic Variations—Ligaments and Muscles

Mastering normal anatomy and its many variations merits ongoing attention with lifelong learning. Anatomic variations in neurovascular structures can be inconspicuous on imaging, but can be associated with serious iatrogenic complications (e.g., arterial transection, limb loss) if the surgeon is not made aware [11].

- For example, the aberrant anterior tibial artery (prevalence, 2–3%) courses along the posterior cortex of the tibia (anterior to the popliteus muscle) and therefore is vulnerable during many procedures on the knee/tibia [12].

Anatomic variations sometimes can be confused with a true derangement or sequelae of tissue trauma.

- With knee MRI, fibrous strands in the infrapatellar fat pad of Hoffa may be misinterpreted as post-arthroscopic scarring, particularly if you are not aware of the variable presence of normal ligaments (secondary patellar stabilizers) in this region [13].
- With ankle MRI, osteochondral lesions are observed more commonly at the talar dome than the tibial plafond. Although osteochondral lesions at the tibial plafond do occur, they are almost never isolated to the anteromedial rim of the tibial plafond. A pseudodefect at the anteromedial rim of the tibial plafond (notch of Harty) is a normal anatomic variant that should be differentiated from a traumatic osteochondral lesion owing to its characteristic location and the absence of subchondral reactive changes [14].

Anatomic variations can sometimes represent an ambiguous "borderland" between "normal" anatomy and a "pathological" derangement. Such anatomic variations include anomalous muscles that are usually incidental findings, but occasionally cause neurovascular entrapment or present clinically as a palpable mass. On MRI, if we are not familiar with these anomalous muscles, they are easily overlooked because they are normally isointense with adjacent muscles. When an anomalous muscle is closely associated with a nerve, the nerve should be scrutinized for findings associated with neuropathy (e.g., abnormal caliber, abnormal signal intensity).

- Examples of anomalous muscles are best known at the elbow (e.g., anconeus epitrochlearis compressing or protecting the ulnar nerve), forearm (e.g., Gantzer's muscle compressing the anterior interosseous nerve), wrist (e.g., palmaris longus variants compressing the median nerve), pelvis (e.g., piriformis variants associated with sciatic nerve entrapment), knee (e.g., third head of the gastrocnemius associated with popliteal neurovascular entrapment), and ankle (e.g., flexor digitorum accessories longus associated with tibial nerve compression in the tarsal tunnel).

17.2.4 Anatomic Variations—Labrum

In the shoulder, morphological variants at the anterosuperior quadrant of the glenoid include the sublabral recess (57%), sublabral foramen (14%), and Buford complex (3%) [15].

A Buford complex is defined as absence of the anterosuperior labrum and a thickened cord-like middle glenohumeral ligament. Recognizing a Buford complex helps avoid misdiagnosis of an anterosuperior labral tear. In a patient with a Bankart lesion at the anteroinferior labrum, the anterosuperior quadrant should be evaluated with care to differentiate true superior extension of the labral tear (can be followed back to the anteroinferior glenoid rim) versus a Buford complex (absent anterosuperior labrum) (Fig. 17.2).

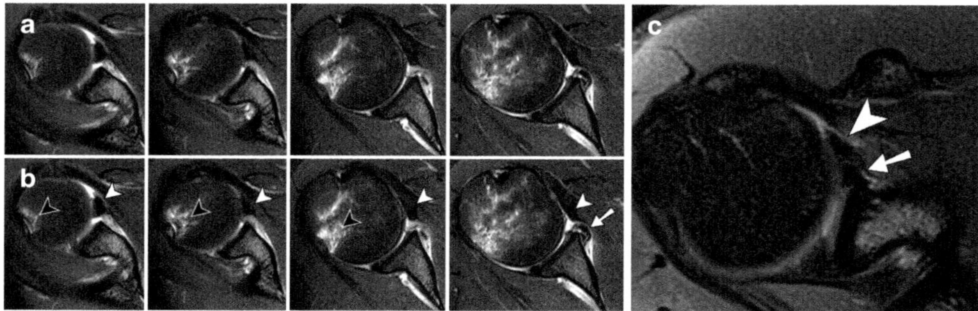

Fig. 17.2 Buford complex misinterpreted as an extensive labral tear. (**a**) Sequential axial intermediate-weighted fat-suppressed MR images of the shoulder in a patient with a history of glenohumeral dislocation. Initial radiological interpretation suggested a large Bankart lesion involving the entire anterior labrum and extending to the superior labrum, associated with a Hill-Sachs lesion. However, intraoperative findings confirmed a Bankart lesion limited to the anteroinferior labrum. The patient presented with a Buford complex, characterized by hyperplasia of the middle glenohumeral ligament and aplasia of the most cranial portion of the anterior labrum. (**b**) Annotated version: white arrowhead—hyperplastic middle glenohumeral ligament; arrow—anteroinferior glenoid labrum tear (Bankart lesion); black arrowhead—Impaction fracture at the posterosuperior aspect of the humeral head (Hill-Sachs lesion) with associated bone marrow edema. (**c**) Normal shoulder for comparison: at the cranial-most portion, both the middle glenohumeral ligament (white arrowhead) and the anterior glenoid labrum (arrow) are typically visible

The Buford complex was historically thought to be an incidental congenital variant. Recent evidence, however, suggests that the Buford complex is an acquired finding developing after childhood that may be related to shoulder instability [16]—including a 2.4× higher risk for superior labral tears (especially SLAP type II lesions) [15]. Therefore, if diagnosing a Buford complex, radiologists should scrutinize the superior labrum for a tear.

Key Point

- We are anatomists for living patients. We therefore need to know relevant normal anatomy (e.g., entheses, apophyses, ossicles) and anatomic variations (e.g., anomalous muscles). Patients with anatomic variants may deserve additional attention to avoid misdiagnosis and determine clinical significance.

17.3 Tip 3: Know Derangement Patterns and Limitations

17.3.1 Common Derangement Patterns

Important perceptual errors can occur when *multiple* abnormalities are present on one examination. Awareness of perceptual errors associated with premature satisfaction of search or excessive speed helps combat these mistakes.

What specific actions can you take? Before finalizing your report, it can be helpful to perform a secondary search to proactively look for associated diagnostic combinations. This process of looking for patterns of injury is second nature to experienced musculoskeletal radiologists.

- With knee MRI, if you see an ACL tear, scrutinize the meniscus posterior horns and posterior roots for a tear that otherwise might be overlooked (Figs. 17.3, 17.4).
- With ankle MRI, if you see pes planovalgus in an adult, a common constellation of findings includes posterior tibial tendon (PTT) tendinopathy/tearing, PTT tenosynovitis, spring (calcaneonavicular) ligament complex attenuation/tearing, sinus tarsi edema, subfibular abutment, and peritalar subluxation. (***News Flash!*** The focus of flatfoot deformity has been on PTT dysfunction for decades, but surgeons aligned with the "International Weight Bearing CT Society" recently have removed the PTT as the defining factor. They instead emphasize peritalar subluxation (i.e., dorsolateral subluxation of the entire foot beneath the talus) as the main driver of symptoms and surgical decisions for the entity they now term "progressive collapsing foot deformity" [17, 18].)

17.3.2 Limitations of Imaging

Limitations of imaging are important to recognize. A common scenario in which the MRI findings have decreased diagnostic accuracy or a discrepant association with symptoms is in the postoperative setting, including after surgery on the rotator cuff in the shoulder, the meniscus in the knee, and the labrum in the hip [19], as well as after hip arthroplasty [20].

Limitations of imaging may also be manifested with small or non-acute derangements; awareness of this issue can improve interpretations.

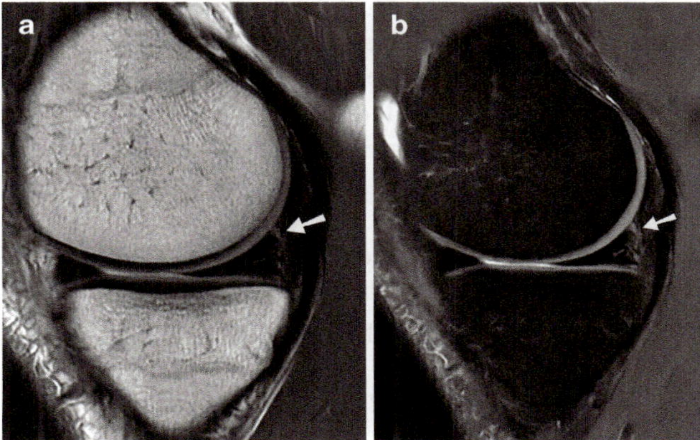

Fig. 17.4 Ramp lesion. Sagittal intermediate-weighted (**a**) and fat-suppressed intermediate-weighted (**b**) MR images of the knee demonstrate a partial vertical tear at the posterior meniscocapsular junction of the medial meniscus (arrows), consistent with a ramp lesion

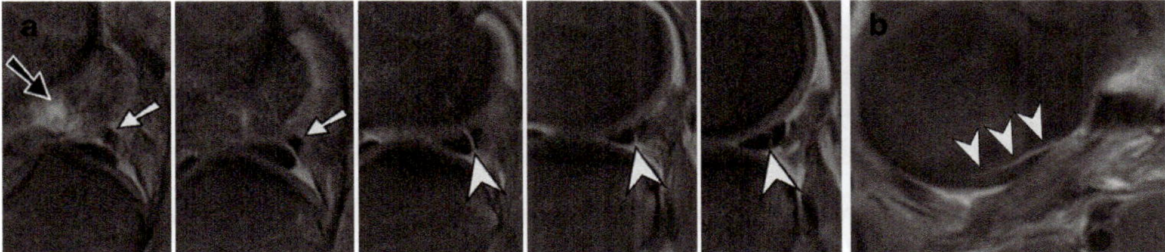

Fig. 17.3 Zip lesion. (**a**) Sequential sagittal and (**b**) axial intermediate-weighted fat-suppressed MR images demonstrate the Wrisberg ligament inserting into the posterior horn of the lateral meniscus (white arrows) and a peripheral vertical longitudinal tear of the lateral meniscus (arrowheads), consistent with a zip lesion. This lesion was not identified in the initial radiological interpretation but was confirmed intraoperatively. An associated anterior cruciate ligament (ACL) tear is also present (black arrow)

- Small calcifications and fragments (e.g., calcific tendinopathy, joint bodies, avulsion fractures) are easily missed on MRI. Correlation with radiography, CT, or sonography is often helpful. Similarly, CPPD deposition as the cause of a retro-odontoid mass and OPLL as the cause of spinal stenosis may be misdiagnosed if a cervical spine MRI is read in isolation [21].
- Cartilage derangements are missed most commonly when they are small or superficial. Vigilance is important because chondral defects can occur in essentially every synovial joint—not just the knee. Remember two helpful pointers here: (1) "conservation of matter" obliges us to look for a joint body if we see a chondral defect (and vice versa) and (2) "anywhere fluid can go, joint bodies can go", indicating that standardized search patterns should include careful inspection of joint recesses.
- Non-acute or partial tears of ligaments and tendons can be subtle, but may be clinically significant. Secondary findings can sometimes be helpful in prompting additional close inspection. Examples include anterior subluxation of the lateral tibial plateau measuring >5–7 mm (prompting evaluation for a chronic ACL tear) or an intramuscular cyst near the rotator cuff (prompting search for a partial-thickness articular-sided delaminating rotator cuff tear).

Partial tears of the ACL can be difficult to diagnose during physical examination, arthroscopy, and MRI (Fig. 17.5) [22]. On MRI, some ACL fibers remain in continuity, but the ACL may show edema, partial discontinuity, attenuation, and bowing. For partial tears involving the posterolateral bundle, helpful MRI findings can include the "footprint sign" (incomplete coverage of the ACL attachment) and the "gap sign" (high T2 signal between the mid-ACL and the lateral wall of the intercondylar notch on coronal or axial images). Supplementary MRI techniques that may help show partial tears include flexion sagittal views, double-oblique images, and 3D high-resolution images [23].

When a partial ACL tear is present on MRI, clinical correlation for functional instability is imperative. Nonoperative care is favored for clinically stable knees, particularly in low-demand patients with isolated injuries. In contrast, a lower surgical threshold is considered in the setting of objective laxity, particularly in high-demand patients (e.g., pivoting athletes) and concomitant arthroscopic indications (e.g., meniscus tear).

Key Point

- When you find an abnormality (e.g., ACL tear, adult flatfoot), a deliberate secondary search for associated derangements before finishing the case can be helpful for picking up inconspicuous imaging findings. With MRI, our diagnostic accuracy can improve when we recognize the potential challenges inherent in perceiving calcifications and joint bodies, as well as some non-acute or partial tears in ligaments and tendons.

17.4 Tip 4: Checklists and Differentials—Expect the Unexpected

Checklists and report templates have become commonplace to re-enforce the need for a systematic approach to interpretation and reporting. In the extremities, a systemic approach that works for most joints covers osteoarticular, ligamentous, musculotendinous, and neurovascular structures, as well as additional relevant findings such as fibrocartilaginous structures (e.g., meniscus, labrum) and space-occupying lesions (e.g., cyst, mass).

Given that our attention is often focused on bones, joints, and muscles, mistakes can occur if we fail to evaluate extra-articular structures, such as nerves and blood vessels.

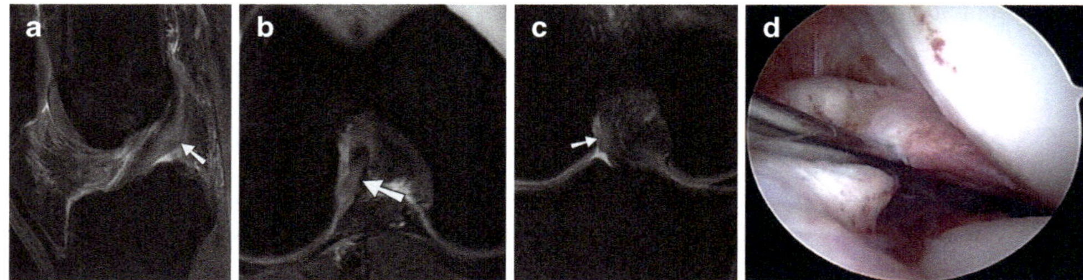

Fig. 17.5 Partial anterior cruciate ligament (ACL) tear. (**a**) Sagittal, (**b**) axial, and (**c**) coronal intermediate-weighted fat-suppressed MR images of the knee in a soccer player who sustained a knee sprain 3 days prior. The initial MRI was interpreted as normal. However, 4 weeks post-injury, the patient continued to experience pain and reported a sensation of knee instability. Clinical examination at that time revealed a grade 1 Lachman test with a soft endpoint. Retrospective MRI analysis demonstrated subtle increased signal intensity in the posterolateral fibers of the ACL across all planes (arrows). Arthroscopic evaluation (**d**) confirmed a partial discontinuity of the posterolateral ACL bundle, with associated ligamentous laxity

17.4.1 Neurovascular Derangements—Vein Thrombosis

Clinicians and radiologists may not suspect important incidental neurovascular abnormalities, such as an arterial aneurysm/pseudoaneurysm (e.g., at abdominal aorta, popliteal artery, ulnar artery) or a vein thrombosis.

With vein thrombosis, symptoms are generally non-specific, such as pain and swelling. Vein thrombosis may develop after musculoskeletal injuries due to venous stasis associated with immobilization and can be easily overlooked. Unlike Doppler ultrasound, routine musculoskeletal MRIs are not optimized for evaluation of vascular derangements.

Using a systematic approach that includes looking at the veins, a vein thrombosis can be suggested on MRI (Fig. 17.6). Characteristic findings include perivascular edema, sometimes accompanied by vein dilatation, wall thickening (>1 mm), and abnormal intraluminal signal (often T1 hypertense). The perivascular edema can result in substantial muscle edema misdiagnosed as a muscle injury or myopathy [24].

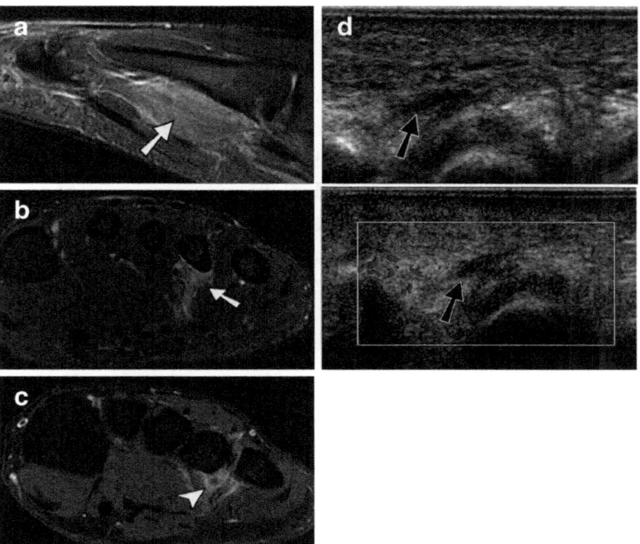

Fig. 17.6 Plantar vein thrombosis. (**a**) Sagittal and (**b**) short-axis T2-weighted fat-suppressed MR images of the forefoot in a patient presenting with metatarsalgia following strenuous hiking. Initial MRI was performed to investigate a suspected stress fracture and revealed soft tissue edema adjacent to the fourth metatarsal (white arrows), suggestive of periosteal stress-related changes. Due to persistent symptoms, a second MRI was performed 1 week later. On the short-axis T1-weighted fat-suppressed post-contrast image (**c**), a tubular structure with central non-enhancement and peripheral enhancement was observed—findings consistent with plantar vein thrombosis. Diagnosis was confirmed by Doppler ultrasound (**d**), which demonstrated an enlarged, non-compressible vein adjacent to the fourth metatarsal without detectable flow (black arrows)

In the lower extremity, vein thrombosis can be seen on routine MRIs of the foot (e.g., plantar or intermetatarsal veins, especially the lateral plantar vein), calf (e.g., peroneal, soleal, posterior tibial, and gastrocnemius veins), knee (e.g., popliteal vein), thigh (e.g., femoral vein), and hip (e.g., iliac, gluteal, and medial femoral circumflex veins) [25].

17.4.2 Differential Diagnosis

Before deciding on a diagnosis for an imaging finding, it can be helpful to ask yourself: *What else could this be?*

Like elite "superforecasters" in other fields, we can best forecast the likelihood of a challenging diagnosis when we practice active open-mindedness with cognitive flexibility and quickly filter out extraneous "noise". Three additional practices of "superforecasters" are intuitively performed by experienced radiologists interpreting an imaging abnormality: account for base-rate prevalence of a diagnosis (e.g., Bayesian pre-test probability affecting diagnostic accuracy), revise the probability of a diagnosis with the use of additional information (e.g., lab results), and then report the imaging diagnosis using explicit probabilistic language.

A broad "universal differential diagnosis" checklist of disease categories can be triggered with the mnemonic "**VINDICATE**" (**V**ascular, **I**nflammatory/**I**nfectious, **N**eoplastic, **D**egenerative, **I**diopathic/**I**atrogenic, **C**ongenital/Anatomic, **A**utoimmune, **T**raumatic, **E**ndocrine/Metabolic).

To avoid mistaken diagnosis of a malignancy (and inappropriate oncologic treatment), non-neoplastic mimics may be considered with some soft tissue masses: atypical infection, heterotopic ossification, hematoma, gouty tophus, tumoral calcinosis, and myonecrosis. Orthopedic tumor surgeons recognize that neoplasm and infection can mimic each other during clinical and imaging evaluations, and therefore they recommend a low threshold for using stains and cultures on some tissue obtained at biopsy for ruling out infection.

Conversely, when a benign fluid collection/cyst is being considered, mistakes can be avoided by ensuring the lesion is isointense with fluid and is located at an appropriate site, ideally with a connection to an underlying joint or tendon sheath (Fig. 17.7). If the lesion does not meet criteria for a simple cyst, the differential diagnosis may include high-water content neoplasms that can mimic a cyst on non-contrast MRI, such as a nerve sheath tumor, synovial sarcoma, and various myxoid neoplasms (e.g., intramuscular myxoma, myxofibrosarcoma).

Post-contrast MRI or sonography is appropriate in such cases to differentiate simple fluid collections from a high-water content neoplasm, and thereby avoid the common problem of unplanned excisions (also known as "whoops surgeries") for soft tissue sarcomas [26].

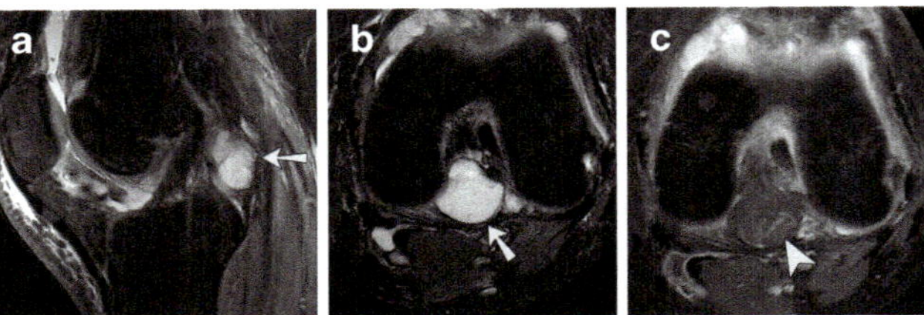

Fig. 17.7 Synovial sarcoma initially mistaken for a ganglion cyst. (**a**) Sagittal and (**b**) axial MR images of the knee demonstrate a cystic lesion in the posterior aspect of the intercondylar notch (arrows), initially interpreted as a ganglion cyst. The patient's symptoms did not resolve despite conservative treatment and corticosteroid injection. A follow-up MRI was performed, and the axial post-contrast T1-weighted fat-suppressed image (**c**) revealed thickened, irregular, and enhancing internal septations within the lesion (arrowhead). Histopathological analysis after surgical excision confirmed the diagnosis of biphasic synovial sarcoma

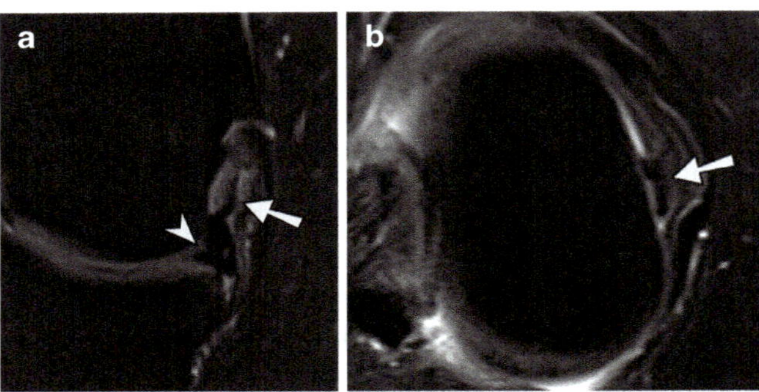

Fig. 17.8 Displaced meniscal fragment. (**a**) Coronal and (**b**) axial intermediate-weighted fat-suppressed MRI images of the knee. A tear is observed at the body of the lateral meniscus, with free edge amputation (arrowhead). The displaced meniscal fragment (arrows) was not identified in the initial MRI report and was confirmed only during arthroscopy

Key Point

- Report templates prompt us to review the entire imaging exam systematically. After identifying an imaging abnormality, keeping an open mind during patient evaluation can be particularly important when considering high-stakes diagnoses with radically different treatments (e.g., neoplasm vs. atypical infection).

17.5 Tip 5: Beware of Gorillas in Our Midst

17.5.1 When Do Checklists Fail?

Even when you conscientiously follow your structured checklist to identify abnormalities, important diagnoses can be missed. We generally only perceive imaging findings that medical training has prepared us to recognize. In other words, we look for what we know and think we might see.

As shown in numerous studies, a gorilla could be right in our midst—even in the middle of our imaging examination [27]—but we won't register it if our cognitive resources are focused on a different task. (Similar "inattentional blindness" occurs when automobile drivers look carefully on a busy road for other cars, but fail to notice bicyclists.) In radiology, mistakes can occur when analysis of complex anatomy and pathology command our attention, especially when a positive finding anchors our attention.

- At the thumb metacarpophalangeal joint, we generally recognize Stener lesions (i.e., interposition of the adductor aponeurosis between a displaced ulnar collateral ligament tear and the subjacent bone); such interposition injuries do not heal normally and are surgical indications. However, despite being clearly visible, radiologists often do not notice less familiar interposition injuries that are surgically important, such as a displaced distal MCL tear in the knee [28] and a tibial plafond fracture with the PTT interposed between the fracture fragments.
- At the knee, meniscus tears with displaced flaps are now well recognized. However, radiologists often miss less familiar patterns of fibrocartilage tears that result in displaced flaps with distinctive appearances involving the labrum of the shoulder [29] and the TFCC of the wrist [30]. Although displaced flaps usually remain connected to the underlying fibrocartilage, these flaps may flip or rotate, making them harder to recognize even when they are clearly visible (Fig. 17.8).

17.5.2 Don't Just Be a Signal Intensity Reader

The best MRI readers are both "morphology readers" and "signal intensity readers". We commonly look at "anatomy" on T1 and PD (intermediate-weighted) MRI and "pathology" on fat-suppressed fluid-sensitive images. However, we sometimes forget to pay sufficient attention to the T1 and PD images for important derangements. This is unfortunate because some derangements are missed if we focus our search for pathology to only hyperintense signal on fat-suppressed fluid-sensitive images.

The Dark Side. Be sure to look at the non-fat suppressed T1 and PD images for abnormalities, because otherwise important diagnostic findings can be missed. Indeed, fat-suppressed images may not conspicuously show some low signal findings, such as fat infiltration in muscle and fibrotic tissue (scarring) after a muscle strain.

- Fibrotic-appearing tissue can be particularly important for recognizing some tumors (e.g., plantar fascia fibromatosis, Morton neuroma). Fibrotic-appearing tissue in the knee can also be an important finding of non-acute injury (e.g., at the medial patellofemoral ligament) or prior surgery (e.g., involving the lateral patellar retinaculum or the infrapatellar fat pad of Hoffa).

Polar Bear in a Snowstorm. Another example of signal intensity failing us occurs when MRI is performed for a soft tissue mass, but we don't see a mass as expected.

- If a patient presents with a soft tissue mass, but no mass is seen at first glance, a common cause is an unencapsulated lipoma in the subcutaneous fat layer. These lesions can be hard to see because the lipoma is similar in signal intensity to the surrounding subcutaneous fat. (Lack of contrast with the surroundings also makes it hard to see a white polar bear in a snowstorm.) Two other causes to consider when a patient presents for evaluation of a soft tissue mass, but you don't see a conspicuous mass: a muscle hernia and an anomalous muscle.

Key Point

- Checklists don't prevent errors if you only see what you expect; stay open to seeing unfamiliar, surgically significant "gorillas", like interposition injuries and displaced flap tears. Complement review of fluid-sensitive images by reviewing images without fat suppression for abnormal fibrotic and fatty tissue.

17.6 Concluding Remarks

Perceptual and cognitive mistakes are common. Acknowledging mistakes are "normal" helps create a nonjudgmental culture that welcomes candid feedback and allows us to focus constructively on opportunities for improvement. Mistakes can then become lessons rather than repeats. With anatomy as a foundation, we can pursue strategies aimed at minimizing errors, including systematically analyzing injury patterns, successfully employing checklists to identify imaging abnormalities, and considering differential diagnostic possibilities when interpreting imaging findings, particularly for high-stakes diagnoses.

Take Home Messages

- Mistakes can be mitigated by acknowledging that errors are common. Focus on collecting and sharing constructive feedback to promote continuous quality improvement.
- Know normal anatomy (e.g., entheses, apophyses, ossicles) and anatomic variations (e.g., anomalous muscles). Patients with anatomic variants often deserve additional attention to avoid misdiagnosis and determine clinical significance.
- Be aware of typical injury patterns. Before finalizing your report, it can be helpful to perform a secondary search to proactively look for associated diagnostic combinations (e.g., posterior horn and root meniscus tears in a patient with an ACL tear).
- Pair a systematic approach with flexible thinking: checklists can guide us, but awareness of biases and attention lapses are important to keep us from missing what we don't expect.

Conflict of Interest I / We declare no competing interests as defined by Springer Nature, or other interests that might be perceived to influence results and/or discussion reported in this manuscript.

References

1. Gunderman RB. Bullshit. J Am Coll Radiol. 2010;7:13–5.
2. Labruto F. The radiology of happiness. Eur J Radiol. 2025;191:112288.
3. Zhang L, Wen X, Li JW, Jiang X, Yang XF, Li M. Diagnostic error and bias in the department of radiology: a pictorial essay. Insights Imaging. 2023;14:163.
4. Kim YW, Mansfield LT. Fool me twice: delayed diagnoses in radiology with emphasis on perpetuated errors. AJR Am J Roentgenol. 2014;202:465–70.
5. Waite S, Grigorian A, Alexander RG, et al. Analysis of perceptual expertise in radiology–current knowledge and a new perspective. Front Hum Neurosci. 2019;13:213.
6. Bruno MA, Walker EA, Abujudeh HH. Understanding and confronting our mistakes: the epidemiology of error in radiology and strategies for error reduction. Radiographics. 2015;35:1668–76.
7. Weber MA. Easily missed pathologies of the musculoskeletal system in the emergency radiology setting. Rofo. 2025;197:277–87.
8. Narayan A, Kaplan RM, Adashi EY. To err is human: a quarter century of progress. J Gen Intern Med. 2025;40:690–3.
9. Rockall A, Visser JJ, Garcia-Villar C, et al. Feedback in radiology: essential tool for improving user experience and providing value-based care. Insights Imaging. 2025;16:132.

10. Tomsan H, Gorbachova T, Fritz RC, Abrams GD, Sherman SL, Shea KG, Boutin RD. Knee MRI: meniscus roots, ramps, repairs, and repercussions. Radiographics. 2023;43:e220208.
11. Albishi W, Albusayes N, Alsabbagh L, et al. Awareness, prevalence, and magnetic resonance imaging landmarks of the aberrant anterior Tibial artery of the knee. Orthop J Sports Med. 2025;13:23259671251374304.
12. Marin-Concha J, Rengifo P, Tapia P, Kaiser D, Siepmann T. Prevalence and characteristics of the aberrant anterior tibial artery: a single-center magnetic resonance imaging study and scoping review. BMC Musculoskelet Disord. 2021;22:922.
13. Zandee van Rilland ED, Payne SR, Gorbachova T, Shea KG, Sherman SL, Boutin RD. MRI of patellar stabilizers: anatomic visibility, inter-reader reliability, and intra-reader reproducibility of primary and secondary ligament anatomy. Skeletal Radiol. 2024;53:555–66.
14. Boutin RD, Chang J, Bateni C, Giza E, Wisner ER, Yao L. The notch of Harty (Pseudodefect of the Tibial plafond): frequency and characteristic findings at MRI of the ankle. AJR Am J Roentgenol. 2015;205:358–63.
15. Benes M, Kachlik D, Kopp L, Kunc V. Prevalence of the anterosuperior capsulolabral anatomical variations and their association with pathologies of the glenoid labrum: a systematic review and meta-analysis. Arch Orthop Trauma Surg. 2023;143:6295–303.
16. Scott JA, Dwek JR, Cheng KY, Bryan TP, Edmonds EW. The Buford complex redefined: a pathologic morphology in sheep's clothing. Orthop J Sports Med. 2024;12:23259671241252834.
17. de Cesar Netto C, Barbachan Mansur NS, et al. From asymptomatic flatfoot to progressive collapsing foot deformity: peritalar subluxation is the main driver of symptoms. J Bone Joint Surg Am. 2025;107:2060–8.
18. Hong VY, Lee DC, Smith RW, Harris TG. So what exactly is progressive collapsing foot deformity? J Am Acad Orthop Surg. 2025;33:e940–8.
19. Kim CO, Dietrich TJ, Zingg PO, Dora C, Pfirrmann CWA, Sutter R. Arthroscopic hip surgery: frequency of postoperative MR Arthrographic findings in asymptomatic and symptomatic patients. Radiology. 2017;283:779–88.
20. Germann C, Filli L, Jungmann PM, et al. Prospective and longitudinal evolution of postoperative periprosthetic findings on metal artifact-reduced MR imaging in asymptomatic patients after uncemented total hip arthroplasty. Skeletal Radiol. 2021;50:1177–88.
21. Kakitsubata Y, Boutin RD, Theodorou DJ, et al. Calcium pyrophosphate dihydrate crystal deposition in and around the atlantoaxial joint: association with type 2 odontoid fractures in nine patients. Radiology. 2000;216:213–9.
22. Volokhina YV, Syed HM, Pham PH, Blackburn AK. Two helpful MRI signs for evaluation of posterolateral bundle tears of the anterior cruciate ligament: a pilot study. Orthop J Sports Med. 2015;3:2325967115597641.
23. Griffith JF, Leung CTP, Lee JCH, Leung JCS, Yeung DKW, Yung PSH. Positional MR imaging of normal and injured knees. Eur Radiol. 2023;33:1553–64.
24. Zandee van Rilland ED, Yao L, Stevens KJ, Chung LS, Fiorentino DF, Boutin RD. Myositis and its mimics: guideline updates, MRI characteristics, and new horizons. AJR Am J Roentgenol. 2024;223:e2431359.
25. Leão RV, Bernal ECBA, Rodrigues MB, et al. Venous thrombosis: a mimic of musculoskeletal injury on MR imaging. Skeletal Radiol. 2023;52:1263–76.
26. Nakamura T, Hasegawa M. Unplanned excision in soft tissue sarcoma: current knowledge and remaining gaps. Diagnostics (Basel). 2025;15:453.
27. Drew T, Võ ML, Wolfe JM. The invisible gorilla strikes again: sustained inattentional blindness in expert observers. Psychol Sci. 2013;24:1848–53.
28. Boutin RD, Fritz RC, Walker REA, Pathria MN, Marder RA, Yao L. Tears in the distal superficial medial collateral ligament: the wave sign and other associated MRI findings. Skeletal Radiol. 2020;49:747–56.
29. Stewart JK, Taylor DC, Vinson EN. Magnetic resonance imaging and clinical features of glenoid labral flap tears. Skeletal Radiol. 2017;46:1095–100.
30. Boutin RD, Fritz RC. Displaced flap tears of the triangular fibrocartilage complex: frequency, flap location, and the "comma" sign on wrist MRI. AJR Am J Roentgenol. 2021;217:707–8.

Peripheral Nerve Imaging

18

Roman Guggenberger and Amelie Lutz

Learning Objectives

- Understand the basic principles and protocols of MRN.
- Describe different fat suppression techniques and their relevance for peripheral nerve imaging.
- Identify characteristic MRI findings in nerve trauma, entrapment, and tumors.
- Apply the MRN-RADS system for standardized reporting of peripheral nerve tumors.
- Appreciate the role of DESS and deep-learning reconstruction in modern MRN.
- Recognize the complementary role of ultrasound in peripheral nerve imaging.

18.1 Introduction

Peripheral nerves have traditionally been difficult to image due to their small size and complex course. Advances in MRI technology, particularly dedicated MRN techniques, have revolutionized the ability to visualize peripheral nerves in vivo [1]. MRI now plays a central role in the evaluation of trauma, entrapment neuropathies, inflammatory conditions, and tumors. While ultrasound offers rapid, dynamic, and cost-effective assessment of superficial nerves, MRI remains indispensable for deep structures, plexus evaluation, and comprehensive pre-surgical planning [2].

R. Guggenberger (✉)
Department of Radiology and Nuclear Medicine, Cantonal Hospital Winterthur, Winterthur, Switzerland
e-mail: roman.guggenberger@ksw.ch

A. Lutz
Department of Radiology, Cantonal Hospital Münsterlingen, Münsterlingen, Switzerland
e-mail: amelie.lutz@team-radiologie.ch

18.2 MRI Techniques

18.2.1 General Considerations

MRN is technically demanding due to their small caliber, long course, and surrounding fat and muscle. Careful optimization of protocols is therefore crucial. Modern scanners (≥1.5 T, ideally 3 T) with dedicated multi-channel coils provide the required spatial resolution. Typical in-plane resolution should be 0.3–0.6 mm, with thin slices (<3 mm) and a high signal-to-noise ratio. Patient positioning should ensure coverage of the region of interest while minimizing motion.

Scan coverage should be tailored to the specific clinical question and may be significantly different from standard MR imaging. As illustrated in Fig. 18.1, coverage of the lumbar spine is different from MRN of pelvic nerves. A larger field-of-view should be applied for the lumbosacral plexus in order to include the L2 nerve root at minimum and the minor trochanters inferiorly.

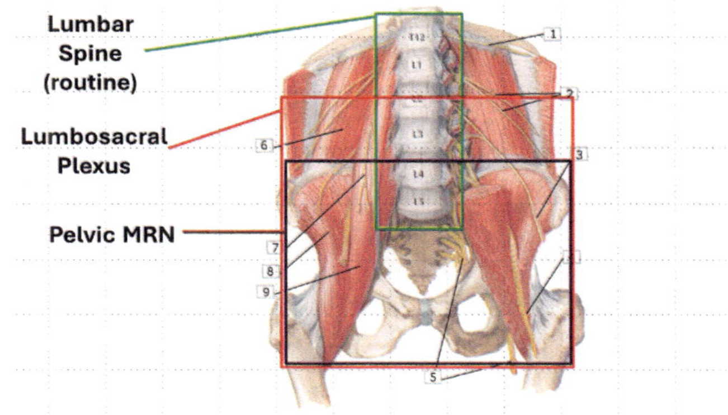

Fig. 18.1 The scan field-of-view should be tailored to the specific clinical questions and body regions. For example, in order to assess the lumbosacral plexus at least the L2 nerve root should be included cranially

18.2.2 Conventional Sequences

- T1-weighted imaging: Provides excellent anatomical detail, depiction of surrounding fat, and continuity with adjacent structures.
- T2-weighted imaging with fat suppression: Essential for detecting pathology, with diseased nerves showing T2 hyperintensity and swelling.
- Proton-density (PD)-weighted imaging: may provide fast anatomic overview, less nerve-specific.
- STIR (Short Tau Inversion Recovery): Robust, homogeneous fat suppression, particularly useful for plexus imaging.
- Gradient echo (GRE): May help detect hemosiderin or calcification in chronic trauma.

18.2.3 Fat Suppression Techniques

Reliable fat suppression is a cornerstone of MRN. Because nerves run adjacent to fat, suppression is essential for contrast. Different methods should be chosen according to anatomy and field strength:

- STIR: Very robust, less sensitive to field inhomogeneities, best for large fields of view but with lower SNR.
- CHESS (frequency-selective): High SNR, fast, but prone to inhomogeneity at 3 T or near implants.
- SPAIR: More homogeneous than CHESS, robust at 3 T, widely used in extremity imaging.
- Dixon techniques: Water-fat separation providing uniform suppression even in difficult regions; versatile, increasingly preferred for MR neurography.

18.2.4 Vascular Suppression Techniques

While larger, fast-flow vessels may be easily identified due to flow-voids, smaller peripheral or low-flow blood vessels have an intrinsically high signal on T2-weighted MR-images and may easily be misdiagnosed as a peripheral nerve. However, there are different options in order to suppress vascular signals each with specific advantages and limitations as listed in Table 18.1. While techniques 1–3 do not require intravenous contrast agent, approaches 4 and 5 are efficient alternatives after intravenous administration of either Gadolinium [3] or superparamagnetic iron oxide (SPIO) particles [4, 5].

18.2.5 MR Neurography (MRN)

Dedicated MRN protocols especially for brachial and lumbosacral plexus imaging use morphologic 3D isotropic fat-suppressed T2-weighted sequences such as 3D STIR images allowing for multiplanar reformats (MPR) and maximum-intensity projections (MIP) with long-segment nerve tracking (Fig. 18.2), in addition to T1-weighted or PD-weighted 2D or 3D sequences.

Functional diffusion-weighted imaging (DWI) highlights nerves due to restricted diffusion and may help in differentiating benign from malignant peripheral nerve sheath tumors, while diffusion tensor imaging (DTI) provides information on fascicular nerve integrity with possible visualization through tractography [6, 7] (Fig. 18.3).

Recent Double Echo Steady State (DESS) and similar steady-state sequences provide high-resolution 3D datasets with strong T2/T1 weighting. They are especially useful for cranial and cervical nerve imaging (Fig. 18.4). Advantages

Table 18.1 There are different options in order to suppress vascular signals each with specific advantages and limitations: while techniques 1–3 do not require intravenous contrast agent, approaches 4 and 5 are efficient alternatives after intravenous administration of either Gadolinium or SPIO particles

Technique	Advantages	Limitations	Best use cases
MSDE (Motion-Sensitized Driven Equilibrium)	Suppresses vascular and CSF flow; improves nerve conspicuity in complex regions	May reduce SNR; sensitive to motion artifacts	Brachial or lumbosacral plexus imaging; cranial/cervical nerves
DP-TSE (Diffusion-Prepared Turbo Spin Echo)	Suppresses vascular flow; provides good nerve-to-background contrast	Longer scan times; less widely available	Plexus imaging requiring strong vessel suppression
SHINKEI (nerve-SHeath signal increased with INKed rest-tissue RARE imaging)	Combines fat and vascular suppression; excellent nerve conspicuity, high contrast	Vendor-dependent availability; longer acquisition times	Advanced clinical MRN of plexus and cranial nerves; high-resolution protocols
IV Gadolinium (post-contrast vascular suppression)	Enhances vessels; with STIR/Dixon suppression, vessels can be distinguished or subtracted from nerves	Requires contrast administration; subtle nerve enhancement may confound interpretation	Differentiation of nerves vs. small vessels; evaluation of inflammatory or tumoral infiltration
Resovist (Peripheral Nerve Imaging Superparamagnetic Iron Oxide, SPIO)	Strong T2* shortening of intravascular signal; near-complete vascular suppression while preserving nerves	Limited clinical availability; regulatory restrictions in many regions	Research MRN protocols where vessel suppression is critical, e.g., plexus and deep nerve studies

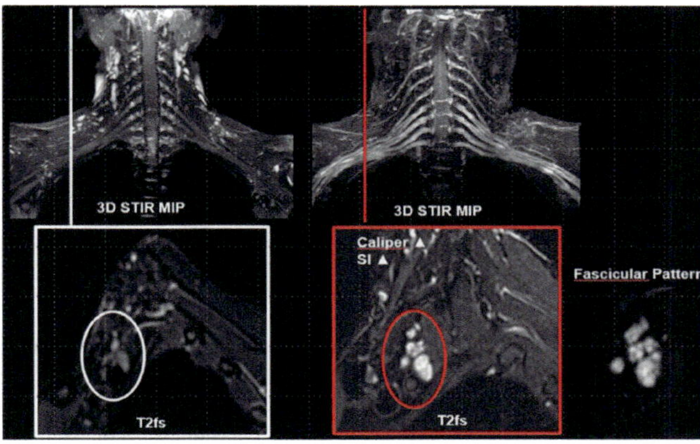

Fig. 18.2 MRN of the brachial plexus in a normal patient (left) and a patient with chronic demyelinating inflammatory polyneuropathy (CIDP, right). Note increased signal intensity and nerve caliper with marked heterogeneity of nerve fascicles that can be perceived by using MPR and MIP techniques of 3D STIR images

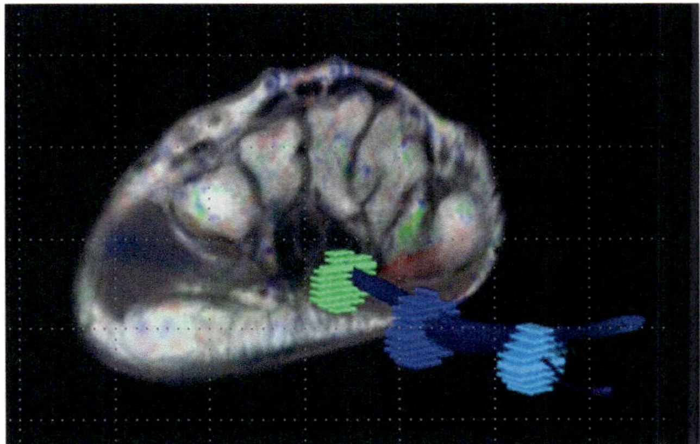

Fig. 18.3 Diffusion tensor imaging (DTI) provides information on fascicular nerve integrity with possible visualization through tractography

include high spatial resolution and relatively fast acquisition, but fat suppression is less robust. Recent studies have shown that DESS with deep-learning reconstruction at 1.5 T can achieve image quality comparable to post-contrast STIR for cranial nerves [8].

18.2.6 Deep Learning–Based Reconstruction

Deep-learning (DL) reconstruction is increasingly applied to MR neurography. These algorithms reduce noise, allow shorter scan times, and enhance nerve conspicuity. Applications include improving the diagnostic quality of DESS and Dixon techniques, especially at 1.5 T, and enabling pediatric and plexus imaging where time is critical. Limitations include vendor variability and the need for standardization [9].

18.2.7 Contrast-Enhanced Imaging

Gadolinium is not routinely required but may be valuable in tumor characterization, inflammatory or infectious neuropathies, and to distinguish recurrent tumor from fibrosis.

18.3 Peripheral Nerve Imaging—What Are We Looking For?

18.3.1 Size/Caliber

A normal peripheral nerve typically has a caliber comparable to adjacent arteries. This is best assessed on axial/nerve-orthogonal slices. Under normal conditions, peripheral

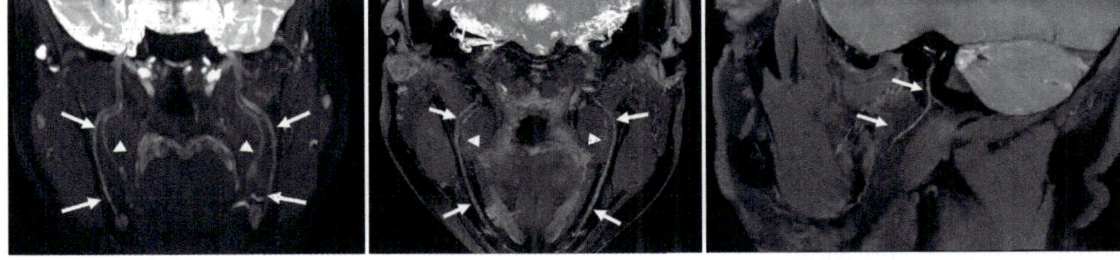

Fig. 18.4 Recent Double Echo Steady State (DESS) and similar steady-state sequences provide high-resolution 3D datasets with strong T2/T1 weighting and nerve conspicuity. The inferior alveolar nerve (arrows) and the lingual nerve (arrowheads) in STIR (left) and DESS (middle) can be nicely delineated on both with slightly higher conspicuity on DESS. The facial nerve can be nicely depicted with DESS (right) at its exit from the skull base and ramifications in the parotid gland (arrows)

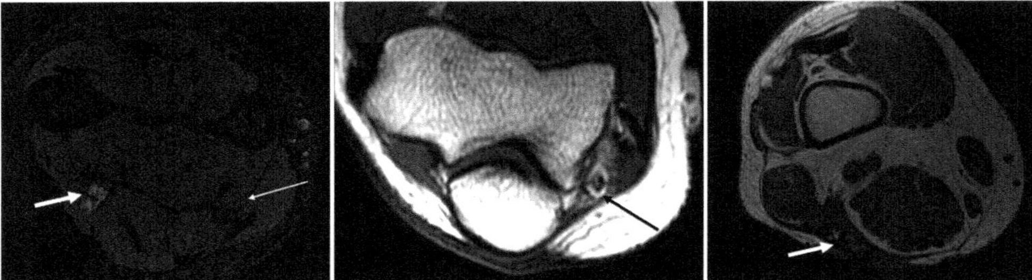

Fig. 18.5 Tra T2-w fat saturated image (left) of a neuropathic ulnar nerve at the level of the distal forearm post neurotmesis injury more proximally. Depicted are the typical T2-signal increase of the nerve fascicles which also show variable caliber sizes, altogether contributing to the enlarged size of nerve (short thick arrow). As a negative internal control the normal median nerve demonstrates normal caliber, uniform fascicle size, and normal T2 signal (long thin arrow). Tra T1-w image (middle) of a normal ulnar nerve at the level of the elbow. The nerve, depicted just below the cubital tunnel, demonstrates a normal, 360-degree fat plane (thin black arrow). This fat plane enables smooth gliding of the nerve with arm movement. Tra T1-w image (right) of a distal sciatic nerve just proximal to its division at the level of the distal femur. The nerve demonstrates an abnormal surrounding thick layer of T1-hypointense fibrosis (thick short white arrow) which developed several years post-neuroplasty during myxoid liposarcoma resection at the distal posterior thigh

nerves gradually taper from proximal to distal. This fundamental principle is often helpful in identifying the site of pathology, particularly in compressive or entrapment syndromes, where nerve diameter may increase proximal to the site of compression. Both focal and diffuse nerve enlargements may indicate underlying pathology. In situations where the nerve remains consistently larger than the adjacent artery over an extended segment, the reader may mistakenly interpret it as a "well-visualized" normal nerve. However, persistent nerve enlargement relative to adjacent arteries is in itself pathological, and such diffuse thickening should raise suspicion for inflammatory or infectious etiologies [10].

18.3.2 Nerve-Intrinsic Signal Intensity

The second key criterion is nerve signal intensity. On T1-weighted and T2-weighted images, a normal nerve appears isointense to skeletal muscle. On T2-weighted fat-suppressed images, the normal signal ranges from isointense to mildly hyperintense. On 3D FSE sequences, normal peripheral nerves appear uniformly and symmetrically hyperintense. Pathology is suggested by more pronounced T2 hyperintensity, approaching the signal intensity of adjacent veins. Any increase in nerve signal intensity should be regarded as suspicious, unless explained by technical artifacts such as in suboptimal fat suppression.

18.3.3 Fascicular Pattern

The fascicular pattern of peripheral nerves can be visualized on high-resolution MR images (Fig. 18.5a–c). This is particularly well seen on axial T1- and T2-weighted sequences. The fascicular pattern should always be identifiable and should never be obliterated. Enlargement or disruption of single or multiple fascicles strongly suggests pathology (Fig. 18.5a–c). Similarly, diffuse loss of fascicular architecture should raise concern. Experienced readers develop an intuitive understanding of normal fascicular patterns across various anatomical locations. Trainees are encouraged to practice evaluating peripheral nerve anatomy and signal characteristics on every scan, even when MR neurography is not the primary indication. For example, while reviewing standard joint MRI examinations, one should assess the size, signal intensity, and fascicular pattern of major nerves within the field of view to develop the understanding of normal nerve imaging appearance.

18.3.4 Course

Normal peripheral nerves exhibit a smooth trajectory without significant deviations. They give rise to relatively few branches, and the major branches of large nerves follow predictable courses toward their target muscles. In contrast, wavy paths, sharp angulations, or diffuse branching are abnormal. A bifid configuration may occur as a normal variant, for example, in the pelvis where the sciatic nerve may divide into two components [11, 12]. Any focal or diffuse deviation or abrupt angulation should be considered suspicious for pathology.

18.3.5 Continuity

A normal peripheral nerve demonstrates uninterrupted continuity. Any discontinuity indicates abnormality. However, artifacts—especially those associated with nearby metallic implants—may mimic discontinuity and should not be misinterpreted. True nerve disruption is usually readily apparent. Nonetheless, precise grading of traumatic nerve injuries according to the Seddon–Sunderland classification remains challenging, even when advanced techniques such as DTI sequences are employed.

18.3.6 Perineural Fat

Peripheral nerves are normally enveloped by a distinct fat plane (Fig. 18.5b–c). Depending on the anatomical site, this layer may be thick or thin and may sometimes be difficult to visualize, for instance, in slender patients or when the nerve courses adjacent to skeletal muscle (e.g., in the forearm). Abnormal findings include perineural stranding on T1- or T2-weighted images or encasement of a peripheral nerve, particularly following surgery or penetrating trauma. Chronic external compression may also result in perineural fibrosis or scarring, which is important to recognize as it may impede spontaneous recovery. Axial/nerve-orthogonal slices are often optimal for detecting perineural fat effacement.

18.3.7 Contrast Enhancement

Under normal conditions, peripheral nerves do not enhance after intravenous administration of gadolinium-based contrast agents due to the integrity of the blood–nerve barrier. Exceptions include sites with physiologic barrier deficiency, such as the dorsal root ganglia. In cases of tumors or infection, disruption of this blood-nerve barrier results in focal or diffuse enhancement. Opinions differ regarding the routine use of gadolinium in MR neurography. Some practitioners reserve contrast for specific indications, such as postoperative assessment or suspected inflammatory/infectious disease. Others advocate routine administration to increase overall sensitivity for neuropathology. While routine use may be advantageous when clinical history is vague or nonspecific, it also increases scan costs and carries the small but real risks associated with gadolinium exposure.

18.3.8 Muscles

Muscle denervation represents a downstream consequence of neurogenic pathology. Identifying the affected muscles and understanding their innervation can help localize the site of nerve injury. In the acute or subacute phase, denervation manifests as muscle edema with increased T2 signal, often without volume loss. With chronicity, progressive fatty infiltration and atrophy develop. Importantly, such changes occur only in neuropathies affecting motor branches; purely sensory neuropathies do not result in muscle denervation. Comprehensive evaluation of muscles within the scan field is therefore critical, though readers should remain mindful that some denervation changes may lie beyond the imaged region.

18.4 Common Clinical Applications

18.4.1 Nerve Trauma

Acute posttraumatic nerve changes include nerve swelling and T2 hyperintensity; chronic changes include fibrosis, discontinuity, and neuroma formation. Traumatic nerve injuries are commonly classified according to the Seddon-Sunderland classification [13]. Class I and II injuries correspond to Seddon's original neuropraxia and axonotmesis, respectively. Class III-V lesions are included in Seddon's neurotmesis. Class III lesions have lesions of the endoneurium but the perineurium and epineurium remain intact. Class IV lesions have damage to the perineurium in addition to Class III lesions. Class V lesions are the most severe lesions with complete nerve transection. Class IV and V lesions typically lead to significant nerve dysfunction and usually require immediate surgical treatment. Class I-III lesions can be treated conservatively. Associated muscle denervation progresses from edema (acute) to fatty atrophy (chronic).

MRI is able to assess pathologic nerve changes associated with all degrees of nerve injury, but may only be able to differentiate low- from high-grade injuries with high inter-reader agreement [14]. Precise differentiation between, e.g., Seddon-Sunderland class III and IV remains challenging. Thus, the most crucial role of MRN is in differentiating low-grade PNI, which have good potential for partial to full recovery and is often managed conservatively with physical therapy, from high-grade PNI in which there is no recovery potential and requires operative management.

18.4.2 Entrapment Neuropathies

MRI complements ultrasound in entrapments such as carpal tunnel, cubital tunnel, and peroneal entrapment. Nerve compression at characteristic anatomical sites results in entrapment neuropathies [12, 15, 16], most commonly chronic in nature. Classic examples include carpal tunnel and cubital tunnel syndromes, but many other sites may be affected, such as the pelvic floor, popliteal fossa, tarsal tunnel, dorsal foot, thoracic outlet, infraclavicular region, quadrilateral space, elbow, forearm, and canal of Guyon. Compression disrupts endoneurial fluid flow and venous drainage, causing vascular congestion and hyperemia at and proximal to the compression site, findings mirrored by MR neurography signal changes. Unlike acute neuropathies, entrapment syndromes evolve through prolonged or repetitive pressure, as peripheral nerves tolerate only minimal external compression. Venous outflow is impaired above 15 mmHg, arterial inflow at >40 mmHg, and irreversible structural damage occurs at ~80 mmHg [17]. Chronic compression may lead to demyelination, axonal loss, Wallerian degeneration, infarction, and fibrosis [18]. Spontaneous recovery in chronic entrapment neuropathies is rare; however, surgical decompression may yield favorable outcomes if performed before irreversible changes occur, typically characterized by fat or fibrous proliferation around axons [19]. Typical findings include nerve enlargement, fascicular loss, T2 hyperintensity, and denervation of target muscles.

18.4.3 Plexus Lesions

MRI is indispensable for brachial and lumbosacral plexus assessment. Traumatic causes include root avulsions and ruptures; tumoral causes include plexus involvement by lymphoma, metastases, or nerve sheath tumors. But plexus involvement is also commonly seen in acute and chronic autoimmune disease-related entities [20]. Contrast-enhanced MRN adds diagnostic value.

18.4.4 Tumors and Tumor-Like Lesions

- Peripheral nerve sheath tumors (schwannomas, neurofibromas) often show fusiform shape, target sign, and continuity with a parent nerve. Malignant peripheral nerve sheath tumors (MPNST) are larger, heterogeneous, and invasive with perilesional edema (Fig. 18.6). DTI can be particularly helpful in the tumor setting. It allows for quantitative analysis of tumor stroma parameters such as mean diffusivity (or ADC) which can help guide the differentiation between non-aggressive and aggressive tumor entities. Furthermore, tractography can help the surgeons conceptualize the expected surgical situs (Fig. 18.7) [21, 22].

18.4.5 MRN-RADS

The MR Neurography Reporting and Data System (MRN-RADS) [10] provides a structured system for peripheral nerve sheath tumor evaluation:

- Score 1: Benign features.
- Score 2: Indeterminate, low suspicion.
- Score 3: Suspicious, follow-up or biopsy indicated.
- Score 4: Highly suspicious for malignancy.

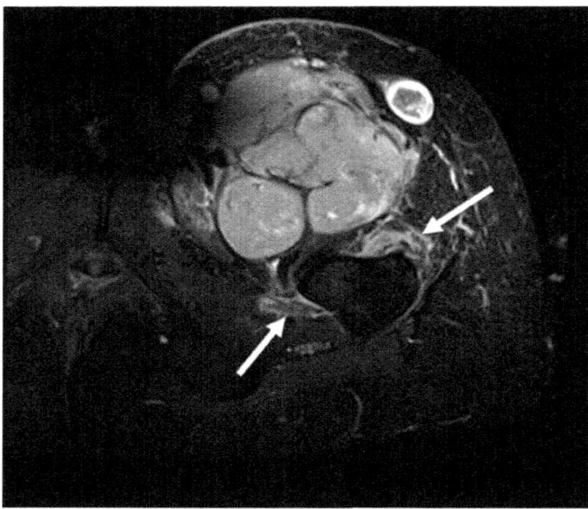
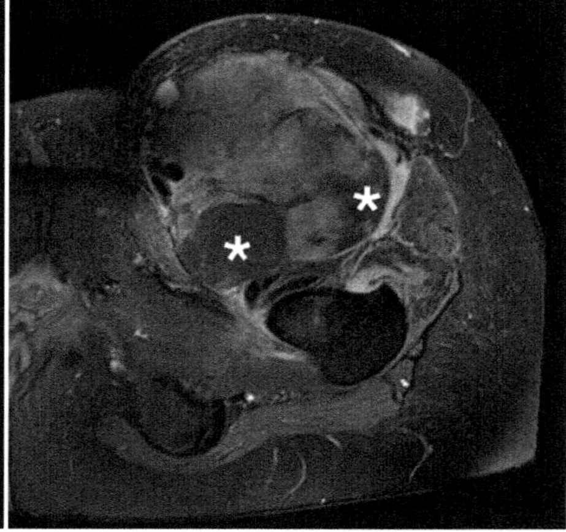

Fig. 18.6 Tra T2-w fat-saturated image (left) and T1-w fat-saturated after iv-Gd image (right) of a malignant peripheral nerve sheath tumor in the left groin. Note substantial heterogeneity of tumor with perilesional edema (arrow) and necrotic areas without contrast uptake (asterisks)

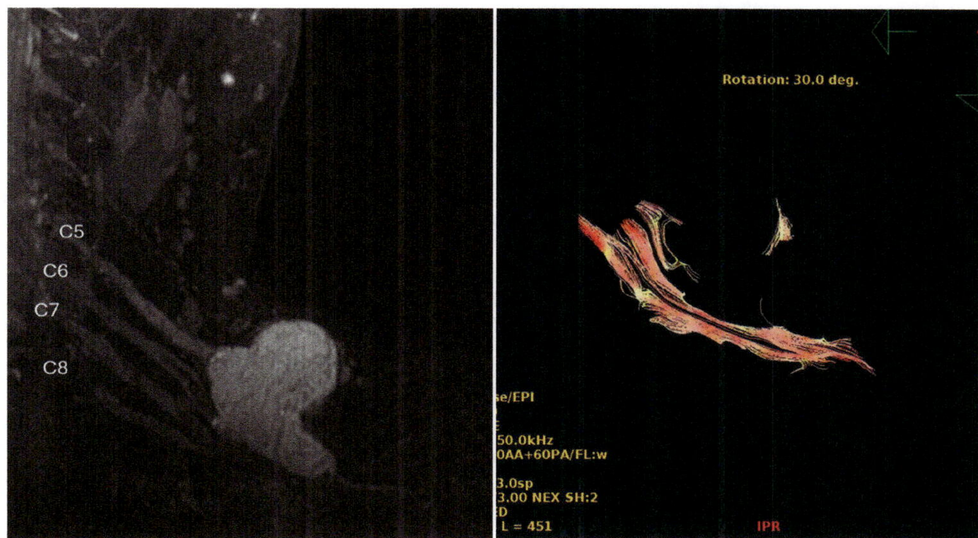

Fig. 18.7 MIP of MSDE-CUBE-FLEX (left) of a recurrent mixed nerve-sheath tumor involving the left brachial plexus in a 47 yo male. Corresponding tractography image from multi-shot EPI (right) to help guiding the surgical approach of the tumor demonstrating nerve damage/involvement of mainly C5 and C6 as well as deviation of C7

18.5 Ultrasound (Brief Overview)

High-resolution ultrasound is valuable for superficial and dynamic nerve evaluation but cannot assess deep structures or plexus lesions. It complements MRI but does not replace it.

18.6 Concluding Remarks

MRI has transformed peripheral nerve imaging, enabling detailed visualization of nerve anatomy and pathology. MR neurography is essential for trauma, entrapments, plexus lesions, and tumors. MRN-RADS supports structured reporting. Ultrasound remains useful for superficial nerves but MRI is the gold standard.

18.7 Future Perspectives

Future developments will further refine MR neurography. Deep-learning reconstruction will enable shorter, higher-quality scans and routine use of advanced 3D sequences such as DESS and Dixon-based techniques, even at 1.5 T. MRN-RADS will enhance reproducibility and clinical integration. The convergence of novel pulse sequences, AI-enhanced reconstruction, and structured reporting will shape the next generation of fast, reproducible, and clinically actionable MR neurography.

Take Home Messages

- MRI is the modality of choice for peripheral nerve imaging, particularly in deep or complex regions.
- Robust fat suppression (STIR, Dixon, SPAIR) is critical for nerve visualization.
- MR neurography with isotropic 3D fat-suppressed sequences is essential for multiplanar evaluation and producing maximum intensity projections for fast side-by-side comparison.
- DESS and deep-learning reconstruction expand imaging capabilities, especially for cranial and cervical nerves.
- MRN-RADS standardizes neuropathy and tumor evaluation with malignancy risk stratification.
- Ultrasound remains complementary but limited to superficial nerves.

Conflict of Interest I/We declare no competing interests as defined by Springer Nature, or other interests that might be perceived to influence results and/or discussion reported in this manuscript.

References

1. Kollmer J, Bendszus M, Pham M. MR neurography: diagnostic imaging in the PNS. Clin Neuroradiol. 2015;25(Suppl 2):283–9. https://doi.org/10.1007/s00062-015-0412-0.

2. Chhabra A, et al. MR neurography: past, present, and future. AJR Am J Roentgenol. 2011;197(3):583–91. https://doi.org/10.2214/AJR.10.6012.
3. Zhang Y, Kong X, Zhao Q, Liu X, Gu Y, Xu L. Enhanced MR neurography of the lumbosacral plexus with robust vascular suppression and improved delineation of its small branches. Eur J Radiol. 2020;129:109128. https://doi.org/10.1016/j.ejrad.2020.109128.
4. Kaniewska M, Deininger-Czermak E, Ensle F, Donati OF, Guggenberger R. Delayed ferumoxtran-10-enhanced magnetic resonance neurography of the lumbosacral plexus: impact on vascular suppression and image quality. J Magn Reson Imaging. 2025;61(4):1677–80. https://doi.org/10.1002/jmri.29604.
5. Pedrick EG, Sneag DB, Colucci PG, Duong M, Tan ET. Three-dimensional MR neurography of the brachial plexus: vascular suppression with low-dose ferumoxytol. Radiology. 2023;307(1):e221087. https://doi.org/10.1148/radiol.221087.
6. Jeon T, Fung MM, Koch KM, Tan ET, Sneag DB. Peripheral nerve diffusion tensor imaging: overview, pitfalls, and future directions. J Magn Reson Imaging. 2018;47(5):1171–89. https://doi.org/10.1002/jmri.25876.
7. Fritz J, Ahlawat S. Getting quantitative diffusion-weighted MR neurography and tractography ready for clinical practice. J Magn Reson Imaging. 2020;51(4):1138–9. https://doi.org/10.1002/jmri.26930.
8. Ensle F, et al. 3D MR neurography of craniocervical nerves: comparing double-echo steady-state and postcontrast STIR with deep learning-based reconstruction at 1.5T. AJNR Am J Neuroradiol. 2025;46(9):1908–16. https://doi.org/10.3174/ajnr.A8750.
9. Ensle F, Kaniewska M, Tiessen A, Lohezic M, Getzmann JM, Guggenberger R. Diagnostic performance of deep learning-based reconstruction algorithm in 3D MR neurography. Skeletal Radiol. 2023;52(12):2409–18. https://doi.org/10.1007/s00256-023-04362-z.
10. Chhabra A, et al. Neuropathy score reporting and data system (NS-RADS): MRI reporting guideline of peripheral neuropathy explained and reviewed. Skeletal Radiol. 2022;51(10):1909–22. https://doi.org/10.1007/s00256-022-04061-1.
11. Bartret AL, Beaulieu CF, Lutz AM. Is it painful to be different? Sciatic nerve anatomical variants on MRI and their relationship to piriformis syndrome. Eur Radiol. 2018;28(11):4681–6. https://doi.org/10.1007/s00330-018-5447-6.
12. Albano D, et al. Imaging of elbow entrapment neuropathies. Insights Imaging. 2025;16(1):24. https://doi.org/10.1186/s13244-025-01901-1.
13. Chhabra A, Ahlawat S, Belzberg A, Andreseik G. Peripheral nerve injury grading simplified on MR neurography: as referenced to Seddon and Sunderland classifications. Indian J Radiol Imaging. 2014;24(3):217–24. https://doi.org/10.4103/0971-3026.137025.
14. Pitman J, Fayad LM, Dabiri M, Ahlawat S. Classification of peripheral nerve injury. Magn Reson Imaging Clin N Am. 2025;33(3):427–36. https://doi.org/10.1016/j.mric.2025.03.003.
15. Andreisek G, Burg D, Studer A, Weishaupt D. Upper extremity peripheral neuropathies: role and impact of MR imaging on patient management. Eur Radiol. 2008;18(9):1953–61. https://doi.org/10.1007/s00330-008-0940-y.
16. Kumar S, Mangi MD, Zadow S, Lim W. Nerve entrapment syndromes of the lower limb: a pictorial review. Insights Imaging. 2023;14(1):166. https://doi.org/10.1186/s13244-023-01514-6.
17. Filler AG, et al. Magnetic resonance neurography. Lancet. 1993;341(8846):659–61. https://doi.org/10.1016/0140-6736(93)90422-d.
18. Beaulieu C, Does MD, Snyder RE, Allen PS. Changes in water diffusion due to Wallerian degeneration in peripheral nerve. Magn Reson Med. 1996;36(4):627–31. https://doi.org/10.1002/mrm.1910360419.
19. Thawait SK, et al. Peripheral nerve surgery: the role of high-resolution MR neurography. AJNR Am J Neuroradiol. 2012;33(2):203–10. https://doi.org/10.3174/ajnr.A2465.
20. Shibuya K, et al. Reconstruction magnetic resonance neurography in chronic inflammatory demyelinating polyneuropathy. Ann Neurol. 2015;77(2):333–7. https://doi.org/10.1002/ana.24314.
21. Ahlawat S, Blakeley JO, Rodriguez FJ, Fayad LM. Imaging biomarkers for malignant peripheral nerve sheath tumors in neurofibromatosis type 1. Neurology. 2019;93(11):e1076–84. https://doi.org/10.1212/WNL.0000000000008092.
22. Debs P, Fayad LM, Ahlawat S. MR neurography of peripheral nerve tumors and tumor-mimics. Semin Roentgenol. 2022;57(3):232–40. https://doi.org/10.1053/j.ro.2022.01.008.

Pediatric and Adolescent MSK Radiology: Top Ten Diagnoses Not to Miss

19

J. Herman Kan and John A. Carrino

Learning Objectives
This review will cover ten important musculoskeletal radiology topics seen in children, including adolescent hip dysplasia, osteomyelitis/septic arthritis, chronic nonbacterial osteomyelitis, chondroblastoma, tenosynovial giant cell tumor, child abuse, slipped capital femoral epiphysis, Salter-Harris injuries, spondylolysis, and osteoid osteoma.

19.1 Introduction

Diagnosis and treatment of musculoskeletal conditions in children requires an understanding of how the growing skeleton may cause or react to stress, inflammation, and tumor-like processes. The purpose of this radiology-focused review is to cover ten important pediatric and adolescent musculoskeletal radiology diagnoses that may be encountered in a routine general radiology practice that should not be missed.

19.1.1 Adolescent Hip Dysplasia

Adolescent hip dysplasia is a frequent and common cause of hip pain [1]. In patients under 50 years of age requiring total hip arthroplasty due to premature hip osteoarthritis, Clohisy et al. found that 48.4% had underlying hip dysplasia [2]. The prevalence of mild hip dysplasia is from 13.4 to 25.6% and for severe hip dysplasia 2.2–10.9% in patients two years and older [3]. The underlying etiology for adolescent hip dysplasia remains controversial. Some cases are due to missed diagnosis during infancy, and others may be due to late-onset development outside the window of hip dysplasia screening programs.

The radiographic diagnosis of adolescent hip dysplasia is challenging because findings may be subtle (Fig. 19.1). Subjective radiographic findings include a shallow and upturned appearance of the acetabular sourcil, irregularity and poorly defined sclerosis of the lateral column of the acetabular sourcil, and femoral head/acetabular fossa mismatch with hip joint incongruity, with the femoral head larger than its acetabular fossa. Secondary osteoarthritic changes are unusual in the adolescent population.

Albar et al. noted that diagnostic accuracy for binomial subjective determination of hip dysplasia among subspecialty-trained pediatric radiologists is 81%, and this statistically improves to 85% when performing lateral center edge angle (LCEA) measurements [4]. Frank hip dysplasia is defined when the LCEA is 18 degrees and under, borderline hip dysplasia is when the LCEA is 18–25 degrees, and normal is 25 degrees and higher (Table 19.1) [5]. When values are >40 degrees, pincer-type impingement should be suggested. Anterior undercoverage of the femoral head is usually present in the setting of hip dysplasia, and this can be quantified by determining the anterior center edge angle (ACEA) based on a properly positioned false profile view of the hip (Fig. 19.1c).

Table 19.1 Lateral center edge angles for the diagnosis of adolescent hip dysplasia

	Lateral Center Edge Angle (LCEA)
Normal	≥25°
Borderline Hip dysplasia	18–25°
Frank hip dysplasia	≤18°

J. H. Kan (✉)
Department of Radiology, Texas Children's Hospital, Baylor College of Medicine, Houston, TX, USA

Department of Radiology, Scottish Rite for Children, Dallas, TX, USA
e-mail: jhkan@texaschildrens.org; j.kan@tsrh.org

J. A. Carrino
Department of Radiology and Imaging, Hospital for Special Surgery, New York, NY, USA
e-mail: CarrinoJ@hss.edu

J. Hodler et al. (eds.), *Musculoskeletal Diseases 2026-2029*, IDKD Springer Series,
https://doi.org/10.1007/978-3-032-17040-8_19

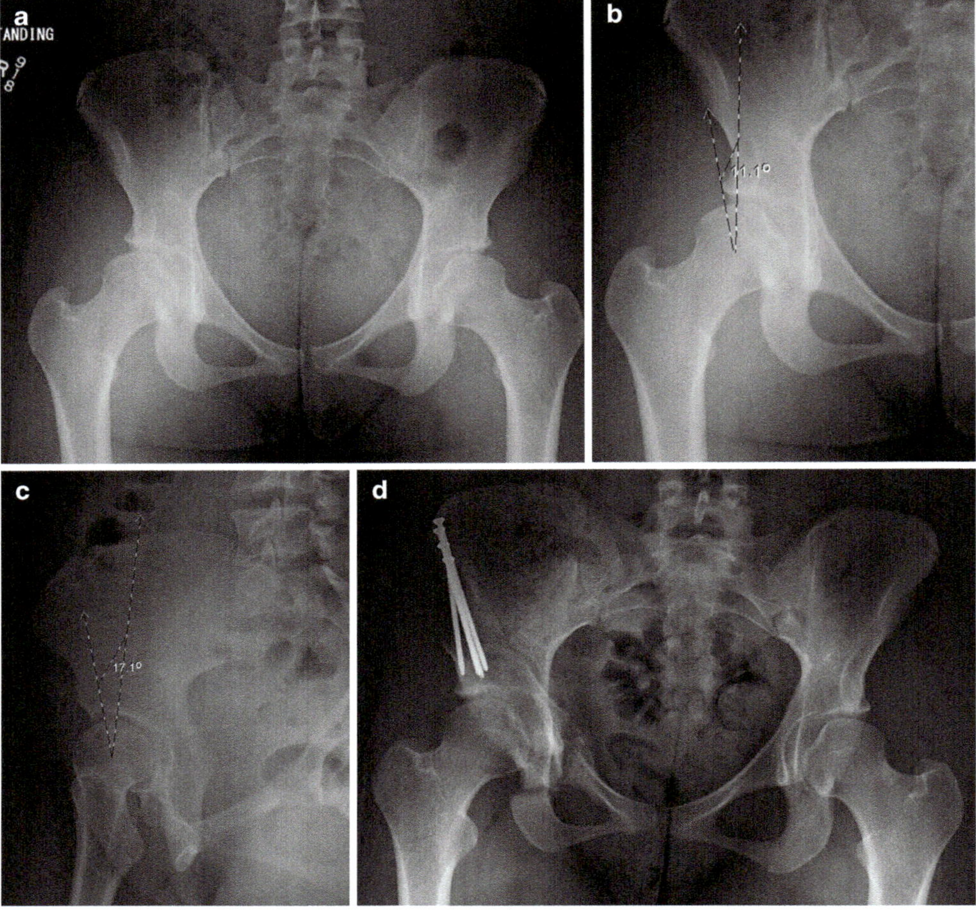

Fig. 19.1 A 17-year-old girl with symptomatic right-sided hip dysplasia. (**a**) AP radiograph and (**b**) AP radiograph of only the right hip demonstrate undercoverage of the right femoral head with LCEA of 11 degrees (normal>25 degrees). (**c**) False profile view demonstrates a ACEA of 17 degrees (normal>25 degrees). (**d**) Postoperative changes related to right-sided periacetabular osteotomy with improved femoral head coverage

The diagnosis of adolescent hip dysplasia is a clinical and radiologic diagnosis. When the diagnosis is in doubt, targeted diagnostic anesthetic injections can be performed to determine if the hip pain is intra- or extraarticular in etiology [6]. When the child responds to an intraarticular anesthetic injection, the diagnosis of a symptomatic dysplastic hip is confirmed, and surgical intervention can be approached with greater confidence. When hip dysplasia is present, it is important to identify coexisting hip pathologies which the surgeon can concomitantly treat, such as CAM-type impingement in the setting of adolescent hip dysplasia (Fig. 19.2).

Key Point

To improve diagnostic confidence, perform a lateral center edge angle measurement when there are subjective radiographic findings that suggest adolescent hip dysplasia.

19.1.2 Osteomyelitis and Septic Arthritis

Hematogenous spread is the most common route for bacterial osteomyelitis and septic arthritis in children [7]. *Staphylococcus aureus* and *Kingella kingae* are the most common pathogens, the latter usually identifiable only by PCR analysis. The clinical presentation of *S. aureus* and most other bacterial pathogens tends to vary based on extent of infection, from nonweight-bearing symptoms to sepsis. *Kingella kingae* is unique compared with other bacterial pathogens for musculoskeletal infection with a typical history of a preceding upper respiratory infection with mild orthopedic symptoms and normal or mildly abnormal inflammatory markers [8].

Once osteomyelitis or septic arthritis is suspected, imaging plays an important role for diagnosis and management. Radiographic workup of the affected osteoarticular region is performed, and findings are usually normal in the acute setting. US may be performed to assess supraphysiologic joint effusions and subperiosteal collections. Early MRI findings

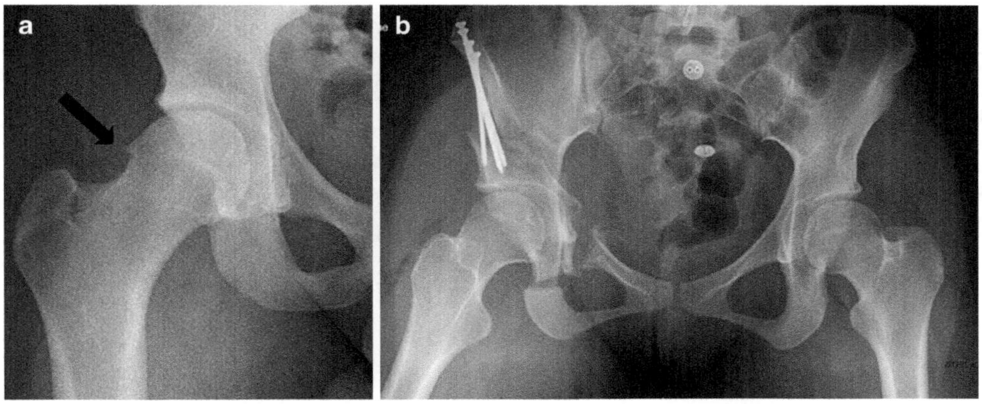

Fig. 19.2 A 17-year-old boy with right hip dysplasia and femoroacetabular impingement. (**a**) AP radiograph demonstrates undercoverage of the right femoral head and focal CAM deformity of the right femoral head-neck junction (arrow). (**b**) AP pelvis postoperative radiographs demonstrate a right-sided periacetabular osteotomy with improved femoral head coverage and femoroplasty for treatment of right-sided CAM deformity

of osteomyelitis include paradoxical T2 hypointense geographic regions (Fig. 19.3), eventually progressing to small pimple-like confluent fluid-like foci (Fig. 19.4) and eventually geographic areas of nonenhancement suggesting phlegmon or developing intraosseous abscess with variable periosteal reaction and subperiosteal fluid. When the metaphysis is involved and there is subjective evidence of a supraphysiologic joint effusion by MRI, coexisting septic arthritis and osteomyelitis is present in 75% (Fig. 19.5) [9]. The presence of any abscess-like intraosseous or soft tissue collection and supraphysiologic joint effusion of the nearby joint should be reported and communicated to the treating physician for potential surgical debridement.

The decision to proceed with MRI in the setting of suspected septic arthritis/osteomyelitis is based on clinical grounds, loosely based on the Kocher criteria, with decreased threshold for proceeding to MRI investigation with higher Kocher scores. The Kocher criteria include temperature > 38.5 C, nonweight-bearing of the affected leg, erythrocyte sedimentation rate > 40 mm/hr., and white blood cell count >12 K cells/mm^3 (Table 19.2) [10]. In the era of MRI, the presence of three or more positive clinical Kocher criteria and the incidence of lower extremity osteomyelitis has been reported to be 47.9% and septic arthritis 22.5% in patients referred for MRI [11].

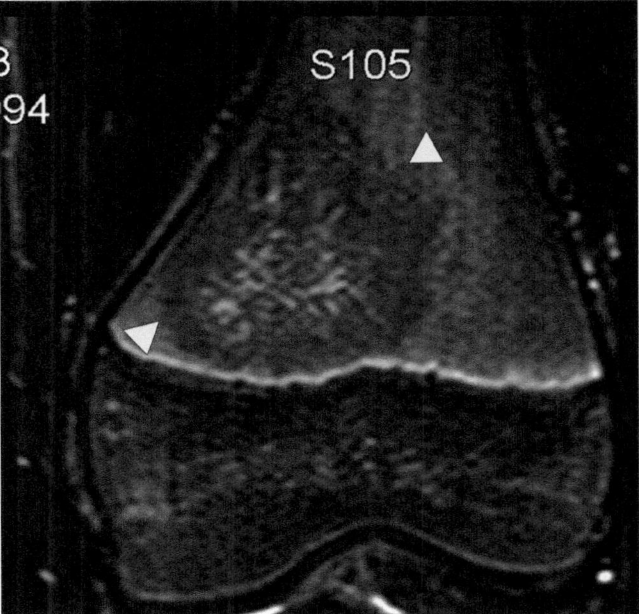

Fig. 19.3 A 13-year-old boy with acute right distal femur osteomyelitis. STIR coronal demonstrates a paradoxical hypointense geographic lesion in the distal femur metaphysis (arrowheads) with small hyperintense serpiginous foci centrally, consistent with acute osteomyelitis

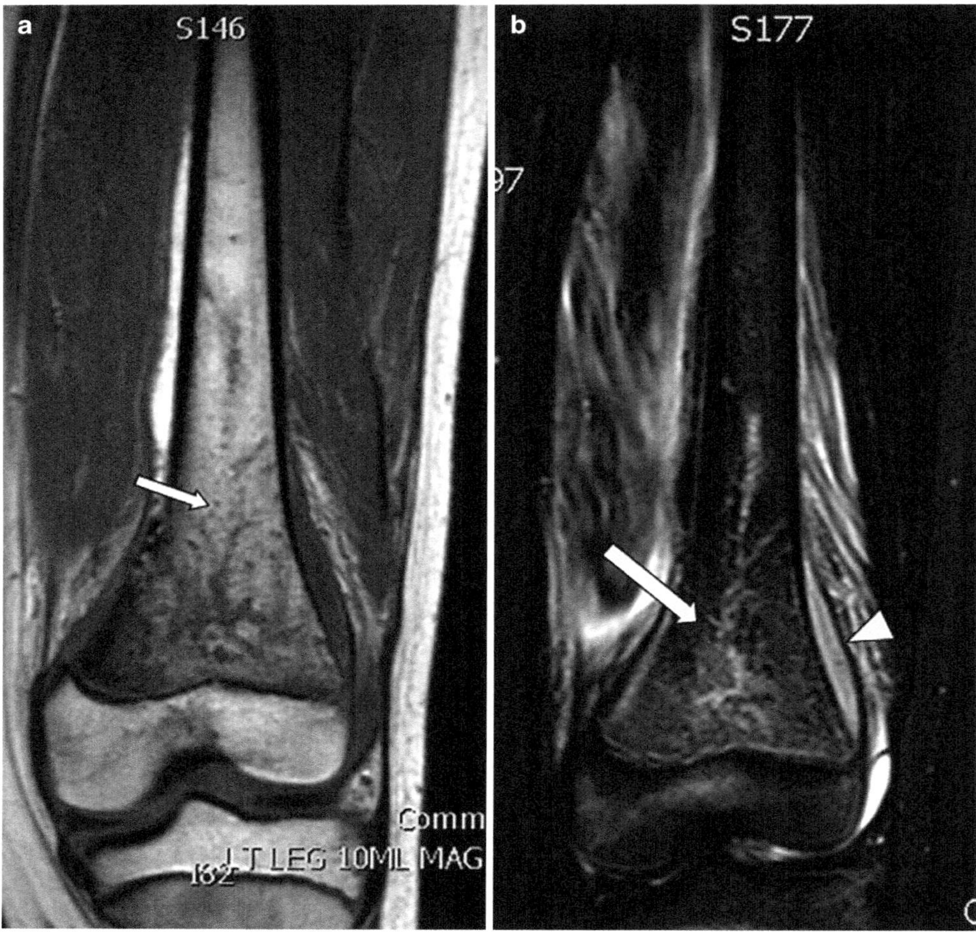

Fig. 19.4 A 12-year-old girl with acute distal femur osteomyelitis. (**a**) T1 coronal demonstrates coalescent hypointense small focal lesions in the distal femur (arrow) which are (**b**) STIR hyperintense (arrow). Note adjacent subperiosteal abscess (arrowhead)

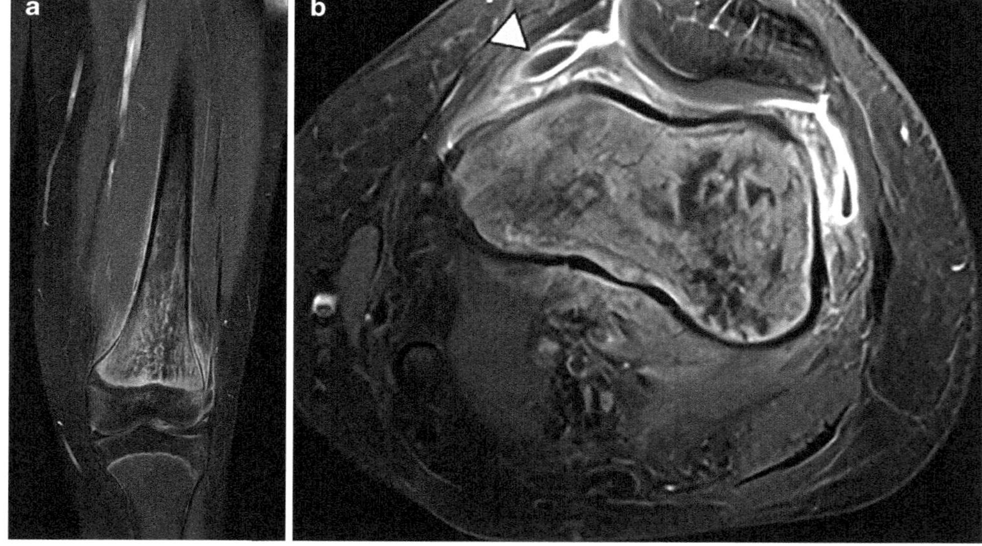

Fig. 19.5 A 12-year-old girl with acute distal femur osteomyelitis and knee septic arthritis. (**a**) T1 FS coronal postcontrast demonstrates heterogeneous enhancement throughout the distal femur inclusive of the lateral juxtaphyseal femoral condylar epiphysis. (**b**) T1 FS axial postcontrast demonstrates intramedullary heterogeneous enhancement of the marrow with supraphysiologic knee effusion with synovitis (arrowhead)

19.1.3 Chronic Nonbacterial Osteomyelitis (CNO)

Chronic nonbacterial osteomyelitis (CNO) is an autoinflammatory disorder affecting bone characterized by osteitis of one or more sites in the appendicular or axial skeleton [12]. The most common age of presentation is 9–10 years of age with female predominance. The disease is like SAPHO (synovitis, acne, pustulosis, hyperostosis, osteitis) seen in adult patients, but CNO less commonly has cutaneous involvement and lower extremity long bones are more commonly affected. The previous term for CNO is chronic recurrent multifocal osteomyelitis (CRMO). CNO is the preferred umbrella term since the process may present as a single lesion or present with multifocal lesions [13].

> **Key Point**
> *Kingella kingae osteomyelitis may present with mild orthopedic symptoms, leading to a delay in diagnosis. Bacteriologic diagnosis requires PCR analysis.*

The most common site of involvement of CNO is the metaphyses or metaphyseal equivalent zones of long bones (Fig. 19.6), preferentially affecting the lower extremities. When the axial skeleton is affected, these regions of osteitis may affect the pelvis, vertebrae, sternum, and clavicles [12]. Unlike bacterial osteomyelitis, disease presentation is mild, gradual with arthritis-like symptoms of the affected osteoarticular regions (40%) and only a minority present with fever (20%) [12].

Table 19.2 Kocher criteria for the diagnosis of septic arthritis

Number of Kocher criteria present	Likelihood of septic arthritis
1	3%
2	40%
3	93%
4	99%

Kocher criteria: Temperature >38.5 C, Nonweightbearing of the affected leg, Erthyrocyte sedimentation rate >40 mm/hr, White blood cell count >12 K cells/mm^3

The radiographic findings of CNO depend on the stage of presentation. Early in the disease process, radiographs may be normal. Subacute and chronic changes include juxtaphyseal metaphyseal osteolysis and sclerosis with variable periosteal reaction with hyperostosis (Fig. 19.6) [14]. These lesions oftentimes may mimic a neoplasm particularly when there is only a single focus and therefore will require biopsy for confirmation (Fig. 19.7). When there are multiple lesions present with typical clinical history for CNO, biopsy usually is not necessary.

MRI changes reflect a juxtaphyseal metaphyseal inflammatory process and will often demonstrate disruptions in metaphyseal ossification and edema (Fig. 19.6). MRI of the specific affected region is advised during the initial workup for primary diagnosis and to exclude pyogenic and neoplastic conditions. After the diagnosis is established clinically or after biopsy, whole body MRI with STIR coronal from head to toe and STIR sagittal of the spine (Fig. 19.7c) is advised to document extent of disease and number of sites involved. The purpose of whole body MRI is to provide a baseline exam that can then be used for reference and follow-up after initiating treatment.

> **Key Point**
> *Unifocal CNO may radiographically mimic a neoplasm or a pyogenic infection; biopsy may be biopsy.*

19.1.4 Chondroblastoma

Chondroblastoma is a rare benign cartilage tumor that can present at all ages, although it preferentially occurs in children with open physis with male predominance [15, 16]. These lesions have characteristic, pathognomonic imaging features that may allow histologic diagnosis but also help

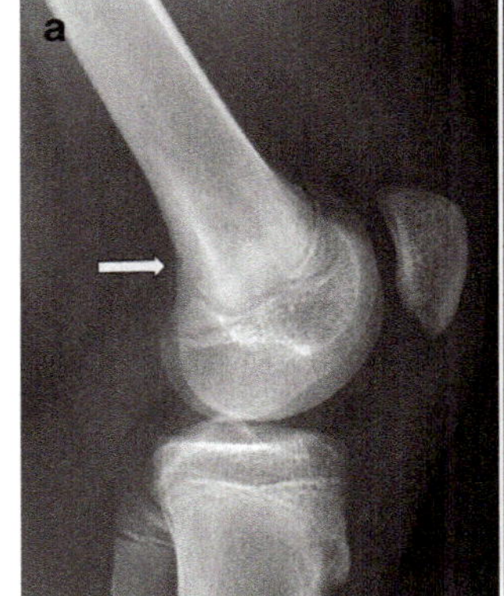

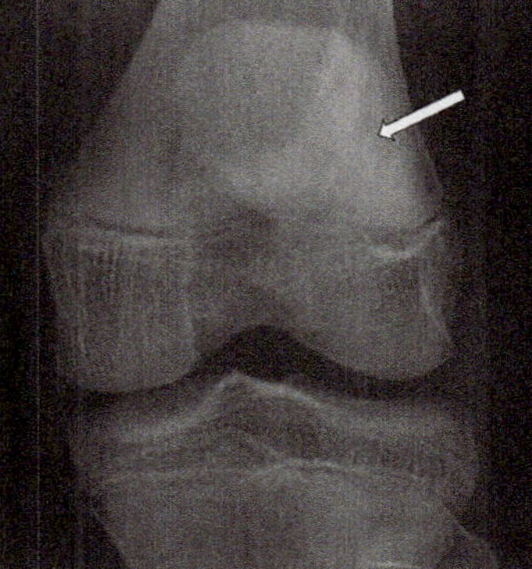
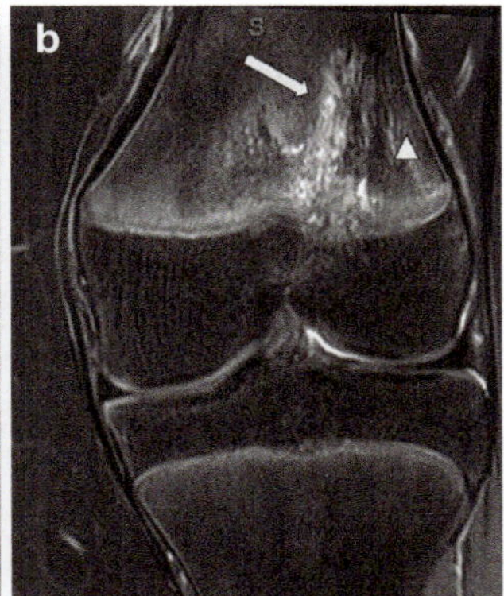

Fig. 19.6 A 13-year-old boy with CNO. (**a**) AP and lateral radiographs of the knee demonstrate focal juxtaphyseal metaphyseal hyperostosis (arrows). (**b**) PD FS coronal demonstrates corresponding regions of edema-like signal (arrow) and also areas that are hypointense (arrowhead), likely corresponding to hyperostotic changes on radiography

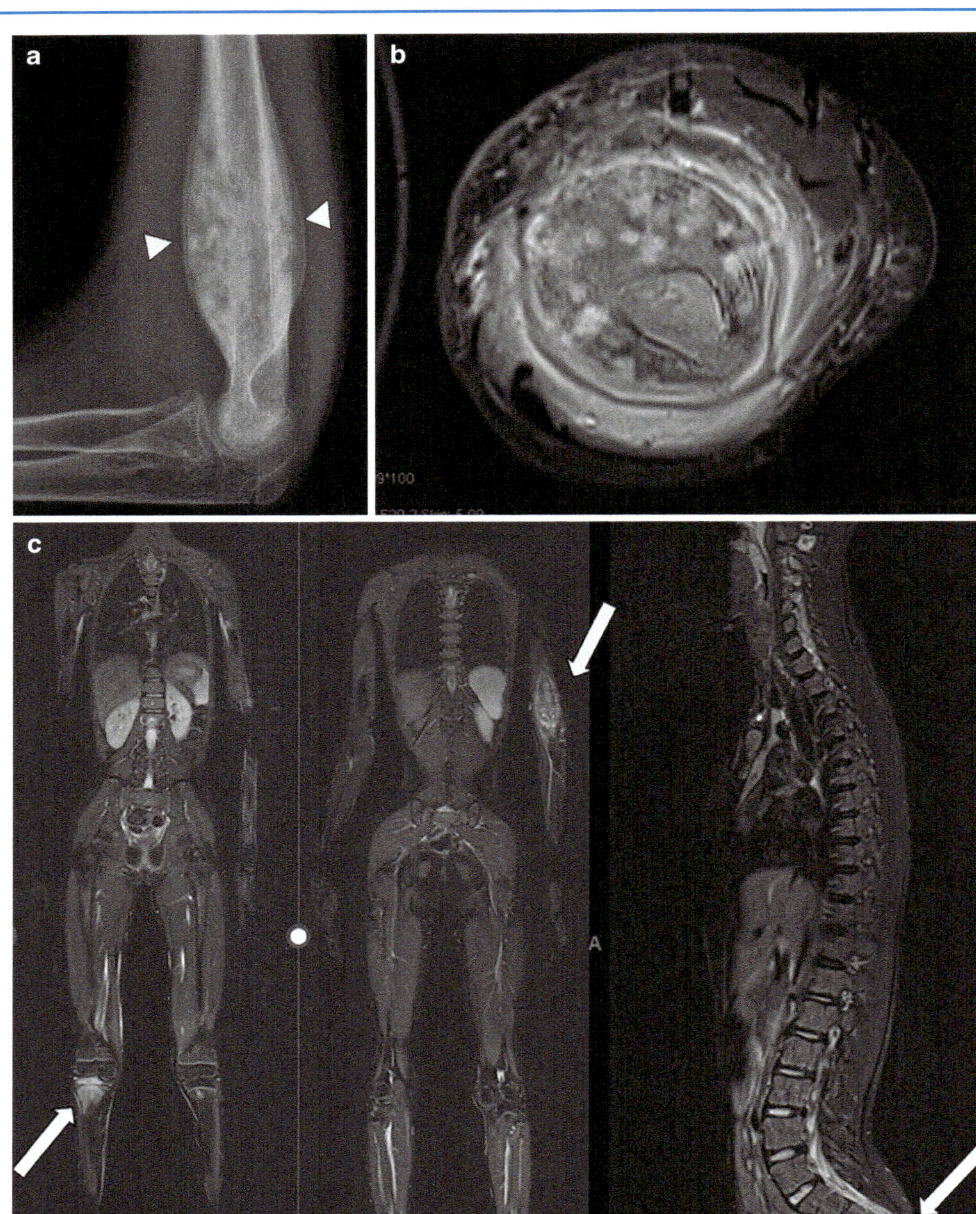

Fig. 19.7 A 12-year-old girl with multifocal osseous changes and CNO, biopsy proven. (**a**) Lateral radiograph of the left elbow demonstrates a hyperostotic expansile mass with laminated periostitis (arrowheads) with multiple intracortical lucencies. (**b**) T1 FS postcontrast axial images demonstrate similar findings with intraosseous and intracortical enhancement with hyperostotic expansion, with associated periostitis. After biopsy confirmation of CNO, whole body STIR (**c**) in coronal and sagittal planes demonstrates several foci of active CNO lesions including right proximal tibia, left distal humerus, and sacrum (arrows)

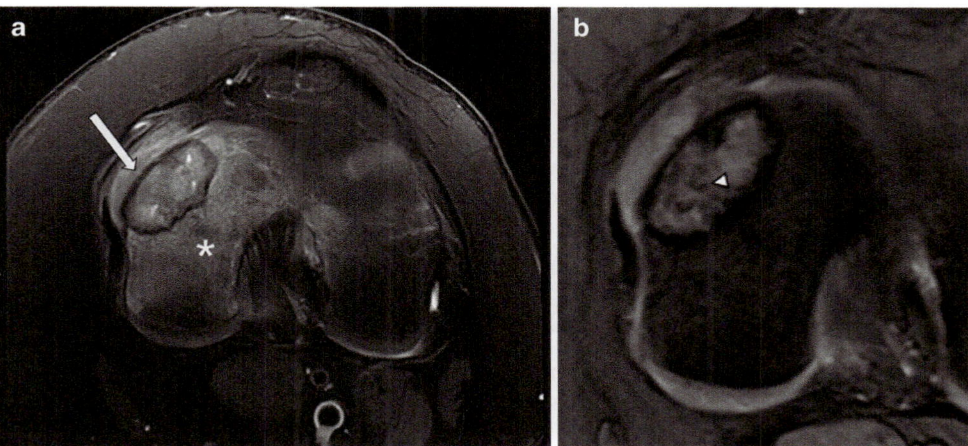

Fig. 19.8 A 9-year-old girl with distal femoral chondroblastoma. (**a**) T2 FS axial of the distal femur demonstrates a well-defined medial femoral condylar mass (arrow) with exuberant perilesional edema (*). (**b**) GRE axial sequence demonstrates internal comma-shaped susceptibility artifact (arrowhead) consistent with chondroid matrix

explain how patients may clinically present. Chondroblastoma usually occurs in long bone epiphysis and is associated with significant perilesional edema (Fig. 19.8). Therefore, symptoms may superficially mimic an inflammatory arthritis given their intraarticular location. Less often, chondroblastomas may occur in the axial skeleton and flat bones, with a tendency to involve the calcaneus and talus [17].

Radiographically, an epiphyseal radiolucent lesion is usually identified in the affected long bone. Although the lesion primarily involves the epiphysis, physeal and juxtaphyseal metaphyseal extension can often be identified related to direct tumor extension or perilesional edema [16, 17]. On CT or MRI, chondroblastomas may have a spiculated architecture related to cartilaginous elements (Fig. 19.9), which helps differentiate this lesion from epiphyseal osteomyelitis which will lack any calcific matrix [18]. MRI will demonstrate exuberant perilesional soft tissue and marrow edema. On postcontrast imaging, central enhancement of the lesion will be present. This will help distinguish chondroblastoma from an epiphyseal Brodie's abscess related to osteomyelitis, the latter which should not demonstrate central enhancement.

Complications related to chondroblastoma include secondary bone cyst formation (Fig. 19.9b), occurring in approximately 15% of lesions [17]. Given that chondroblastomas are benign, curettage is often attempted with a reported incidence of local recurrence of 9% [19].

Key Point

Epiphyseal chondroblastomas may superficially mimic a nonpyogenic inflammatory arthritis because they are intraarticular and cause significant perilesional inflammation.

19.1.5 Tenosynovial Giant Cell Tumor

Tenosynovial giant cell tumor (TGCT) is the updated umbrella term for pigmented villonodular tenosynovitis and giant cell tumor of the tendon sheath [20]. TGCT terminology is applied when these lesions involve tendon sheath or arise from within the synovium of a joint. TGCT represents a benign but locally aggressive synovial neoplasm containing a mixture of macrophages, stromal and fibroblast proliferation, with variable hemosiderin deposition [20]. These synovial-based masses usually occur in adult patients and less commonly occur in children including in the first decade of life [21]. The knee is most commonly affected.

TGCT is usually a diagnosis of exclusion, and its diagnosis is often delayed due to symptom overlap with juvenile idiopathic arthritis. Due to the locally aggressive nature of TGCT, they may present with regional osseous erosions which are frequently seen in less capacious joints such as the hip (Fig. 19.10). On MRI, mass-like synovium with frond-like architecture is appreciated (Fig. 19.10b). Due to the presence of fibroblastic and fibrous elements, these lesions tend to be intermediate-signal intensity on fluid-sensitive sequences. In children, hemosiderin lining with susceptibility artifact may be present (Fig. 19.11), although in the authors' experience, hemosiderin-related susceptibility artifact is less frequently seen compared with adult patients with TGCT. TGCT should be differentiated from secondary hemosiderin deposition from trauma, bleeding diathesis, or JIA with hemorrhagic synovitis. On postcontrast imaging, diffuse mass-like enhancement is appreciated. When identified, these lesions should be subcategorized as diffuse (Fig. 19.10) or focal (Fig. 19.11). Erosions can be seen with either subtype, although they are more frequently seen with the diffuse-type TGCT.

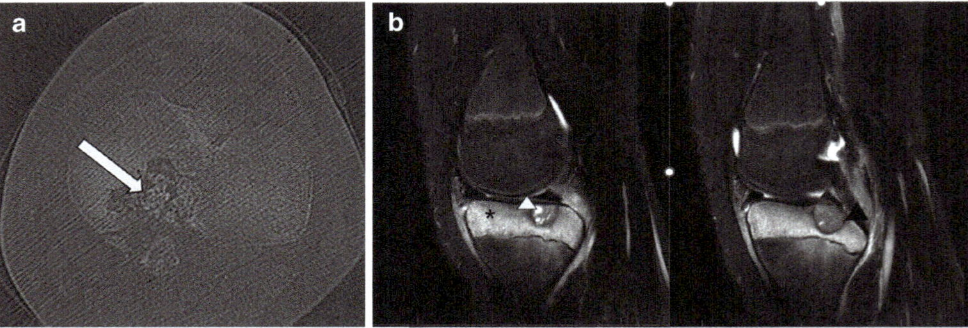

Fig. 19.9 A 14-year-old boy with proximal tibial chondroblastoma. (**a**) CT axial of the proximal tibial epiphysis demonstrates exuberant chondroid matrix (arrow) within the lesion, consistent with a chondroblastoma. (**b**) T2 FS sagittal demonstrates secondary cyst-like changes within the lesion (white arrowhead) and that the primary lesion is predominantly hypointense (black arrowhead). Note diffuse regional edema-like signal throughout the epiphysis (*)

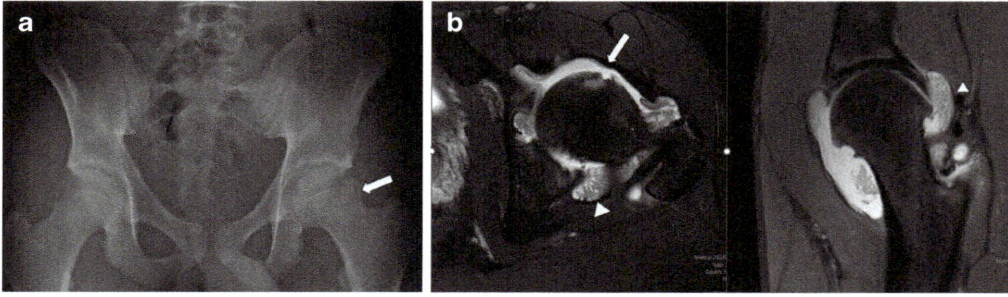

Fig. 19.10 A 17-year-old boy with left hip tenosynovial giant cell tumor. (**a**) AP radiograph demonstrates asphericity of the left hip with subtle lateral femoral head erosions (arrow). (**b**) T2 FS axial and sagittal demonstrates erosion (arrow), marginal femoral head osteophytes, and frond-like synovial proliferation (arrowheads)

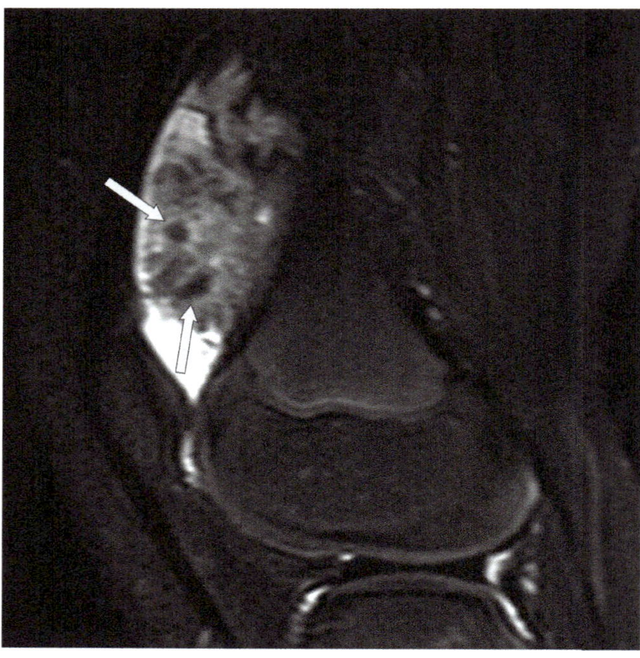

Fig. 19.11 A six-year-old boy with focal left knee tenosynovial giant cell tumor. T2 FS sagittal demonstrate focal intermediate mass with hypointense central irregularly round lesions centrally which may represent either fibrous elements and/or blood (arrow)

Definitive treatment requires complete resection/synovectomy. MRI is important for presurgical planning to identify extent of involvement of the affected joint. The recurrence rate is similar between open and arthroscopic techniques [20].

> **Key Point**
>
> *Synovial proliferation from JIA and TCGT may be difficult to distinguish by MRI when hemosiderin staining is absent. When there is concern for TCGT, biopsy of the synovium is necessary.*

19.1.6 Nonaccidental Injury (NAI)/Child Abuse

Imaging plays a critical role in detecting signs of child abuse, particularly fractures in specific locations or with unusual patterns. According to the AAP (American Academy of Pediatrics), fractures that are more concerning for abuse include fractures in a nonambulatory child, fractures that are not consistent with the history provided or for which no history of injury is given, and fractures that have a high or moderate specificity for abuse [22]. In the absence of major trauma such as a motor vehicle injury, femoral shaft fractures are extraordinarily rare in preschool children. Therefore, child abuse should be considered for any femoral shaft fracture in a preschool child even if there is a history of mild trauma like a fall from a bed or playground injury.

Careful examination for occult or healing fractures is essential in cases of suspected child abuse. A head CT is recommended in children up to six months of age to rule out intracranial injury or calvarial fracture; a skeletal survey is recommended up to two years of age to evaluate for any clinically unsuspected fractures, although the survey may be performed up to five years of age in certain situations. All children with concern for abuse will also need a follow-up skeletal survey two weeks after the initial evaluation to assess for interval healing [23]. Certain fracture patterns, especially in infants, have a high specificity for child abuse (Table 19.3). Posteromedial rib fractures and classic metaphyseal lesions (CMLs) of long bones are particularly concerning (Fig. 19.12), and child abuse should be raised even if there is coexisting metabolic bone disease. The CMLs are caused by indirect injury related to torsional and tractional shearing forces, often from vigorous pulling or twisting of an infant's extremity.

Table 19.3 Specificity of radiologic findings in infants and toddlers in NAI (nonaccidental injury)

High specificity (highest specificity applies in infants)	Classic metaphyseal lesions (CMLs) Rib fractures, especially posteromedial Scapular fractures Spinous process fractures Sternal fractures
Moderate specificity	Multiple fractures, especially bilateral Fractures of different ages Epiphyseal separations Vertebral body fractures and subluxations Digital fractures Complex skull fractures
Common, but low specificity	Subperiosteal new bone formation Clavicular fractures Long-bone shaft fractures Linear skull fractures

Adapted from Kleinman [36]

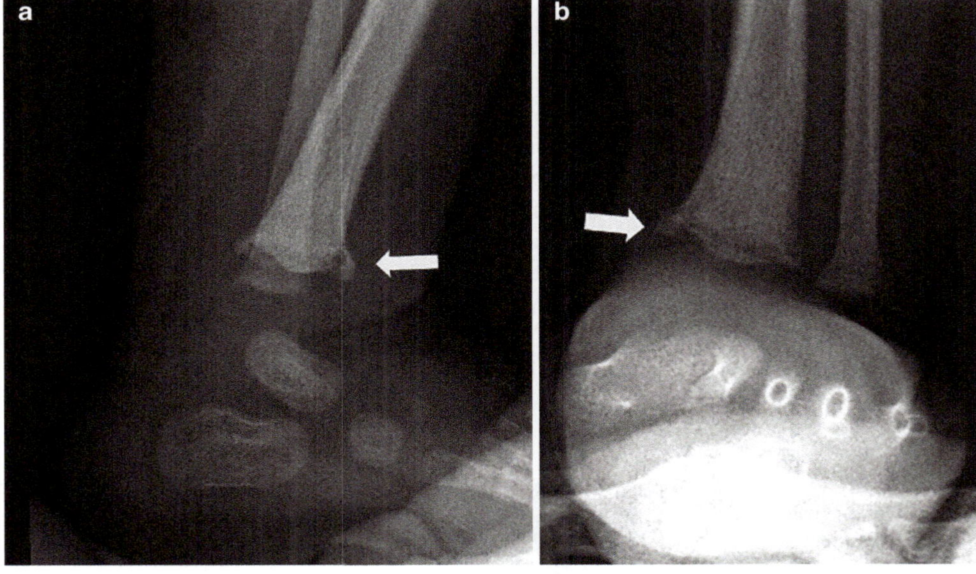

Fig. 19.12 A two-month-old g2-month-olding with facial bruising. (**a**) Left ankle lateral and (**b**) AP views demonstrate classic metaphyseal lesion (arrow) of child abuse

Key Point
A follow-up skeletal survey is advised 11–14 days after the initial survey for suspected child abuse.

19.1.7 Slipped Capital Femoral Epiphysis (SCFE)

SCFE is a chronic proximal femoral physeal injury affecting the adolescent hip and may manifest with physeal widening and/or displacement, with the femoral head displacing medially and posteriorly with respect to the femoral neck. Risk factors include obesity and metabolic bone disorders. The blood supply to the femoral head is mainly from the deep medial circumflex artery, and SCFE with displacement may potentially compromise blood flow to the femoral head, potentially leading to osteonecrosis. SCFE is usually an emergency and must be diagnosed and treated early, particularly if the child is unable to bear weight (unstable slip). Radiography (frontal pelvis and frog-lateral projections including both hips) is the initial imaging modality (Fig. 19.13).

Radiological signs on the frontal projection of the pelvis can be subtle and include widening of the growth plate, decreased epiphyseal height, Trethowan sign (positive Klein's line), Blanch sign, Capener sign, and Sham sign (Table 19.4): while several of the imaging features on the frontal projection are subtle, nonetheless, early slips are readily diagnosed on the frog leg lateral projection, which is more sensitive for detection of posterior slips [24].

MRI is more sensitive for detecting early signs of SCFE like physeal widening and bone marrow edema. MRI is particularly useful for detecting early changes in the preslip stage and evaluating complications like osteonecrosis. Ultrasound can demonstrate epiphyseal displacement, often with concomitant joint effusion. Early diagnosis is crucial to prevent complications such as osteonecrosis of the femoral head and premature osteoarthritis. While this lesion involves the physis, it is not considered in the same category as an acute Salter-Harris fracture as it is typically related to a chronic insult. While standard radiography is the first-line imaging modality for patients with suspected SCFE, advanced imaging modalities of ultrasound and MRI may aid in surgical planning, diagnosis of complications, and treatment follow-up [25].

There is a grading system based on the severity of the slip: Grade I, slip less than 30% of the width of the femoral neck; Grade II, slip between 30% and 60% of the width of the femoral neck; and Grade III, slip greater than 60% of the width of the femoral neck.

Key Point
SCFE is a condition that needs urgent attention, and early diagnosis is best made by having both frontal and frog lateral projection radiography.

Table 19.4 SCFE: Radiological signs on frontal projection

Widening of the growth plate, which becomes irregular compared to the contralateral hip with an accentuated lucency medially
Decrease of the epiphyseal height
Positive Klein's line (Trethowan sign): there is a slip of the capital epiphysis when the line drawn along the superior border of the femoral neck does not intersect the epiphysis
Blanch sign: the opacity overlying the metaphysis adjacent to the physis is increased due to the capital epiphysis which is posteriorly displaced
Capener sign: the posterior displacement of the capital epiphysis leads to a decrease of the overlapped opacity between ischium and femoral head
Sham sign: the normal adolescent hip shows an opaque triangle formed by the overlap of the inferomedial femoral neck on the posterior wall of the acetabulum. In SCFE, the reduction of this opaque normal triangle occurs

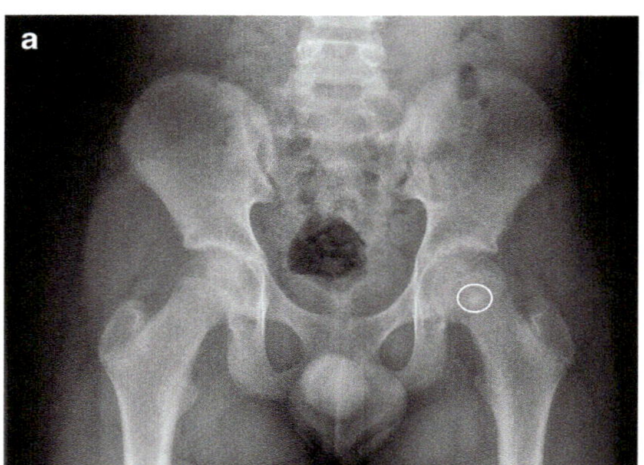

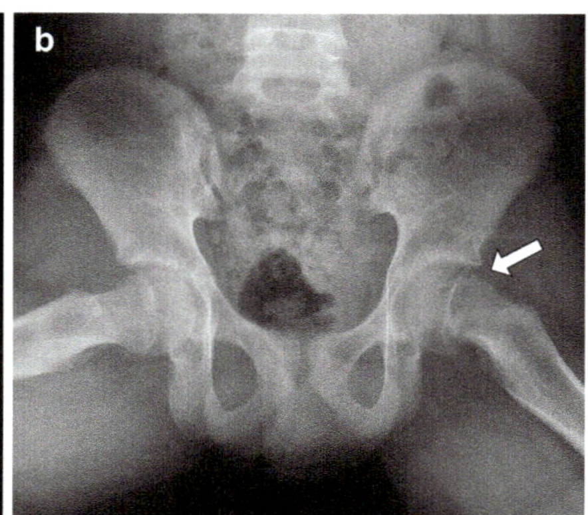

Fig. 19.13 An 11-year-old boy with left hip pain with slipped capital femoral epiphysis (SCFE). (**a**) Frontal projection radiograph of the pelvis shows focal sclerosis along the metaphyseal side of the left proximal femur (oval). (**b**) However, the posterior displacement of the left capital femoral epiphysis is only visualized on the frog-leg lateral projection (arrow). The right hip is normal

19.1.8 Occult Salter-Harris Injuries

Physeal fractures are common in children. Physeal or growth plate injuries comprise approximately 15–30% of all pediatric long bone fractures, with Salter Harris type II as the most common type of fracture injury pattern observed in about 61% of patients [26]. The incidence of growth arrest is quite variable depending on physeal location, type of injury, and treatment received [27].

The Salter-Harris classification system is a widely used method for describing and categorizing fractures involving the growth plate (physis) in children (Fig. 19.14). It helps predict the potential for growth disturbances and guides treatment decisions. The system categorizes fractures into five types [28]. A type I fracture is a separation through the physis. A type II fracture enters in the plane of the physis and exits through the metaphysis. The resulting metaphyseal fragment is called the Thurston-Holland fragment. A type III fracture enters in the plane of the physis and exits through the epiphysis. A type IV fracture crosses the physis, extending from the metaphysis to the epiphysis. A type V fracture is a crush injury resulting in injury to the physis. There have been extensions to the traditional Salter-Harris classification that include modified types. A type VI is an avulsion fracture, and a type VII is an open fracture with partial physeal loss.

While most physeal fractures can be obvious on projection radiography, certain physeal fractures, particularly Salter-Harris type I, can be very subtle or even radiographically occult. The main MRI findings in an occult Salter Harris type I injury are increased physeal thickness and signal intensity on fluid-sensitive sequences, perichondrial disruption with elevation of the periosteum, and intracartilaginous fracture with associated periphyseal marrow edema.

Additional indication for MRI referral for radiographically identified Salter-Harris fractures is when there are challenges related to fracture reduction and the surgeon is excluding soft tissue interposition including entrapped periosteum, tendons, or ligaments (Fig. 19.15) [29]. Soft tissue interposition may cause delayed fracture healing and reduction. MRI is also useful after a Salter-Harris fracture is healed and there is symptomatic premature physeal growth disturbance. When a physeal bar is present, it is important to document location (central/peripheral/global) and percentage area involvement of the physis for potential surgical decision making for physeal bar resection.

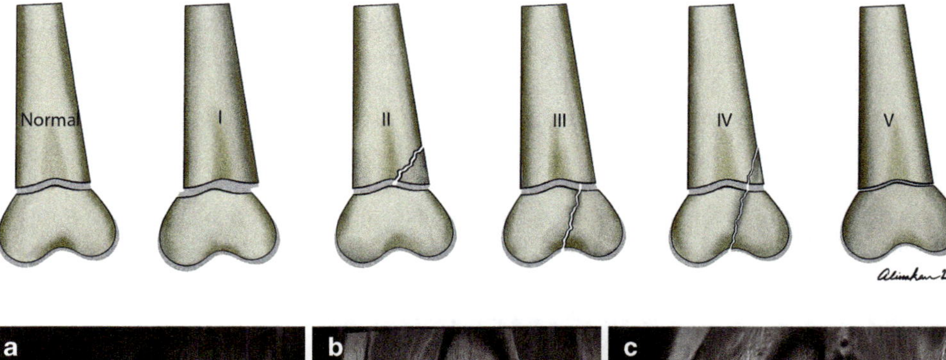

Fig. 19.14 Salter-Harris classification

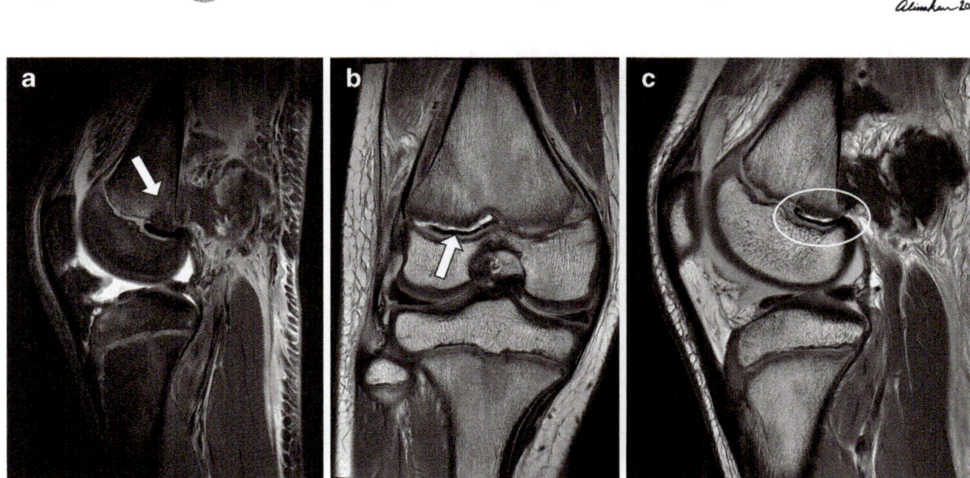

Fig. 19.15 A nine-year-old girl after a trampoline injury with Salter-Harris fracture with periosteal entrapment. (**a**) Sagittal STIR demonstrates Salter-Harris type II distal femoral fracture, with metaphyseal component without displacement. (**b**) Coronal IW-weighted FSE image (arrow) and (**c**) sagittal IW-weighted FSE image show widening of the physis with lateral side interposition of linear low-signal intensity periosteum (oval)

Key Point
Displacement of torn periosteum into the growth plate is an uncommon pediatric entity following trauma, can be detected on MRI as low-signal intensity physeal interposition on all pulse sequences, and may require open surgical reduction, as it may lead to growth plate bridging and subsequent extremity length discrepancy.

19.1.9 Spondylolysis

Spondylolysis, a stress fracture of the pars interarticularis, is a common cause of low back pain in children and adolescents, particularly athletes, and the most common level is at L5. The incidence of a par stress injury in the active adolescent population presenting with mechanical lower back pain ranges from 8 to 50% with males four times more likely than females [30]. Although multiple factors may be involved in its pathogenesis, spondylolysis is generally considered to arise from mechanical stress applied to that portion of the neural arch as a result of repetitive extension and/or rotation activities. Spondylolysis generally responds well to conservative treatment including activity modification, physical therapy, and cessation of sports until the patient is pain-free. The progression of active spondylolysis from stress reaction to incomplete fracture to complete fracture to nonunion has been associated with an increased incidence of spondylolisthesis. It is important to recognize that spondylolysis represents the endpoint of an injury continuum comprising adaptive physiological bone remodeling, maladaptation, stress reaction, and progressive bone failure at the pars interarticularis and possible nonunion (Fig. 19.16).

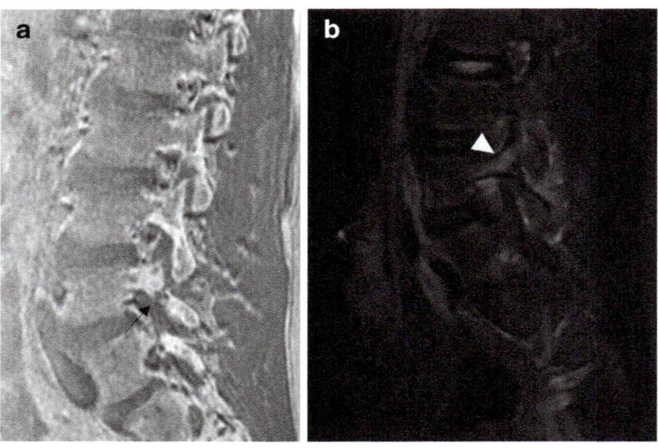

Fig. 19.16 An 11-year-old boy with back pain. (**a**) UTE and (**b**) T2 FS sagittal sequence at the level of the left pedicle demonstrates pars and pedicle edema (arrowhead) with juxtacortical soft tissue edema present

Table 19.5 Hollenberg MRI classification of spondylolysis

Grade	MRI findings at Pars interarticularis
0	No abnormality
1	Marrow edema only; no fracture
2	Marrow edema; partial/incomplete pars fracture
3	Marrow edema; complete pars fracture
4	Un-united fracture

Adapted from Hollenberg et al. [31]

Hollenberg et al. devised a five-grade classification system [31] to provide the framework for standardized reporting and grading (Table 19.5), with an additional goal of supplying prognostic information on fracture healing potential to help guide management. However, there are additional factors that influence healing response such as fracture orientation, anatomical location (zones of injury), spine level, and systemic factors, which are being elaborated.

Early diagnosis is crucial, and MRI can detect stress reactions before a complete fracture is visible on radiography or CT. MRI can also assist in differentiating from other causes of back pain. With regard to imaging techniques, the protocol should include a fluid-sensitive sequence (fat-suppressed T2-WI or STIR) in the sagittal and axial planes. The addition of bone MRI technique, typically gradient based such as UTE MR sequence to generate a CT-like image, is superior in performance and confidence to detect a fracture line over just using conventional MRI pulse sequences and provides classification similar to CT imaging (Fig. 19.16a) [32].

Key Point
MRI exams in young athletes with low back pain should ideally include fluid-sensitive and bone-specific techniques to optimize detection and characterization of the spectrum of spondylolysis lesions.

19.1.10 Osteoid Osteoma

Diagnosing an osteoid osteoma in a pediatric patient who is athletic can be confusing because its symptoms can overlap with common sports injuries like stress fractures, overuse strains, and joint inflammation. The location of the tumor and sometimes atypical presentation make differentiating it from these other conditions challenging [33]. Osteoid osteoma is commonly classified according to its location: intracortical (75%), medullary (20%), subperiosteal (4%), and endosteal (4%).

There may be location-dependent symptoms. While classic osteoid osteoma presents with pain that is worse at night and relieved by NSAIDs, this can change depending on where the nidus is located. Osteoid osteomas near a joint, such as the hip, can cause nonspecific joint pain, swelling, and stiffness that mimics an arthritis. The classic nighttime pain may be absent or less prominent in these cases. An osteoid osteoma in the femoral neck can be easily mistaken for a femoral neck stress fracture, a critical injury in athletes. Both can cause groin pain that worsens with activity. The definitive diagnosis is often delayed because of this confusion. Lesions in the hands or feet can cause swelling and joint pain, often mimicking sprains or an arthritis [34].

Athletes frequently experience bone pain from the repetitive stress of their sport. A clinician may initially attribute the pain to common overuse injuries before considering a bone tumor, particularly if the initial imaging is inconclusive. Standard radiography can miss osteoid osteoma, especially if it is small, intraarticular, or intramedullary, since these areas may not produce the characteristic surrounding reactive bone sclerosis. In these cases, an MRI or CT scan is necessary to locate the small central tumor nidus. An MRI can show extensive bone marrow edema around the lesion, which can be mistaken for a stress reaction, especially in weight-bearing bones like the femur. This edema can be the only abnormality seen on initial imaging, leading to a misdiagnosis [35]. When standard imaging is inconclusive, cross-sectional imaging with thin section CT is used to identify the small central nidus that is characteristic of an osteoid osteoma (Fig. 19.17).

Key Point

A delay in diagnosis of osteoid osteoma is not uncommon in pediatric athletes; a high index of suspicion, especially when symptoms do not improve with conservative care for a suspected sports injury, is crucial.

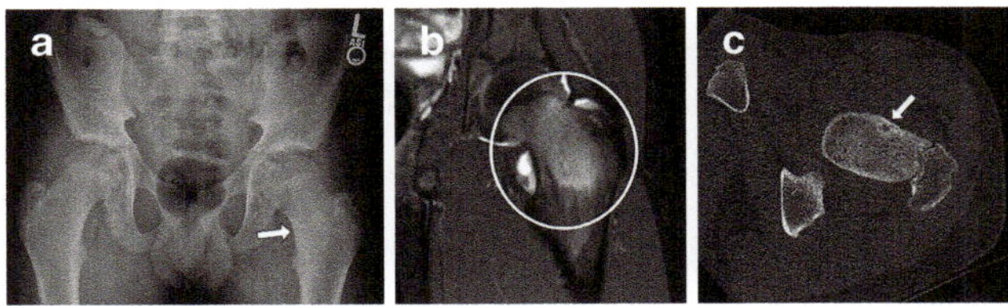

Fig. 19.17 A 12-year-old boy baseball player with left hip pain with an osteoid osteoma. (**a**) Frontal projection radiograph shows subtle inconspicuous thickening of the femoral neck (arrow). (**b**) Coronal STIR demonstrates a prominent bone marrow edema pattern of the femoral neck simulating a stress reaction (oval). (**c**) CT bone algorithm MPR parallel to the femoral neck reveals the characteristic features of an intracortical osteoid osteoma with a lucent nidus (arrow)

19.2 Conclusion

In summary, we have reviewed ten important not to miss conditions that may be seen in children that may present in a general radiology practice. Understanding orthopedic pathophysiologic processes in children, clinical symptomatology, and knowing what the surgeon needs to know will help improve strategies for imaging workup and arriving at a correct diagnosis.

Acknowledgment Figure 19.14 original illustration by Alissa Kan

Conflict of Interest Statement I/We declare no competing interests as defined by Springer Nature or other interests that might be perceived to influence results and/or discussion reported in this manuscript.

References

1. Bixby SD, Millis MB. The borderline dysplastic hip: when and how is it abnormal? Pediatr Radiol. 2019;49:1669–77.
2. Clohisy JC, Dobson MA, Robison JF, et al. Radiographic structural abnormalities associated with premature, natural hip-joint failure. J Bone Joint Surg Am. 2011;93(suppl 2):3–9.
3. de Vos-Jakobs S, Boel F, Bramer WM, et al. Prevalence and radiological definitions of acetabular dysplasia after the age of 2 years: a systematic review. J Pediatr Orthop B. 2023;33:334–9.
4. Albar A, Sher AC, Rosenfeld S, et al. Improved identification of adolescent hip dysplasia using a screening method based on lateral center edge angle measurements. Acad Radiol. 2023;30:2140–6.
5. Sinha R, Morris WZ, Ellis HB, et al. Radiographic evaluation of the painful adolescent and young adult hip. J Pediatr Soc North Am. 2024;3(7):100039.
6. Tran E, Rosenfeld S, Ngan E, et al. Clinical impact of diagnostic image-guided injections for musculoskeletal pain work-up in adolescent and adult patients at a children's hospital: initial results. Skeletal Radiol. 2024;53(8):1573–82.
7. Hannon M, Lyons T. Pediatric musculoskeletal infections. Curr Opin Pediatr. 2023;35(3):319–5.
8. Restrepo R, Park HJ, Karakas SP, et al. Bacterial osteomyelitis in pediatric patients: a comprehensive review. Skeletal Radiol. 2024;53:2195–210.
9. Schallert EK, Kan JH, Monsalve J, et al. Metaphyseal osteomyelitis in children: how often does MRI-documented joint effusion or epiphyseal extension of edema indicate coexisting septic arthritis? Pediatr Radiol. 2015;45:1174–81.
10. Kocher MS, Zurakowski D, Kasser JR. Differentiating between septic arthritis and transient synovitis of the hip in children: an evidence-based clinical prediction algorithm. JBJS. 1999;81(12):1662–70.
11. Nguyen A, Kan JH, Bisset G, et al. Kocher criteria revisited in the era of MRI: how often does the Kocher criteria identify underlying osteomyelitis? J Pediatr Orthop. 2017;37:e114–9.
12. Handa A, Restrepo SB, Restrepo R, et al. Imaging evaluation of rheumatologic musculoskeletal disorders in children. Skeletal Radiol (prepress). 2025;54(11):2357–71.

13. Zhao Y, Ferguson PJ. Chronic nonbacterial osteomyelitis and chronic recurrent multifocal osteomyelitis in children. Pediatr Clin North Am. 2018;65(4):783–800.
14. Sheikh Z, Bhatt D, Chowdhury M, et al. Challenges in the imaging and diagnosis of chronic non-bacterial osteomyelitis (CNO). Clin Radiol. 2025;85:106905.
15. Douis H, Saifuddin A. The imaging of cartilaginous bone tumours. I. Benign lesions. Skeletal Radiol. 2012;41:1195–212.
16. Karhbari A, Vijan A, Janu AK, et al. Retrospective study of multimodality imaging features of chondroblastoma. Indian J Orthop. 2025;58:1303–9.
17. Bloem JL, Mulder JD. Chondroblastoma: a clinical and radiological study of 104 cases. Skeletal Radiol. 1985;14:1–9.
18. El-Ali AM, Coblentz A, Degnan AJ. Solitary long-bone epiphyseal lesions in children: radiologic-pathological correlation and epidemiology. Pediatr Radiol. 2020;50:1724–34.
19. Hirozane T, Sekita T, Kobayashi EK, et al. Clinical characteristics and outcomes of patients with chondroblastoma undergoing surgery with various adjuvant procedures: a retrospective study of 59 cases. BMC Surg. 2025;25(1):40.
20. Kemp AK, Brigman B, Siegel G, et al. Tenosynovial giant cell tumor and pigmented villonodular synovitis. J Am Acad Orthop urg. 2025;33(11):e593–602.
21. Inarejos Clemente EJ, Moreno Romo D, Barber I, et al. Tenosynovial giant cell tumor and its differential diagnosis in children. Peditr Radiol (Online ahead of print). 2025;55(10):1992–2008.
22. Haney S, Scherl S, DiMeglio L, Perez-Rossello J, Servaes S, Merchant N, And the Council on Child Abuse and Neglect; Section on Orthopaedics; Section on Radiology; And Section on Endocrinology; And the Society for Pediatric Radiology. Evaluating young children with fractures for child abuse: clinical report. Pediatrics. 2025;155(2):e2024070074. https://doi.org/10.1542/peds.2024-070074. PMID: 39832712
23. Colleran GC, Fossmark M, Rosendahl K, Argyropoulou M, Mankad K, Offiah AC. ESR Essentials: imaging of suspected child abuse-practice recommendations by the European Society of Paediatric Radiology. Eur Radiol. 2025;35(4):1868–80. https://doi.org/10.1007/s00330-024-11052-4. Epub 2024 Sep 18. PMID: 39289300; PMCID: PMC11914366
24. Bomer J, Klerx-Melis F, Holscher HC. Painful paediatric hip: frog-leg lateral view only! Eur Radiol. 2014;24(3):703–8. https://doi.org/10.1007/s00330-013-3038-0. Epub 2013 Oct 8
25. Hesper T, Zilkens C, Bittersohl B, Krauspe R. Imaging modalities in patients with slipped capital femoral epiphysis. J Child Orthop. 2017;11(2):99–106. https://doi.org/10.1302/1863-2548-11-160276. PMID: 28529656; PMCID: PMC5421351
26. Mizuta T, Benson WM, Foster BK, Morris LL. Statistical analysis of the incidence of physeal injuries. J Pediatr Orthop. 1987;7(5):518–23.
27. Mann DC, Rajmaira S. Distribution of physeal and nonphyseal fractures in 2650 long-bone fractures in children aged 0–16 years. J Pediatr Orthop. 1990;10(6):713–6.
28. Cepela DJ, Tartaglione JP, Dooley TP, Patel PN. Classifications in brief: Salter-Harris classification of pediatric physeal fractures. Clin Orthop Relat Res. 2016;474(11):2531–7. https://doi.org/10.1007/s11999-016-4891-3. Epub 2016 May 20. PMID: 27206505; PMCID: PMC5052189
29. Chen J, Abel MF, Fox MG. Imaging appearance of entrapped periosteum within a distal femoral Salter-Harris II fracture. Skeletal Radiol. 2015;44(10):1547–51. https://doi.org/10.1007/s00256-015-2201-x. Epub 2015 July 3. PMID: 26138340.
30. Michali LJ, Wood R. Back pain in young athletes: significant differences from adults in causes and patterns. Arch Pediatr Adolesc Med. 1995;149(1):15–8. https://doi.org/10.1001/archpedi.1995.02170310017004.
31. Hollenberg GM, Beattie PF, Meyers SP, Weinberg EP, Adams MJ. Stress reactions of the lumbar pars interarticularis: the development of a new MRI classification system. Spine (Phila Pa 1976). 2002;27(2):181–6. https://doi.org/10.1097/00007632-200201150-00012. PMID: 11805665
32. Okuyama K, Aoki Y, Maki S, Matsushita Y, Toyooka T, Orita S, Inage K, Sugiura S, Inoue M, Sakai T, Shiga Y, Hozumi T, Ohtori S, Nishikawa S. Staging lumbar spondylolysis in adolescents: can MR bone imaging replace CT? Spine (Phila Pa 1976). 2025; https://doi.org/10.1097/BRS.0000000000005416. Epub ahead of print. PMID: 40458988
33. Carneiro BC, Da Cruz IAN, Ormond Filho AG, Silva IP, Guimarães JB, Silva FD, Nico MAC, Stump XMGRG. Osteoid osteoma: the great mimicker. Insights Imaging. 2021;12(1):32. https://doi.org/10.1186/s13244-021-00978-8. PMID: 33683492; PMCID: PMC7940467
34. Napora J, Wałejko S, Mazurek T. Osteoid osteoma, a diagnostic problem: a series of atypical and mimicking presentations and review of the recent literature. J Clin Med. 2023;12(7):2721. https://doi.org/10.3390/jcm12072721. PMID: 37048803; PMCID: PMC10095250
35. Cordova CB, Dembowski SC, Johnson MR, Combs JJ, Svoboda SJ. Osteoid osteoma of the femoral neck in athletes: two case reports differentiating from femoral neck stress injuries. Sports Health. 2016;8(2):172–6. https://doi.org/10.1177/1941738115614263. Epub 2015 Oct 28. PMID: 26517936; PMCID: PMC4789927
36. Kleinman PK. Diagnostic imaging of child abuse. Cambridge University Press; 2015.

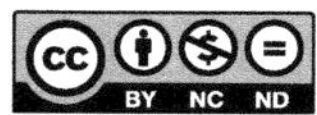

Small Joints: Imaging of the Hand and Forefoot

20

Christine B. Chung and Viviane Khoury

Learning Objectives

- Describe the relevant anatomy of small joints in the hands and feet with emphasis on structures commonly affected in traumatic and degenerative conditions.
- Differentiate among arthritic and nonarthritic conditions affecting small joints using imaging features across imaging methods.
- Evaluate soft tissue abnormalities and space-occupying lesions, and apply imaging strategies for assessment of osseous pathology in the hands and feet.

20.1 MCP and CMC Joint Anatomy of the Thumb

The metacarpophalangeal (MCP) joint of the thumb is a condylar, ellipsoid-type synovial joint formed by the articulation between the first metacarpal head and the base of the proximal phalanx. Although structurally similar to the MCP joints of the lesser digits, the thumb MCP joint is functionally more restricted, primarily permitting flexion and extension, with limited abduction and adduction. The MCP joint stability is provided by robust radial and ulnar collateral ligaments, taut in flexion, and the volar plate, a fibrocartilaginous thickening of the joint capsule that reinforces the palmar aspect and resists hyperextension. Dorsally, the extensor pollicis longus (EPL) and brevis (EPB) tendons contribute to joint extension and are stabilized by sagittal bands, which center the tendons over the MCP joint [1] (Fig. 20.1).

The carpometacarpal (CMC) joint of the thumb is a saddle-shaped articulation between the base of the first metacarpal and the trapezium. This joint is highly mobile, enabling the thumb to perform a wide range of movements, including flexion, extension, abduction, adduction, opposition, and circumduction—essential for precision grip and hand dexterity. The CMC joint is stabilized by a complex of ligaments, of which the most important is the anterior oblique ligament (with deep and superficial components), also known as the beak ligament, which prevents dorsal dislocation and subsidence of the metacarpal base. Additional supporting ligaments include the dorsoradial ligament, crucial for resisting dorsal translation, as well as the intermetacarpal, posterior oblique, and ulnar collateral ligaments [2].

Complementing the osseous and ligamentous structures, the flexor pulley system of the thumb plays a vital role in efficient tendon biomechanics and joint stability. The thumb contains two annular pulleys (A1 and A2) and one oblique pulley. The A1 pulley overlies the MCP joint and is a frequent site of stenosing tenosynovitis or trigger thumb. The oblique pulley, located between the A1 and A2 pulleys along the proximal phalanx, is essential for maintaining the flexor pollicis longus (FPL) tendon close to the bone during flexion. The A2 pulley, more distal, is less clinically significant than in the fingers but still contributes to tendon excursion [1].

20.2 Commonly Encountered Lesions of the Thumb

20.2.1 Gamekeeper and Stener Lesions

Gamekeeper's thumb refers to an injury of the ulnar collateral ligament (UCL) of the first metacarpophalangeal (MCP). This injury most commonly occurs following a valgus force applied to the abducted thumb. The UCL is a key stabilizer of the thumb MCP joint, particularly during pinching or grasp-

C. B. Chung
Radiology, University of California, San Diego, CA, USA
e-mail: cbchung@health.ucsd.edu

V. Khoury (✉)
Radiology, Imagerie Medvue, Montreal, Canada
e-mail: vkhoury@imagixmedical.com

J. Hodler et al. (eds.), *Musculoskeletal Diseases 2026-2029*, IDKD Springer Series,
https://doi.org/10.1007/978-3-032-17040-8_20

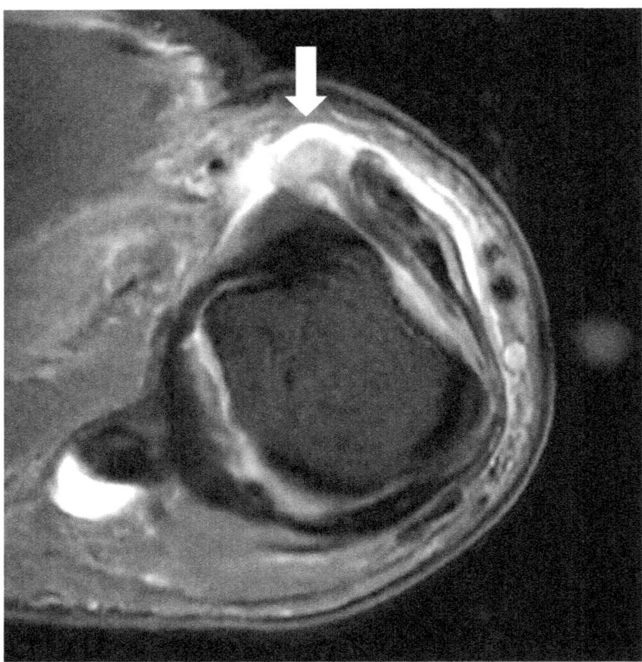

Fig. 20.1 Axial T2-weighted fat-suppressed image demonstrates a partial tear of the ulnar limb of the sagittal band of the thumb

ing. Disruption of the UCL can be either partial or complete and the result of a single acute event or chronic repetitive trauma. Its clinical presentation includes pain and swelling over the ulnar aspect of the MCP joint, reduced grip strength, and joint instability on valgus stress testing. MRI is the modality of choice to evaluate UCL injuries, allowing precise visualization of the ligament and its attachments as well as adjacent structures. Imaging findings include discontinuity, thickening, or abnormal signal within the UCL, as well as surrounding soft tissue edema. Occasionally, a small osseous avulsion at the UCL insertion may be identified on radiographs or CT.

A Stener lesion represents a specific type of complete UCL tear in which the torn, retracted ligament becomes displaced superficial to the adductor aponeurosis, preventing the ligament from reapproximating to its normal insertion and thus precluding natural healing. This complication is critical to recognize because Stener lesions require surgical intervention, in contrast to some complete UCL tears that may be treated conservatively if no interposition is present. On MRI, a Stener lesion is diagnosed by identifying the torn UCL displaced superficial to the adductor aponeurosis, sometimes seen as the so-called yo-yo on a string sign [1] (Fig. 20.2).

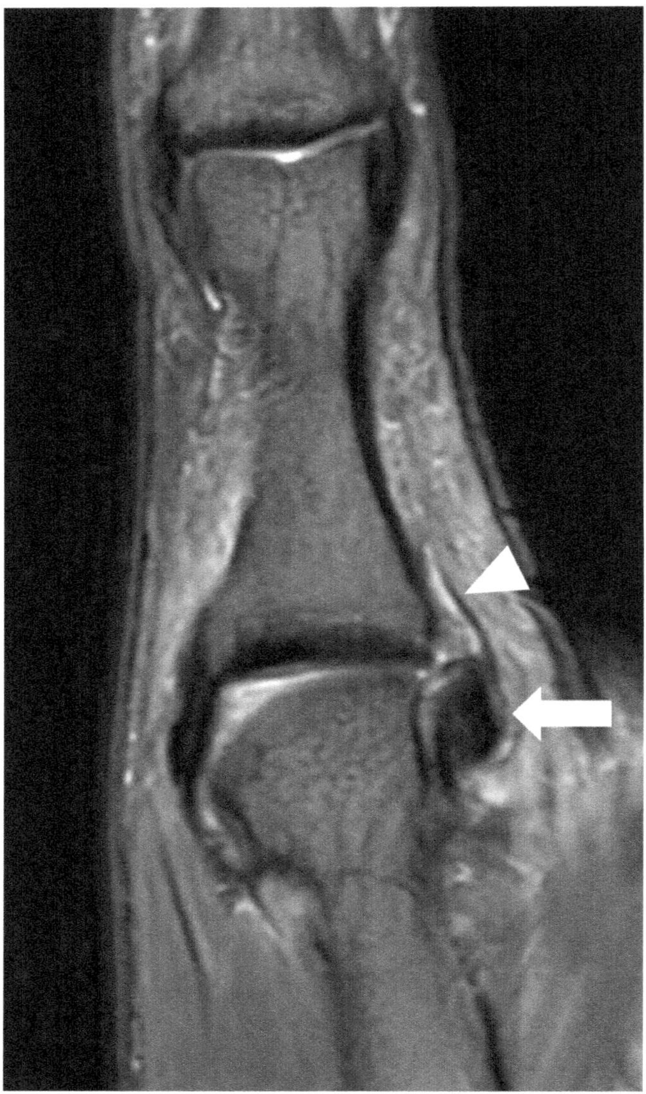

Fig. 20.2 Coronal PD-weighted fat-suppressed image of the MCP joint of the thumb shows a torn and proximally retracted ulnar collateral ligament (arrow) with a preserved relationship deep to the adductor pollicis aponeurosis (arrowhead)

20.2.2 Bennett Fracture

A Bennett fracture is the most common type of fracture involving the base of the first metacarpal. This fracture results from an axial load transmitted through a partially flexed thumb, which causes an intraarticular fracture-dislocation at the base of the first metacarpal. The fracture typically extends obliquely into the carpometacarpal (CMC) joint, resulting in a two-part configuration. A small triangular fragment on the ulnar side of the metacarpal base remains anchored by the anterior oblique (volar beak) ligament, while the larger radial fragment is pulled proximally and dorsally due to the action of the abductor pollicis longus and adductor pollicis muscles [2].

On imaging, the diagnosis is often made using standard radiographs, which reveal an oblique intraarticular fracture with subluxation or dislocation of the metacarpal shaft from the trapezium. Anteroposterior, oblique, and lateral views are useful for characterizing the fracture and displacement. While MRI is less commonly used in acute trauma settings for Bennett fractures, it may provide useful information about associated ligamentous injuries, bone marrow edema, or articular cartilage damage in cases where the diagnosis is uncertain or in subacute presentations.

20.2.3 Osteoarthritis of the First CMC

Osteoarthritis (OA) of the first carpometacarpal (CMC) joint, also known as basal joint arthritis, is a highly prevalent condition, particularly among postmenopausal women (accounting for up to 60% of hand OA cases in women over 55) and individuals engaged in repetitive thumb activity. It is the most common site of osteoarthritis in the hand, responsible for a significant portion of hand pain and dysfunction in older adults. This high degree of mobility in the first CMC predisposes the joint to instability and degenerative change [2].

Pathophysiologically, degeneration of the anterior oblique ligament plays a central role in the development of OA at the first CMC joint. Ligamentous laxity leads to dorsoradial subluxation of the metacarpal base and progressive cartilage loss.

Radiographic evaluation is the first-line imaging modality. Typical findings include joint space narrowing, subchondral sclerosis, osteophyte formation (often dorsoradial), and metacarpal base subluxation.

Key Points

- Thumb injuries often involve ligamentous or intraarticular disruption that compromise joint stability.
- MRI and radiographs play complementary roles in diagnosis of thumb injuries.
- The thumb CMC joint is a common site of degenerative change with a predictable progression of soft tissue and osseous changes.

20.3 Articular and Soft Tissue Anatomy of the Fingers

The fingers are composed of complex and interdependent articular and soft tissue structures. These joints are synovial, lined by articular cartilage, and enclosed in fibrous joint capsules that provide mechanical stability. The collateral ligaments on either side of the joints and the volar plate on the palmar side are key stabilizers, particularly against lateral and hyperextension stresses [3].

The flexor and extensor tendon systems traverse each finger and are held in alignment by fibrous pulley systems that anchor the tendons to the bone. Annular (A1–A5) and cruciform (C1–C3) pulleys maintain tendon proximity to the bone and facilitate efficient flexion. On the dorsal aspect, the extensor tendons trifurcate distal to the metacarpophalangeal joints and include the central slip attachment to the dorsal base middle phalanx and two lateral slips that extend to the distal phalanx and contribute to a terminal tendon attachment. The triangular ligament, sagittal bands, and retinacular ligaments coordinate balanced extension and digit alignment [3–5].

20.4 Commonly Encountered Traumatic Lesions of the Fingers

20.4.1 Central Slip Rupture and Boutonniere Deformity

A central slip injury involves disruption of the central band of the extensor mechanism at the dorsal aspect of the proximal interphalangeal (PIP) joint, which inserts on the base of the middle phalanx. This injury may result from direct trauma or forced flexion of an extended PIP joint. If left untreated, it can progress to a Boutonnière deformity, characterized clinically by PIP flexion and distal interphalangeal (DIP) joint hyperextension. This occurs due to volar subluxation and fibrosis of the lateral bands and unopposed flexor digitorum superficialis activity at the PIP joint [4–6].

Imaging findings include PIP joint soft tissue swelling on radiographs, while ultrasound and MRI provide more definitive assessment. MRI demonstrates central slip disruption, lateral band displacement, and secondary synovitis or tenosynovitis.

20.4.2 Palmar Plate Injury

A palmar plate injury involves damage to the fibrocartilaginous structure located at the volar aspect of the proximal interphalangeal (PIP) joint, which provides stability by preventing hyperextension. These injuries typically result from forced hyperextension or axial loading trauma and can range from isolated soft tissue tears to avulsion fractures at the volar base of the middle phalanx.

Soft tissue injuries may involve attenuation, partial tears, or complete rupture of the palmar plate. These are best visualized with MRI, which shows discontinuity, edema, and thickening of the volar plate.

Osseous injuries include avulsion fractures seen on lateral radiographs as small bony fragments at the volar base of the middle phalanx. These fractures are sometimes subtle and better appreciated on CT or confirmed by MRI if soft tissue assessment is also warranted. Dorsal displacement or rotation of the middle phalanx relative to the proximal phalanx can be seen [3, 6, 7].

20.4.3 Mallet Finger

Mallet finger is a common injury of the terminal extensor mechanism of the distal interphalangeal (DIP) joint, usually caused by sudden forced flexion of an extended fingertip. This results in either a soft tissue disruption of the extensor tendon insertion or an avulsion fracture at the dorsal base of the distal phalanx. Clinically, patients present with an inability to actively extend the DIP joint, which remains in a flexed posture.

Imaging plays a key role in diagnosis. Standard radiographs typically demonstrate a triangular dorsal avulsion fragment at the base of the distal phalanx if a bony mallet injury is present. In purely tendinous injuries, radiographs may appear normal, though soft tissue swelling may be seen [3, 6, 7].

Key Points

- Arthritis is a major cause of hand symptoms, with OA, RA, PsA, and gout showing distinct joint preferences and imaging patterns.
- Soft tissue tumors outnumber bone tumors in the hand.
- Metabolic bone diseases show distinctive radiographic signs.

20.5 Miscellaneous Conditions of Fingers

20.5.1 Arthritides

The most common arthritides affecting the hand include osteoarthritis (OA), rheumatoid arthritis (RA), psoriatic arthritis (PsA), and gout, with OA being the most prevalent overall. OA particularly targets the first carpometacarpal (CMC) and distal interphalangeal (DIP) joints. RA, the most common inflammatory arthropathy, characteristically involves the metacarpophalangeal (MCP) and proximal interphalangeal (PIP) joints in a bilateral, symmetric distribution, with imaging showing marginal erosions, periarticular osteopenia, and synovial thickening (Fig. 20.3). PsA, although less common, frequently involves the DIP joints and presents with erosions, soft tissue swelling, and periostitis (Fig. 20.4). It may also cause the classic "pencil-in-cup" deformity. Gout, while less frequent in the hand, can lead to soft tissue tophi and juxtaarticular erosions with overhanging edges (Fig. 20.5); dual-energy CT (DECT) can aid in identifying urate deposition. Early recognition of these patterns is crucial for accurate diagnosis and management [8–10].

20.5.2 Soft Tissue or Osseous Tumors

Soft tissue tumors are far more common than osseous lesions in the hand, with the ganglion cyst being the most prevalent. These benign, mucin-filled cysts typically arise adjacent to joints or tendon sheaths, especially around the dorsal wrist and volar radial aspects of the fingers. Imaging with ultrasound often reveals an anechoic or hypoechoic mass with posterior acoustic enhancement, while MRI demonstrates a well-circumscribed T2 hyperintense lesion with thin rim enhancement. Other common soft tissue lesions include giant cell tumor of the tendon sheath (GCTTS), which presents as a lobulated, hypointense soft tissue mass on both T1 and T2, and lipomas, which show homogeneous fat signal and suppress on fat-saturated sequences. Glomus tumors, though rare, should be considered in cases of fingertip pain and show intense enhancement on MRI [11–13].

Among osseous tumors in the hand, enchondromas are the most common benign lesions. These are typically central, expansile, and lucent lesions often found in the phalanges, frequently discovered incidentally or after a pathologic fracture. On imaging, enchondromas may contain stippled or arc-and-ring calcifications, and MRI shows T2 hyperintensity with possible chondroid matrix. Malignant tumors are rare but include chondrosarcoma, which may arise from pre-

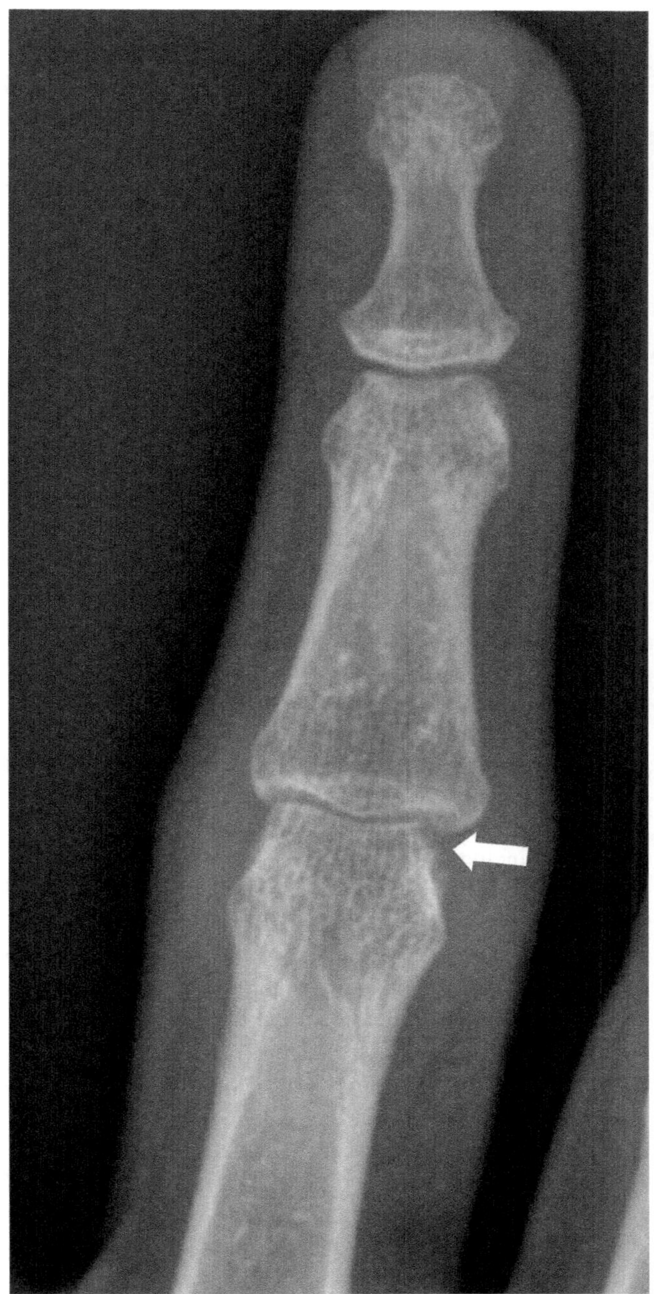

Fig. 20.3 Frontal radiograph of the long finger shows circumferential soft tissue swelling about the PIP joint with a subtle erosion (arrow)

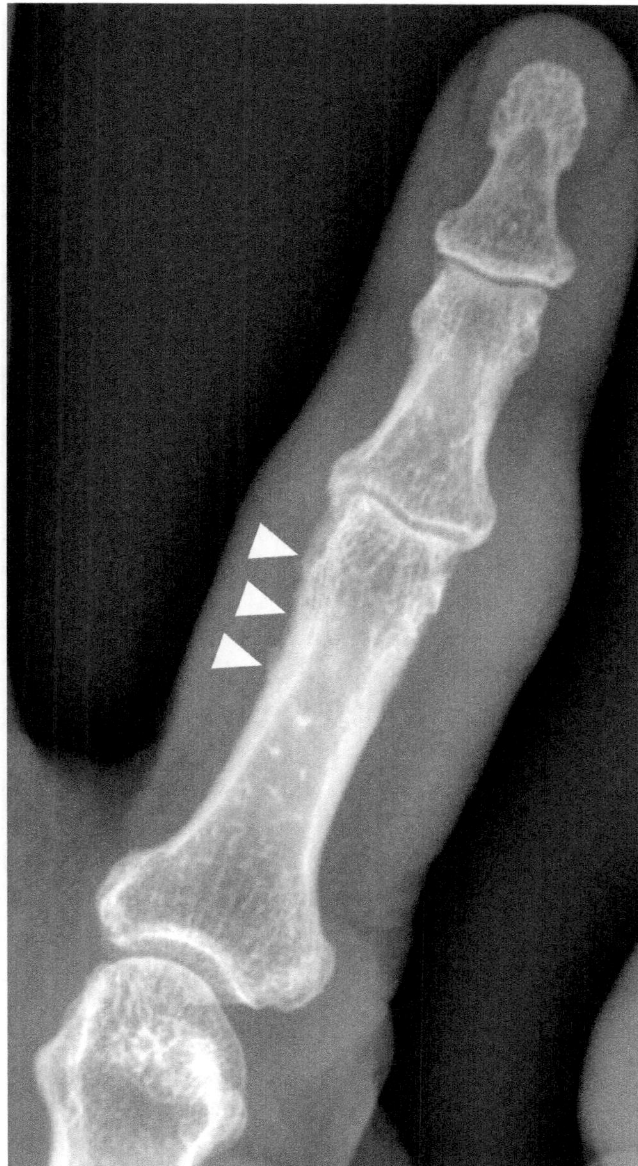

Fig. 20.4 Frontal radiograph of the index finger demonstrates long segment soft tissue swelling about the ray with entheseal periosteal reaction along the proximal phalanx (arrowheads) in a patient with psoriasis

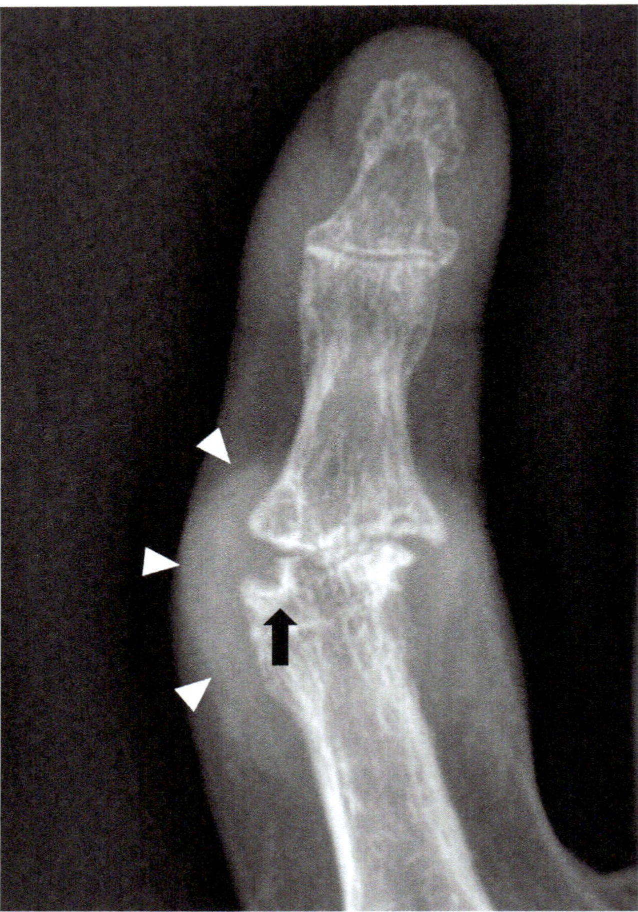

Fig. 20.5 Frontal radiograph of the index finger shows focal periarticular tophus (arrowheads) with increased density with an underlying erosion with overhanging edges (arrow) characteristic of gout

existing enchondromas and display aggressive features such as cortical destruction or soft tissue extension.

20.5.3 Metabolic Disorders

The most common metabolic bone disorder affecting the hand is osteoporosis, which manifests as generalized trabecular bone loss, cortical thinning, and increased radiolucency on radiographs, particularly in postmenopausal women and individuals with chronic illness. Another frequently encountered condition is primary hyperparathyroidism, with hallmark radiographic findings of subperiosteal bone resorption, especially along the radial aspects of the middle phalanges, as well as acroosteolysis and Brown tumors in more advanced disease. Renal osteodystrophy, due to secondary hyperparathyroidism in chronic kidney disease, shows similar features and may include soft tissue vascular and periarticular calcifications. A less common but highly distinctive condition is thyroid acropachy, typically associated with autoimmune thyroid disease, most often Graves' disease. It presents with periosteal new bone formation along the mid-diaphyses of the metacarpals and phalanges, often bilateral and symmetric, accompanied by soft tissue swelling, mimicking hypertrophic osteoarthropathy. Recognition of these imaging patterns is essential for suggesting an underlying systemic disorder and guiding appropriate clinical evaluation [14].

Key Points

- Finger injuries frequently involve damage to the extensor or volar stabilizers of interphalangeal joints, requiring prompt recognition to prevent chronic deformities.

20.6 MTP Joint Anatomy of the First Toe

The anatomy of the first metatarsophalangeal joint (MTPJ) is complex because of its sesamoid apparatus and its integration with multiple musculotendinous structures, making it different than that of the lesser MTPJs. The plantar plate complex is a functional unit that envelops the sesamoid bones and includes the plantar capsule itself, the intersesamoid ligament (transversely oriented between medial and lateral sesamoids), paired metatarsosesamoid ligaments (MTSLs) (linking each sesamoid to the plantar crest of the metatarsal head), and paired sesamoid-phalangeal ligaments (SPLs) (from each sesamoid to the base of proximal phalanx). Medial and lateral collateral ligaments extend from the metatarsal head to the proximal phalanx, blending with the capsule and further reinforcing the joint [15].

The plantar plate complex also includes several musculotendinous structures that provide dynamic stabilization of the MTPJ. These include the medial and lateral heads of the flexor hallucis brevis, attaching to the medial and lateral sesamoids, respectively; the flexor hallucis longus, coursing between the sesamoids and inserting on the base of the distal phalanx; the abductor hallucis tendon, inserting on the medial sesamoid and blending with the medial capsular structures; and the adductor hallucis tendon (formed from both medial and transverse heads), inserting on the lateral sesamoid and blending with the lateral capsular structures.

On the dorsal aspect, the extensor hallucis longus tendon inserts onto the distal phalanx and reinforces the dorsal capsule, while the thinner extensor hallucis brevis inserts at the base of the proximal phalanx.

20.7 Lesions of First MTP Joint Instability

Instability of the first MTPJ is typically the result of an acute traumatic event to the joint involving the plantar plate complex and less commonly the dorsal capsular structures. A substantial number of athletes with capsuloligamentous injury of the first MTPJ will continue to experience persistent or chronic disabling symptoms that can hinder their return to competition [16]. Early surgical intervention in selected cases can restore function and return to play.

20.7.1 Turf Toe

"Turf toe" is a term used to describe a spectrum of acute traumatic injuries to the plantar aspect of the first MTPJ that typically occur due to hyperextension, commonly with a valgus component, which classically occur when playing on artificial turf. They range from mild sprains to partial and complete tears of the plantar plate complex [16].

Mild (grade I) injuries are sprains and appear as abnormally increased signal on fluid-sensitive sequences about the plantar ligaments and/or other capsulo-tendinous structures of the plantar aspect of the MTPJ. They present clinically as point tenderness and slight swelling. Grade II injuries represent partial tears of the plantar plate complex, most commonly of the SPLs, with more marked surrounding soft tissue edema on MRI. Movement of the toe is limited and painful. In grade III injuries, there is complete disruption of the plantar complex and/or diastasis or fracture of the sesamoids, with marked surrounding soft tissue edema on MRI. There is instability of the joint clinically, pain with toe movement, marked tenderness, and ecchymosis.

Management of turf toe is typically conservative, with varying length of time before returning to activity, typically 3–5 days for grade I lesions, at least two weeks for grade II lesions, and a prolonged period for grade III lesions that can be of up to sxi months. Surgical intervention may be indicated for certain grade III injuries, such as when there is persistent instability, large capsular avulsions, sesamoid fractures with diastasis, intraarticular bodies, chondral damage, or failure of conservative management [16].

20.7.2 Other First MTP Joint Injuries

"Skimboard toe" is a traumatic lesion happens when skimboarding when the board slips backward under the foot, forcing the toe(s) into acute hyperextension. There is injury of the dorsal sagittal bands, with the plantar plate typically not affected. On MRI, there is edema of the dorsal soft tissues and absence of an intact extensor hood around the MTP joint [17].

Hyperflexion injuries of the first MTPJ sustained during beach volleyball are commonly referred to as "sand toe" and typically result in dorsal capsular injury [18].

Key Points

- The first MTPJ possesses a plantar plate complex, in contrast to the lesser MTPJs, which exhibit a single dominant fibrocartilaginous thickening. This complex surrounds the sesamoids and merges with the plantar capsule, ISL, MTSLs, SPLs, and surrounding musculotendinous structures, forming a functional unit.
- Management of turf toe is typically conservative, with surgery performed uncommonly for certain grade III injuries.

20.8 Anatomy of the Lesser MTP Joints

The lesser MTPs, like the first, must withstand large forces during weight-bearing and ambulation. The most important static stabilizer of the lesser MTPJ is the plantar plate, a thick, strong fibrocartilaginous structure at the plantar aspect of each MTPJ, lying just deep to the flexor digitorum tendon. It extends from the base of the proximal phalanx to the neck of the metatarsal, to which it loosely attaches by fibrosynovial tissue. Laterally, the plantar plate attaches to the medial and lateral accessory collateral ligaments [19, 20]. Other contributors to lesser MTPJ stability include the plantar fascia, the accessory and phalangeal collateral ligaments, flexor digitorum longus (FDL), flexor digitorum brevis (FDB) tendons, and the extensor hood and sling mechanism.

20.9 Lesser Plantar Plate Tears

Degeneration or rupture of a lesser plantar plate can lead to progressive MTPJ instability, most commonly involving the second MTPJ. This lesion may lead to medial deviation, lateral deviation, or dorsal subluxation of the MTPJ, as well as to hammer toe deformity.

Lesser plantar plate tears typically occur close to their phalangeal insertion, most commonly inferolaterally at the attachment to the accessory ligaments.

On US and MRI, the plantar plate should be examined in both longitudinal and transverse planes. On US, tears appear as hypoechoic defects of variable extent within the substance of the plantar plate and may be partial or complete [19]. On MRI, partial and complete tears are seen as defects within the substance of the plantar plate, typically as a hyperintense abnormality [21] (Fig. 20.6). With a chronic complete tear

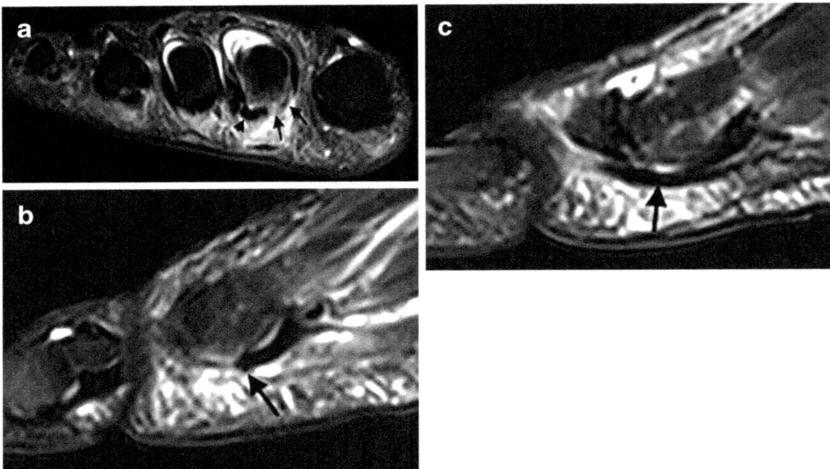

Fig. 20.6 42-year-old woman with a plantar plate tear of the second MTP joint. (**a**) Coronal FS T2-weighted MR image shows focal discontinuity of the plantar plate (arrows). Note associated lateral subluxation of the flexor digitorum tendon (arrowhead). Sagittal FS T2-weighted images showing in (**b**) discontinuity of the plantar plate at its distal insertion (arrow), and in (**c**), abnormal apposition of the flexor digitorum tendon to the metatarsal head)

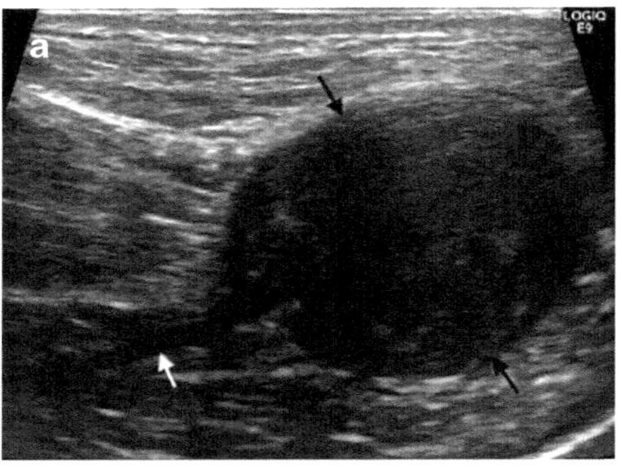

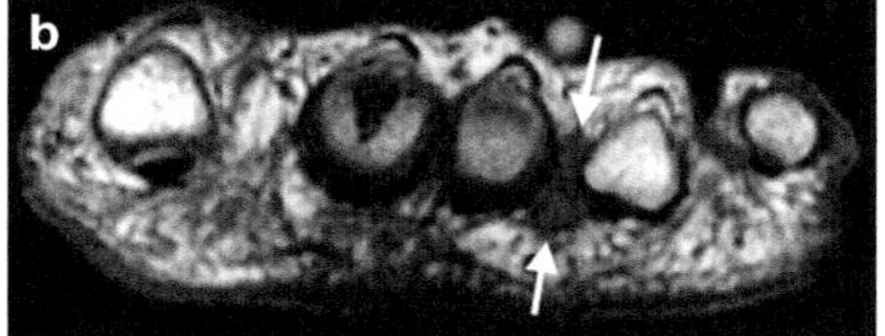

Fig. 20.7 Morton neuroma. (**a**) Longitudinal US image in the intermetatarsal space showing a rounded hypoechoic mass (black arrows) in continuity with the interdigital nerve (white arrow). (**b**) Coronal T1-weighted image of the forefoot in a different patient showing a hypointense soft tissue lesion in the third intermetatarsal space (arrows)

and loss of substance of the plantar plate, the flexor digitorum tendon is seen on imaging to be directly apposed to the metatarsal head (Fig. 20.6c). Degeneration may also lead to diffuse thinning of the plate.

A diagnostic pitfall in assessing plantar plate tears relates to the presence of a normal recess in the midline of the plantar plate, which is due to the distal insertion of the plantar plate being thicker medially and laterally, with relative thinning centrally. This recess appears as a hyperintense zone on MRI and a hyperechoic cleft on US and should not be mistaken for a tear [19, 20].

On ultrasound, dynamic evaluation during dorsiflexion can improve tear detection as well as allowing for visualization of MTPJ subluxation [19]. On MRI, prone positioning has been described as potentially improving evaluation of the plantar plate [21]. Associated findings of plantar plate tears on MRI may include MTP joint effusion, edema of the surrounding soft tissues, reactive subchondral marrow edema, and flexor tenosynovitis.

With chronic disease, reparative pericapsular fibrosis may develop, a condition that is likely underdiagnosed. It appears as a broad soft tissue thickening at the inferomedial or inferolateral aspect of the MTP joint, on both US and MRI (see Fig. 20.6b). This lesion may potentially be confused with a Morton neuroma [21]. On US evaluation, pain directly over the MTPJ and a negative Mulder maneuver can be helpful distinguishing features of pericapsular fibrosis [22].

20.10 Other Commonly Encountered Lesions of the Forefoot

20.10.1 Intermetatarsal Bursitis and Morton (Interdigital) Neuroma

Intermetatarsal bursae are synovial-lined sacs located in the superior intermetatarsal spaces, dorsal to the intermetatarsal ligament, reducing friction between the metatarsal heads and surrounding soft tissues [19, 23]. The neurovascular bundle courses inferior to the transverse intermetatarsal ligament, but distally it deviates superiorly, curving around the ligament and lying adjacent to the bursa [24].

Key Points

- Morton neuroma represents perineural fibrosis of the interdigital nerve, most often in the third intermetatarsal space, caused by chronic compression beneath the transverse intermetatarsal ligament and frequently associated with intermetatarsal bursitis.
- US and MRI show plantar plate tears as hypoechoic/hyperintense defects near the inferolateral phalangeal insertion; beware of the normal central recess, which mimics a tear. Dynamic dorsiflexion on US and prone MRI positioning improve detection.

Morton neuromas are not true tumors but consist of perineural fibrosis and degenerative changes of the interdigital nerve [25], most commonly occurring in the third and less commonly the second intermetatarsal space. (It is now preferable to use the term "Morton neuroma" rather than "Morton's neuroma," in line with recommendations against using possessive eponyms in medical terminology [26].) The etiology is likely chronic compression of the nerve against the transverse intermetatarsal ligament. Predisposing factors include shoe wear that is too narrow at the toe box and/or high-heeled shoes, as well as obesity. Clinically, Morton neuroma presents with forefoot pain, worsened by weight-bearing and often likened to "walking on a pebble," sometimes with numbness, burning, or tingling of the toes.

A distended intermetatarsal bursa is often an associated finding. In fact, there is likely progression from intermetatarsal bursitis to neuroma with continued microtrauma. Intermetatarsal bursitis may also be an early manifestation of rheumatoid arthritis, before clinical joint swelling [23].

Ultrasound and MRI both detect neuromas with high sensitivity [27]. US is cost-effective and allows for dynamic evaluation and guidance of therapeutic injections. US is performed from the dorsal and/or plantar aspect, with interdigital pressure and correlation with the site of pain increasing sensitivity and specificity. Mulder's maneuver can also accentuate findings by displacing the lesion and eliciting a palpable click. Morton neuroma appears as a well-defined hypoechoic mass, with contiguity with the interdigital nerve in the longitudinal plane (Fig. 20.7a). It may contain a central echogenic focus that corresponds histologically to the true neuroma, with the surrounding hypoechoic component representing perineural fibrosis, vascular proliferation, and thickened bursa [28]. On MRI, Morton neuroma appears as a rounded or fusiform mass of intermediate T1 and low T2 signal in the inferior intermetatarsal space, with possible contrast enhancement [27]. The coronal T1-weighted sequence is especially helpful in detection (Fig. 20.7b). Intermetatarsal bursitis alone presents as a cystic lesion in the superior intermetatarsal space with subtle peripheral enhancement.

20.10.2 Sesamoid Disorders

The hallux sesamoids, particularly the medial, are the most frequently injured bones of the forefoot. Acute trauma may result in fracture or diastasis of a bipartite sesamoid. Repetitive strain injury due to repetitive axial loading may result in "sesamoiditis." This is a clinical diagnosis and descriptive umbrella term that encompasses several causes of chronic pain arising from the hallux sesamoid complex. Lesions include stress reaction, fracture, osteonecrosis, or capsular inflammation.

Radiography—including sesamoid views—play an important role in the diagnosis of sesamoid disorders. CT may be indicated for a more sensitive examination if radiographs are not conclusive. Irregular, jagged margins are seen with fracture, whereas smooth, rounded margins are typical for bipartite sesamoid. Increased sclerosis with or without fragmentation may be seen in sesamoiditis (Fig. 20.8). MRI will detect marrow changes including edema and cystic changes.

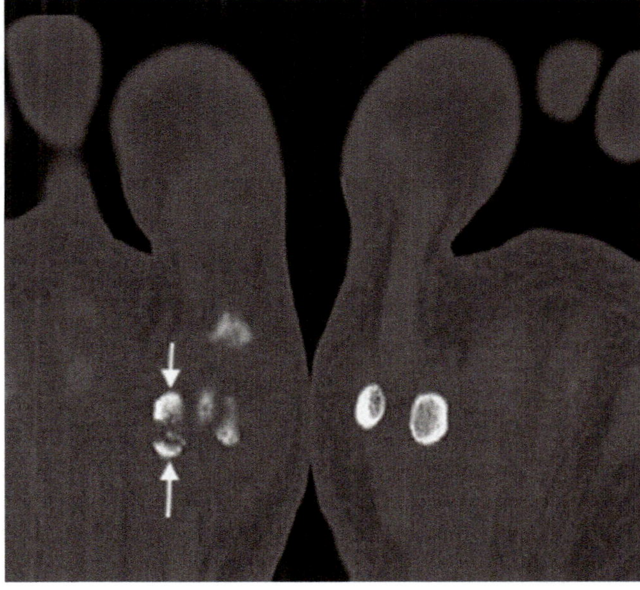

Fig. 20.8 Lateral "sesamoiditis" in a patient with chronic plantar first MTPJ symptoms. Axial CT image of the forefoot shows fracture versus diastasis of a bipartite lateral sesamoid (arrows) with fragmentation and sclerosis. Normal contralateral lateral sesamoid is shown for comparison

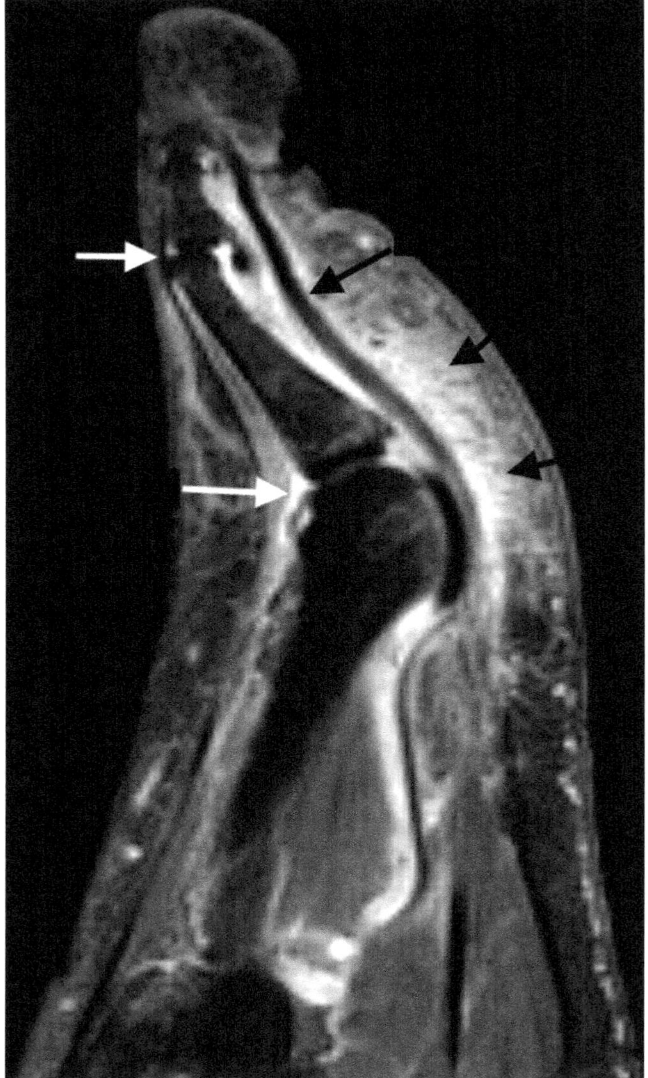

Fig. 20.9 Sagittal fat-saturated T2-weighted image of the third ray showing flexor tenosynovitis and submetatarsal edema (black arrows) and synovitis of the MTPJ and proximal interphalangeal joint (white arrows) in this patient with known psoriatic arthritis

20.10.3 Hallux Valgus

Hallux valgus is an excessive adduction of the first MTP joint, diagnosed clinically and supported by standing radiographs, which show a hallux angle of greater than 15°. Hallux valgus starts with medial metatarsal head migration and lateral sesamoid subluxation and then valgus drift of the proximal phalanx. Progressive capsular and ligamentous tearing, tendon displacement, and osteophyte formation eventually cause attrition of the plantar plate and surrounding soft tissues. US may be helpful in showing associated joint effusion, osteoarthrosis, or adventitial bursitis medially.

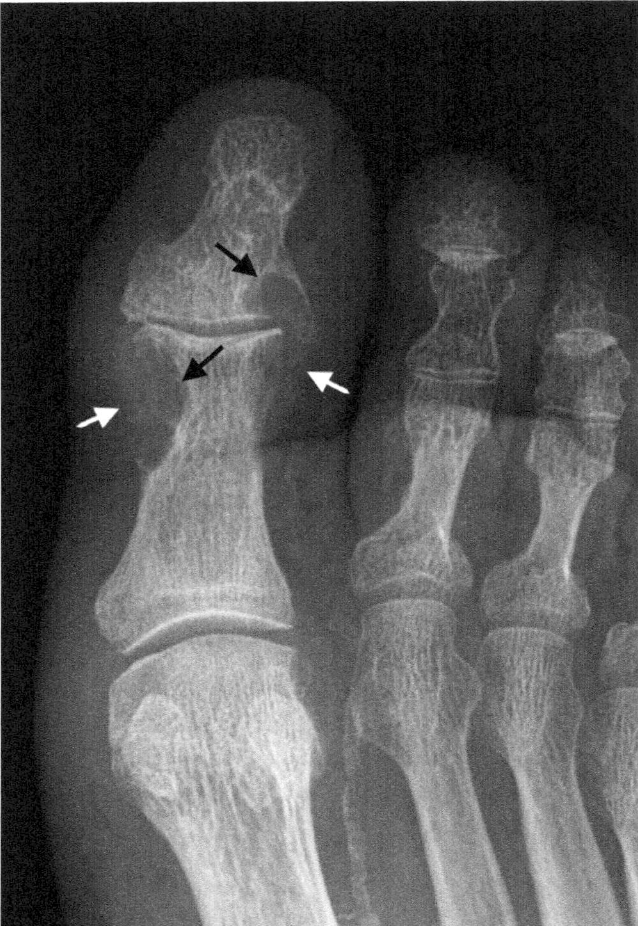

Fig. 20.10 Frontal radiograph of the foot shows faintly calcified periarticular tophi (white arrows) with adjacent large erosions with overhanging edges (black arrows) of the interphalangeal joint of the first toe, typical for gouty arthritis

20.11 Miscellaneous Conditions of the Forefoot

20.11.1 Arthritides

The same arthritides affecting the hand already described affect the forefoot. Radiography remains the primary tool for assessing joint space narrowing, marginal osteophytosis, marginal erosions, subchondral sclerosis, deformity, and soft tissue calcifications. US and MRI are powerful adjuncts due to their high sensitivity in detecting joint effusions, marginal erosions, synovial thickening, and active synovitis.

OA in the forefoot particularly targets the first MTPJ, typically manifesting as hallux rigidus ("stiff big toe"). Dorsal osteophyte formation restricts dorsiflexion of the joint, contributing to the pain and stiffness characteristic of this condition.

RA affecting the forefoot typically affects the MTPJs, with the fifth MTPJ frequently being the earliest and most severely affected. Imaging shows marginal erosions and synovial thickening and/or inflammation. Other findings in RA of the MTPJs may include adjacent tenosynovitis, intermetatarsal bursitis, and submetatarsal bursitis [23]. Similar findings may be seen with PsA of the forefoot (Fig. 20.9). Additionally, PsA may affect the DIP joints of the foot and IP joint of the big toe with distinctive fluffy periostitis on joint surface margins and phalangeal tufts. The characteristic finding of an "ivory phalanx" in PsA—classically the involving the distal phalanx of the first toe—is related to periosteal and endosteal bone formation leading to increased bone density of the entire phalanx.

The classic and most common site of gout in the body is at the first MTPJ ("podagra"), noting that other joints of the forefoot may be affected. Soft tissue tophi (best seen radiographically or sonographically) and juxtaarticular erosions with overhanging edges are characteristic (Fig. 20.10). US may reveal the "double contour" sign of urate crystal deposition. As previously mentioned, dual-energy CT (DECT) can be helpful by identifying monosodium urate crystals.

Given advances in medication for inflammatory arthritides, advanced imaging has become increasingly important for early disease detection.

20.11.2 Soft Tissue Masses and Osseous Tumors

The most common soft tissue masses in the forefoot are pseudotumoral lesions [29]. Cystic lesions include synovial cysts, ganglia, adventitial bursae, or abscesses. Noncystic lesions include calluses, rheumatoid nodules, and the previously discussed Morton neuroma.

Plantar fibromas, or Ledderhose disease, present as nodular thickening that may occur anywhere along the plantar fascia including in the forefoot. On ultrasound they appear hypoechoic and fusiform with minimal vascularity in contiguity with the plantar fascia, while MRI demonstrates low to intermediate T1 signal and variable T2 signal along the fascia with variable enhancement.

The forefoot is a common site of penetrating foreign bodies. Foreign body granuloma is a tissue reaction to objects penetrating soft tissue. On US, it appears as a nonspecific mass surrounding an echogenic foreign body, the latter typically showing posterior shadowing.

Adventitious bursae develop in subcutaneous tissues at sites of pressure or friction. Adventitial bursitis commonly occurs under the metatarsal heads (also termed submetatarsal bursitis) or medial to a hallux valgus. Repeated stress causes small fluid collections to merge into well-defined, synovium-like cavities lacking a mesothelial lining (the latter in contrast with native bursae). On US, they appear as compressible, ill-defined, or focal fluid collections and as low T1/high fluid-sensitive lesions on MRI, sometimes with rim enhancement and adjacent soft tissue stranding.

Osseous tumors of the forefoot are exceedingly rare, occurring mostly in the metatarsals [30]. Common benign lesions include osteoid osteoma, giant cell tumor, and enchondroma, while malignant lesions most often are Ewing's sarcoma, chondrosarcoma, and osteosarcoma.

20.11.3 Metabolic Disorders

The metabolic disorders that were described in the Hand section can also occur in the forefoot.

In diabetes mellitus, the forefoot is a frequent site of pathology. Lesions can include callus formation, adventitious bursitis, skin ulcers, and bone involvement such as Charcot arthropathy and osteomyelitis, particularly beneath the first and fifth metatarsal heads. These conditions frequently coexist and carry significant morbidity. The imaging literature provides comprehensive coverage of this topic. The radiologist plays a central role in accurate diagnosis and early detection, essential for timely treatment and prevention of progression

Key Points

- Arthritides are a major cause of forefoot symptoms, with hallux rigidus, RA, PsA, and gout being most prevalent and showing pathognomonic imaging findings.
- The most common soft tissue masses in the forefoot are pseudotumoral lesions, including synovial and ganglion cysts, adventitial bursae, calluses, rheumatoid nodules, plantar fibromas, and Morton neuroma/neuroma-bursitis complex.

20.12 Conclusion

The complex anatomy of the thumb, fingers, and forefoot—encompassing specialized joints, capsuloligamentous stabilizers, tendon, and pulley systems—underpins the hand and foot's exquisite balance of mobility and stability. These structures, however, are vulnerable to injury, arthritides, and systemic disease. Traumatic lesions, from UCL tears and Bennett fractures in the thumb to central slip injuries of the fingers to plantar plate injuries of the forefoot, can compromise function if not promptly recognized. Likewise, degenerative and inflammatory arthritides, along with soft tissue and osseous tumors or metabolic disorders, follow characteristic patterns that imaging plays a central role in detecting. A thorough understanding of normal anatomy, common pathologies, and their characteristic imaging features is essential for accurate diagnosis, timely treatment, and preservation of function in these complex and vital small joints.

Conflict of Interest Statement I/We declare no competing interests as defined by Springer Nature or other interests that might be perceived to influence results and/or discussion reported in this manuscript.

References

1. Udit R, Pierce JL, Evans S, et al. High-resolution MR imaging and US anatomy of the thumb. Radiographics. 2016;36:1701–16.
2. Bouredoucen H, Abs B, Ferreira BD, et al. Trapeziometacarpal joint imaging: normal high-resolution MRI, US and CT compared with cadaveric specimens and pathologic imaging findings. Eur J Radiol. 2024;177:111561.
3. Gupta P, Lenchik L, Wuertzer S, et al. High-resolution 3-T MRI of the fingers: review of anatomy and common tendon and ligament injuries. AJR. 2015;204(3):W314–23.
4. Clavero JA, Golano P, Farinas O, et al. Extensor mechanism of the fingers: MR imaging—anatomic correlation. Radiographics. 2003;23(3):593–611.
5. Hauger O, Chung CB, Lektrakul N, et al. Pulley system in the fingers: normal anatomy and simulated lesions in cadavers at MR imaging, CT, and US with and without contrast material distention of the tendon sheath. Radiology. 2000;217(1):201–12.
6. Pilania K, Jankharia B. A pictorial essay on focused magnetic resonance imaging of the normal anatomy and various injuries of the finger. Can Assoc Radiol J. 2018;69(4):437–49.
7. Petchprapa C, Vaswani D. MRI of the fingers: an update. AJR. 2019;213:534–48.
8. Tins BJ, Butler R. Imaging in rheumatology: reconciling radiology and rheumatology. Insights Imaging. 2013;4(6):799–810.
9. Shiraishi M, Fukuda T, Igarashi T, et al. Differentiating rheumatoid and psoriatic arthritis of the hand: multimodality imaging characteristics. Radiographics. 2020;40(5):1339–54.
10. Haugen IK, Boyesen P. Imaging modalities in hand osteoarthritis-status and perspectives of conventional radiography, magnetic resonance imaging, and ultrasonography. Arthritis Res Ther. 2011;13(6):248–56.
11. AbuMoussa S, Roshan MP, Souza FF, et al. Soft tissue masses of the hand: a review of clinical presentation and imaging features. Durr Oncol. 2023;30(2):2032–48.
12. Yue KLC, Lans J, Castelein RM, et al. Benign hand tumors (part I): cartilaginous and bone Tumors. Hand. 2022;17(2):346–53.
13. Lans J, Yue KLC, Castelein RM, et al. Benign hand tumors (part II): soft tissue Tumors. Hand. 2022;17(3):519–28.
14. Scullion S, Grainger AJ, Greenspan A. Radiologic imaging of metabolic and endocrine disorders as they affect the hand and wrist. Semin Musculoskelet Radiol. 2021;25(2):246–59.
15. Hallinan JTPD, Statum SM, Huang BK, Bezerra HG, Garcia DAL, Bydder GM, Christine B. Chung high-resolution MRI of the first metatarsophalangeal joint: gross anatomy and injury characterization. Radiographics. 2020;40(4):1107–24.
16. Anderson RB. Turf toe injuries of the hallux metatarsophalangeal joint. Tech Foot Ankle Surg. 2002;1(2):102–11.
17. Donnelly LF, Betts JB, Fricke BL. Skimboarder's toe: findings on high-field MRI. AJR Am J Roentgenol. 2005;184(5):1481–5.
18. Frey C, Andersen GD, Feder KS. Plantar flexion injury to the metatarsophalangeal joint ("sand toe"). Foot Ankle Int. 1996;17(9):576–81.
19. McCarthy CL, Thompson GV. Ultrasound findings of plantar plate tears of the lesser metatarsophalangeal joints. Skeletal Radiol. 2021;50(8):1513–25. https://doi.org/10.1007/s00256-020-03708-1.
20. Umans H, Elsinger E. The plantar plate of the lesser metatarsophalangeal joints: potential for injury and role of MR imaging. Magn Reson Imaging Clin N Am. 2001;9(3):659–69.
21. Mann TS, Nery CAS, Baumfeld D, Fernandes EÁ. Degenerative injuries of the metatarsophalangeal plantar plate on magnetic resonance imaging: a new perspective. Foot Ankle Orthop. 2022;7(4):2473011421S00768.
22. Reijnierse M, Griffith JF. High-resolution ultrasound and MRI in the evaluation of the forefoot and midfoot. J Ultrason. 2023;23(95):e251–71.
23. Dakkak YJ, Jansen FP, De Ruiter MC, Reijnierse M, van der Helm-van Mil AHM. Rheumatoid arthritis and tenosynovitis at the metatarsophalangeal joints: an anatomic and MRI study of the forefoot tendon sheaths. Radiology. 2020;295(1):146–54.
24. Bossley CJ, Cairney PC. The intermetatarsophalangeal bursa—its significance in Morton's metatarsalgia. J Bone Joint Surg. 1980;62(2):184–7.
25. Addante JB, Pericott PS, Wong KY, et al. Interdigital neuromas: results of surgical excision of 152 neuromas. J Am Podiatr Med Assoc. 1986;76(9):493–5.
26. Christiansen S, Iverson C, Flanagin A, et al. AMA manual of style: a guide for authors and editors. 11th ed. Oxford University Press; 2020.
27. Bignotti B, Signori A, Sormani MP, Molfetta L, Martinoli C, Tagliafico A. Ultrasound versus magnetic resonance imaging for Morton neuroma: systematic review and meta-analysis. Eur Radiol. 2015;25(8):2254–62.
28. Cohen SL, Miller TT, Ellis SJ, Roberts MM, DiCarlo EF. Sonography of Morton neuroma: what are we really looking at? J Ultrasound Med. 2016;35(10):2191–5.
29. Van Hul E, Vanhoenacker F, Van Dyck P, De Schepper A, Parizel PM. Pseudotumoural soft tissue lesions of the foot and ankle: a pictorial review. Insights Imaging. 2011;2(4):439–52.
30. Ritchie DA. Tumors of the foot. In: Mark Davies A, Murali S, James Steven J, editors. Imaging of bone tumors and tumor-like lesions: techniques and applications. Berlin Heidelberg: Springer; 2009. p. 647–64.

GPSR Compliance

The European Union's (EU) General Product Safety Regulation (GPSR) is a set of rules that requires consumer products to be safe and our obligations to ensure this.

If you have any concerns about our products, you can contact us on ProductSafety@springernature.com

In case Publisher is established outside the EU, the EU authorized representative is:

Springer Nature Customer Service Center GmbH
Europaplatz 3
69115 Heidelberg, Germany

Batch number: 10371057

Printed by Printforce, the Netherlands